THE ESSENTIALS OF PÆDIATRIC SURGERY

H. H. NIXON
M.A., F.R.C.S.

Consultant Surgeon, The Hospital for Sick Children, Great Ormond Street,
London, W.C.1
Consultant Pædiatric Surgeon, Paddington Green Children's Hospital,
St Mary's Hospital Group, Paddington
Hunterian Professor, Royal College of Surgeons, England

and

BARRY O'DONNELL
M.Ch., F.R.C.S., F.R.C.S.I.

Consultant Surgeon, Our Lady's Hospital for Sick Children, Dublin

Foreword by
SIR DENIS BROWNE, F.R.C.S.

SECOND EDITION

WILLIAM HEINEMANN MEDICAL BOOKS LTD

First published .   . 1961
Second Edition .   . 1966
Reprinted .   . 1968

Printed by The Whitefriars Press Ltd
London and Tonbridge

FOREWORD

THIS book deals with one of the rapidly developing sections of surgery, that concentrating on the young. A similar concentration, apparently permanent, has been established, in pædiatric medicine; but it should be remembered that this speciality was bitterly opposed when it was first suggested, as pædiatric surgery is being opposed at the present time. There is no cause for complaint in this; it is part of the invariable reaction of mankind to new ideas. It is, however, worth examining the arguments against such specialism. No one suggests that children do badly among their contemporaries in institutions specially built, equipped and staffed for them; nor that it is to their disadvantage to be watched continuously by those who have studied their rapid changes of condition. The opposition is from those working in other specialities, who complain that pædiatric surgeons are treating cases which "belong" to them. The division of the human body into its systems, each to be treated by a closed corporation dedicated to one of them, is perhaps inevitable given the immense and constantly increasing amount of knowledge to be absorbed and applied. But there are certain disadvantages to this, apart from such obvious ones as the difficulty of deciding whether a diaphragmatic hernia belongs to the specialist in respiratory diseases or to him who works in the abdomen. One of the most important is that no one looks at the patient as a whole—the neurologist, called to a case of spina bifida and hydrocephalus, takes no interest in any deformities of the feet; the orthopædist leaves the pregnancy history of congenital dislocation of the hip and arthrogryposis to the obstetricians, who respond by ignoring the subsequent history of the child whom they have assisted into the world.

In order to understand the principles upon which pædiatric surgeons work it is most important to realize that they have no ambition whatever to establish another "closed shop" to add to those already in existence; they gladly admit progress in the surgery of the young which comes from those outside their ranks, such as the first successful treatment of œsophageal atresia. And they would also welcome comparisons between their results in such conditions as deformities of the bowel and anus with those gained elsewhere. But as a corollary to claiming no monopoly they also recognize none, and follow their work into any region of the body into which it may lead them.

Besides the advantages of looking at a child as a whole, and not as a collection of systems, there is another contribution which pædiatric surgery can make to the science of surgery; that of preserving the competition between different methods and hypotheses which is an indispensable factor in progress. Specialization of the conventional sort leads to a great early improvement in efficiency; this is liable to be succeeded by a period of comparative stagnation, when the elders have settled down to set ways, and the prospects of a junior are apt to be damaged if he departs from them.

This particular textbook is designed to give a general impression of the work that has been done and the problems that remain to be solved in the future: it makes no attempt to cover any subject completely, but gives an excellent picture of the whole child from the surgeon's point of view which should be most valuable to those at the start of careers in medicine and general practice as well as in surgery. Any who doubt the need of a book of this sort are recommended to look up such subjects as Hirschsprung's disease or deformities of the anus in the textbooks of general surgery which instruct students; or to take an instance from a speciality, try to find any definition of such a common term as "talipes" in a textbook of orthopædic surgery. In this latter instance the relations between moulding deformities of the feet, congenital dislocation of the hip, spinal deformities and pregnancy history form a fascinating and complicated field for study, at present largely untouched.

As a purely personal note, I had the good fortune to be among those early workers who found this field opening before them almost unexplored, and I feel the greatest satisfaction in finding from this book how much of what I have to teach has been learnt, and how much further certain studies have been carried than I was able to take them myself.

SIR DENIS BROWNE.

PREFACE TO THE FIRST EDITION

THERE are several good textbooks of Pædiatrics which comment on surgical aspects and several good textbooks of Surgery which comment on pædiatric aspects. We felt that a short book on the surgery of children would be useful in giving an idea of the scope of this expanding field where the disciplines overlap. The book is intended mainly for the senior student but it is hoped that others such as D.C.H. candidates, surgeons with a part time pædiatric interest and General Practitioners may also find it of use.

We have tried to approach the subject in the form of a discussion of problems as they present to the clinician. This has meant some repetition to reduce the need to refer to several parts of the book to find the answer to a problem, but it is hoped that increased convenience will justify this.

Common conditions have been given prominence but a number of rarities are described in some detail when they have been thought to be of particular intrinsic interest or to illustrate embryological and other underlying principles. Some are mentioned because though uncommon their curability or serious nature make their diagnosis important.

It is our hope that we have kept the book to a reasonable size for reading in the heavily loaded curriculum of today without missing out anything of real importance, remembering that the surgery of children constitutes at least a fifth of all surgery. The resources of a modest hospital library have been in our minds in selecting references. This has meant the exclusion of many excellent papers in specialist journals.

September 1961

H. H. N.
B. O'D.

PREFACE TO THE SECOND EDITION

IT has been gratifying to find a second edition necessary within five years and it is encouraging to realize that advances in the subject have made extensive rewriting necessary. Our object remains the same, the book being primarily directed to the senior student. We are particularly concerned that he should make the correct decision in emergencies and that his advice to anxious parents on less urgent matters should be accurate. However, the interest shown by pædiatricians, surgeons and general practitioners has persuaded us to make more use of small type sections to include material of less importance to students. No chapter is completely unchanged. Some have been rearranged to clarify certain sections, more have been altered to bring them up to date. The chapters on urology and spina bifida are amongst those most extensively rewritten.

August 1966

H. H. N.
B. O'D.

ACKNOWLEDGMENTS

WE are indebted to our many Senior and Junior colleagues who have been so helpful with advice and discussion. It would be impossible to overstate the value of these free and informal talks in shaping our opinions. We have also been helped by the constructive comments of several reviewers of the first edition.

We were fortunate in having Mr. Derek Martin, Assistant Curator of the Museum, The Hospital for Sick Children, Great Ormond Street, and Mr. Geoffrey Lyth, Medical Artist, to supply the illustrations.

The late Mr. Johnston Abraham and Mr. Owen R. Evans of Heinemanns have borne with us most patiently and understandingly. Their experience and advice have been invaluable.

CONTENTS

CONTENTS

CHAPTER 1

THE CAUSES OF CONGENITAL MALFORMATIONS

CONGENITAL malformations are responsible for about a quarter of all infant deaths and about one in forty infants is born with a major defect.

The causes of congenital malformations are still little understood. In the last century malformations were widely attributed to accidents to the developing fœtus—intra-uterine infections, maternal falls and frights and intercourse during pregnancy were all invoked. Then, with the rise in the science of genetics, unusual formations of the chromosomes—abnormal genes or mutations—were recognized as causing malformations which ran in families. The importance of these genetic factors was perhaps overstressed. Now it is considered that, whilst some congenital abnormalities have a *genetic* and some an *environmental* cause, the great majority are *multifactorial*, i.e. they have genetic and environmental factors. It is important to realize that the same defect may arise in more than one way—perhaps by genetic or environmental factors. For example, a genetic factor is recognizable only in a proportion of cases of isolated cleft palate.

GENETIC CAUSES

About 4 per cent of infants are born with a genetically determined anomaly, though many of these are unimportant. For centuries it has been realized that certain conditions tended to run in families. Achondroplasia (the type of dwarfism seen in the typical circus dwarf) and hare lip are such conditions.

The science of genetics was based on the rediscovery of the work of Abbott Mendel on the breeding of garden peas. It was subsequently recognized that the chromosomes carried genes determining the character of the individual, such as eye colour, height and build, and that from time to time changes (*mutations*) in the genes would cause abnormalities such as those mentioned above. When the abnormality was incompatible with life (lethal genes) the change was self-limiting. Less severe abnormalities were repeated in two main ways. *Dominant* genes were expressed in the offspring when only one partner passed on the gene—the *hereditary* abnormalities such as achondroplasia which recur in successive generations. *Recessive* genes were expressed only if the same abnormal gene was passed on by both partners—the *familial* abnormalities such as cystic fibrosis which recur in siblings. Probably one in twenty-five people are *carriers* for cystic fibrosis, i.e. have one abnormal gene in their make up (heterozygous). They show no abnormality but should they mate with another carrier the chances are one in four that an offspring will receive the gene from both parents (homozygous) and will manifest the disease.

If the factor is carried on the sex chromosome (*sex linked*), there will be a different incidence in the sexes, e.g. hæmophilia which is carried by females but manifest only in males.

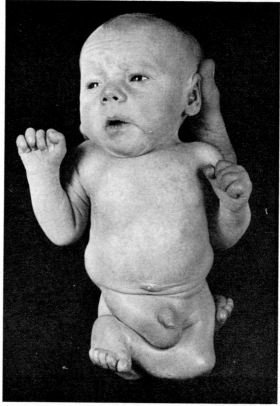

Fig. 1. This malformed baby shows the effects of malposition and increased uterine pressure.

The pattern of inheritance is often confused by *incomplete penetrance* in which only a proportion of those carrying the necessary genes show the clinical abnormality. An additional environmental factor may be necessary for manifestation.

A recent break through has revealed a different group of abnormalities caused by chromosomes. During meiotic nuclear division of the cells forming the sperm or ovum *nondisjunction* may result in a cell having an extra or a missing chromosome. Certain types of intersex (e.g. Turner's syndrome, XO and Klinefelter's syndrome, XXX) arise in this fashion, the sex chromosomes being the ones involved. In Down's syndrome (Mongolian idiocy) there is an extra somatic chromosome.

In other instances a part of a dividing chromosome may be lost during the cell division or a part remain attached to its neighbour forming an unusually large chromosome (*translocation* during metaphase). An abnormal division after the first may produce a "*mosaic*" individual with two sets of cells with differing chromosomal patterns.

ENVIRONMENTAL FACTORS

It is perhaps a truism to point out that the baby has been alive for nine months before birth and that it can suffer infection, physical trauma and even neoplasia and degenerations during that time. Tissues are most vulnerable when they are developing rapidly so that the *timing* of an insult is more important than its nature in deciding the result. The first three months constitute the period of organogenesis and damage at this time may produce developmental arrest. The embryo is most sensitive during the first six weeks after conception— when the mother may not even realize she is pregnant.

A good example of this sensitivity is the association between maternal rubella (German measles) and congenital defects including cataracts. If contracted during the first month of pregnancy the fœtus is malformed in about 50 per cent of cases; if in the second month 25 per cent are affected; in the third month 10 per cent. Maternal rubella after the third month leaves the fœtus unaffected.

Infections

Congenital syphilis used to be the common example of intra-uterine infection. Modern treatment of syphilis has made it rare in these islands.

VIRUSES. Gregg first recognized the association between maternal rubella and congenital cataract and it was later noticed that many of those affected were deaf and had congenital heart disease. It has also been shown serologically that the fœtus may be affected without any clinically recognizable manifestations of German measles in the mother and that second attacks of rubella are possible. Recently some work has suggested that rubella some weeks *before* conception might cause abortion or an affected fœtus.

The search for other teratogenic viruses has gone on from that time but in the past twenty-four years there has been little to show any other association between maternal viral infections and congenital malformations. Infective hepatitis, mumps, measles and, until recently, poliomyelitis have all occurred in well documented epidemics and if these viruses were causing defects the evidence should be to hand by now.

TOXOPLASMA. The protozoon toxoplasma passing through the placental barrier causes toxoplasmosis in which mental defect, due to hydrocephalus, and a typical retinitis occur.

Drugs

In 1961 Lenz of Hamburg observed the association between mothers taking thalidomide in early pregnancy and the subsequent birth of babies with severe symmetrical defects of the limbs often amounting to complete absence, sometimes with other associated defects. This tragedy touched off a big enquiry into the effects of drugs taken early in pregnancy and some useful products were put under a cloud on scanty evidence. No similar hazard from any other drug has been revealed but the importance of caution in prescribing in the first trimester is evident. So is the importance of including tests for teratogenicity in the investigation of new drugs.

Progesterone and testosterone, given for habitual abortion, have caused local but reparable masculinization of the genitalia of female babies.

Physical Agents

INTRA-UTERINE MALPOSITION AND PRESSURE. Denis Browne has revived interest in the old Hippocratic concept of intra-uterine pressure. He attributes talipes to intra-uterine moulding of feet displaced into a cross-legged position and congenital dislocation of the hip to pressure on the knee in the fœtal flexed position. Associated findings are cited as evidence for this hypothesis such as the presence of pressure dimples on the convexities of the baby; mutual deformities which fit one into the other (e.g. bizarre valgus and varus talipes in opposite feet), and the association of abnormalities which could all have arisen from pressure (e.g. postural torticollis, congenital postural scoliosis and a hip with limited abduction).

Much opposition has been aroused by the simplicity of these concepts. To the authors it seems that clinical observation of malformed babies reveals again and again groups of lesions which fit the hypothesis too well for them to be disregarded as *one* of the factors influencing the production of deformities. For example there is clearly a genetic factor in the production of congenital dislocation of the hip, but its occurrence does not fit a simple genetic factor. Additional environmental factors such as hormone induced and inherited joint laxity are now recognized and it may well be that intra-uterine pressure is the mechanism of dislocation in some hips which are genetically shallow. Others may remain in joint but be recognizably dysplastic and give arthritic trouble in adult life.

Browne has divided these *mechanical* forces into three types.

Malposition. The baby is folded up the wrong way. The cross-legged position (Fig. 2) results in clubfoot (talipes total varus). The outer of the two feet is more severely affected.

Increased mechanical pressure. The mother may have noticed she was unusually small whilst carrying the infant which may have severe clubfeet with severely affected legs (Fig. 1). The upper limbs are less affected as they are largely protected by the size of the head.

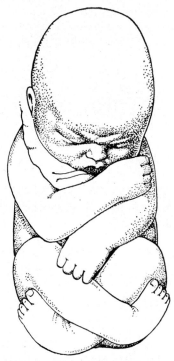

Fig. 2. Malposition *in utero*. The cross-legged position thought to cause talipes total varus ("equino varus").

Increased Hydrostatic Pressure. Increased hydrostatic pressure is thought to produce compression dysplasia in which all four limbs are malformed with poor development of the muscles, due to interference with blood flow which would be more severe towards the ends of the limbs. This may be a cause of arthrogryposis congenita multiplex.

Recently Browne has suggested that some congenital amputations and ring constrictions of the limbs may arise from the part being pushed through a hole in the amniotic membranes.

These mechanical concepts are only hypotheses but they are helpful in explaining certain conditions and the observed groupings of these conditions. It seems rational to use them at least until further evidence alters the situation.

X RADIATION. X-rays, even a single film very early in pregnancy, *may* be harmful to the developing fœtus though it is difficult to prove that it is the only factor in subsequently malformed infants.

ANÆSTHESIA. Hypoxia may arise during even trivial surgical procedures under general anæsthesia and placental anoxia may be a factor in, for example, limb malformations.

INTRA-UTERINE ACCIDENTS. It has been assumed until recently that intestinal atresia was due to agenesis or primary failure of development. Evidence is accumulating that this view is much too narrow. For instance skilful intra-uterine surgery has shown that ligature of blood vessels to the ileum causes typical ileal atresia in dogs, and some cases of human atresia have recognizable remnants of a fœtal intussusception, one obvious cause of interference with the blood supply of the fœtal bowel, though probably not the usual one. It must not be assumed that parts absent at birth were never formed—in the sterile conditions *in utero* complete resorption can occur. (The mechanism by which genetic defects are produced is unknown and it may be that alteration of the fœtal blood supply is a final common path.)

Experimental Teratogens

In experimental work a large number of chemical substances and physical agents have been shown to cause malformations. Four Nobel prize-winning drugs, insulin, penicillin, streptomycin and cortisone, have caused malformation in animals. But many experimental animals, and particularly insects, have natural mutation rates far in excess of the human and it is very difficult to assess the relevance of such work to the human.

Geographic

Certain anomalies have a distinct seasonal variation in incidence. Spina bifida is one such. The question is further complicated by the fact that the peak season is not the same in different parts of the country.

Social Class

An association between social grade and some malformations seems to exist, but in general malnutrition affects prematurity and abortion rate rather than that of malformations.

Hydramnios. Practically every malformation has been described with hydramnios from time to time without evidence of cause and effect. There is an established association between hydramnios and atresia in the alimentary tract, apparently due to inability of the fœtus to swallow, absorb and recirculate the fluid. As would be expected the incidence of hydramnios is greater the higher in the alimentary tract the atresia occurs.

Spina bifida and anencephaly are often associated with hydramnios, possibly as a result of excretion of cerebrospinal fluid into the amniotic cavity.

ANATOMICAL CLASSIFICATION OF MALFORMATIONS

We have discussed the ætiology of malformations. It is of some interest to consider an anatomical classification of these anomalies. The fœtal arrest concept fits many of the situations.

1. *Failure of Formation.*
2. *Excessive Formation.*
3. *Failure of Fusion.*
4. *Excessive Fusion.*
5. *Failure of Migration.*
6. *Failure of Atrophy.*

Syndactyly is a good example of failure of formation. There may be a simple webbing of the skin between two normal fingers in a mild case. In a severe one the hand is represented by ill-formed digital rays in a block of soft tissue, usually with an attempt at separation of a thumb. It clearly recalls the early stage of fœtal development of the hand. Excessive formation can also be exemplified in the hand. The development of an extra digit, usually protruding from the ulnar side of the carpus, is a fairly common deformity.

Failure of fusion is typified by harelip and cleft palate. Some recent work suggests that inadequate invasion by the mesodermal processes causes subsequent breakdown of the already formed primary lip and palate. Other animal work suggests a primary failure of fusion in isolated cleft palate. Excessive fusion is seen in the anomaly of anal development called covered anus. The site of the anus is hidden by an epithelial excrescence. Further forward in the perineum meconium may be seen shining through the perineal raphe. If the raphe is split back it is found that a complete anus underlies the epithelial tissues. The fusion of the anal tubercles and of the genital folds has been so excessive as to cover the anus.

Failure of migration is seen in the common type of undescended testis called "superficial inguinal ectopic". This organ can easily be felt in the groin in front of the inguinal canal. It cannot be pushed into the scrotum. Operation demonstrates that this is because the testis has got into an inguinal pouch which has a fascial floor preventing further descent. Most of the other types of undescended testis are in the correct line of descent but have not completed the journey. They will probably be inside the canal where the intact overlying external oblique muscle prevents their palpation. Thus we see that undescended testis may result from incomplete or erratic migration, leading to the clinical types of incomplete descent and ectopic testis.

Failure of atrophy of the processus vaginalis which descends with the testis is the cause of the common condition of inguinal hernia of childhood.

ADVICE TO PARENTS

Many are understandably anxious to know "if it will happen again". In the majority of conditions the mode of inheritance is as yet incompletely worked out and it is possible only to give an empirical statement as to the risk of recurrence. In counselling, the parents should not so much be advised as to whether or not to have more children but should have the facts presented, so far as these are known, and be allowed to make up their own minds.

A feeling of guilt is common and it may help to explain that the factors causing the defect are not due to anything the parents have done or failed to do. The fact that the chance of a pregnancy producing a defective child is one in forty in the general population is little realized.

A second interview should always be arranged and a much more careful enquiry into the family history will be required than is obtained at first. For instance, the parents may be genuinely unaware of the existence of affected babies in their families until they make further enquiries.

REFERENCES

Browne, Denis (1955) Congenital deformities of mechanical origin, *Arch. Dis. Childh.* **30**, 37.

Carter, C. O. (1963) "Clinical Genetics" Chapter in *Recent Advances in Pædiatric Surgery.* J. & A. Churchill, London.

Carter, C. O. (1962) *Human Heredity.* Penguin Books Ltd., Middlesex.

Congenital abnormalities (1963) *Practitioner* August 191.1142. (An entire issue.)

Congenital malformations, *Ciba Foundation Symposium.* J. & A. Churchill, London (1960).

Reed, Sheldon (1963) *Counselling in Medical Genetics.* W. B. Saunders, Philadelphia & London.

Roberts, J. Frazer (1963) *An Introduction to Medical Genetics.* Oxford University Press, London.

CHAPTER 2

BIRTH INJURIES

BIRTH injuries most often follow a difficult delivery. Primiparity, prolonged labour and disproportion between the passages and the passenger are all possible factors in the mechanism of injury. The premature baby is unduly vulnerable and the precipitate delivery may be just as injurious as a prolonged labour. Obstetrical accidents still occur even in the best hands, and they may cause permanent damage. The most serious birth injuries are those involving the *brain* and the commonest are probably the *birth fractures*.

Birth injuries may be considered in this order:

HEAD

LIMBS

VISCERA

HEAD

DEPRESSED FRACTURE OF THE SKULL. A distinctive form of birth fracture occurs in the vault of the skull. The bone is driven in to form a pond fracture, so called because of the rounded depression which results from pressure on the supple bone. The dura is usually left intact and mild depressions under 6 mm. can be left to correct spontaneously with growth. Deeper depressions should be elevated to avoid any risk of late sequelæ to the underlying brain. Elevation can be done simply by making a burrhole at one edge of the depression, sliding in a flat elevator under the bone and levering it up.

CEPHALHÆMATOMA. This is a collection of blood under the pericranium caused by pressure of the presenting part on the resisting os. It usually occurs over the presenting parietal bone, and is limited by the pericranial attachment around the bone. The edge of the hæmatoma forms a firm ridge while the centre remains fluid. The immediate impression on palpation is that a depressed fracture has occurred, and unnecessary alarm may be caused if the condition is not recognized. The temptation to aspirate the swelling should be resisted. The condition will resolve if left alone, and the introduction of infection could be serious.

CEREBRAL INJURIES. *Anoxia* during a difficult labour may damage the brain so that groups of cells die and are replaced by gliosis or porencephalic cysts. In this way cerebral palsy may occur and this particular mechanism is more likely to produce the athetoid type.

Hæmorrhage may block the aqueduct of Sylvius or the basal cisterns

9

and interfere with the flow of cerebrospinal fluid. The pressure in the ventricles rises compressing the brain and expanding the skull at the unfused sutures of the vault and hydrocephalus develops (see Chapter 8). Hæmorrhage over the surface of the brain (commonly subdural, or less commonly extradural) may cause progressive compression. Clearly all three types of brain injury may coexist.

Overlying scalp bruising or hæmatoma may be an early clue to deeper injury, but usually these external signs will be absent. Brain damage must be suspected in a baby who is unduly hypotonic, with perhaps intermittent twitchings of the limbs, cyanotic attacks, irregular respiratory and pulse rates, vomiting and inability to suck properly. The infant is often restless, hyperirritable and resents being handled. All these are

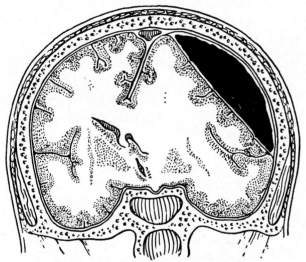

Fig. 3. Subdural hæmatoma compressing and displacing the brain.

signs of failure of central control. There may be neck stiffness and a tense fontanelle or a third nerve palsy, but often distinctively neurological signs are absent. The general state of the baby should arouse suspicion and a lumbar puncture will confirm the presence of blood. In such circumstances the subdural spaces should be tapped by a needle through the coronal sutures, well lateral to the fontanelle. A subdural hæmatoma or hygroma may require evacuation. Local signs such as twitching of one arm, or differences in tone between the two sides may give a clue to such collections. But again localizing signs may be absent. Such a brain-damaged baby may progress to normality or may develop cerebral palsy, often of the spastic hemiplegic type.

Subdural Hæmatoma. There are two types in infancy, the *acute* condition which is seen in the first week of life is often associated with a unilateral third nerve palsy. It can almost always be treated satisfactorily by a few subdural taps without resort to operation. The *chronic subdural hæmatoma* may present later with a gradual increase in head size. It is usually a more stubborn condition and may not respond to conservative measures. Drainage by needle should be repeated each day on alternate sides until the condition clears. The collection is usually bilateral but more extensive on one side than the other. A short bevel short lumbar puncture needle is satisfactory for the withdrawal of the subdural fluid. There should be no attempt at aspiration of the fluid, which should be allowed to drip out. Not more than 20 ml. should be withdrawn at any one time. The withdrawal of larger quantities may precipitate further hæmorrhages. Usually one side becomes dry after about two taps. The remaining side continues to be tapped daily. Normally, as the fluid is drawn off daily, it becomes lighter in colour, due to the influx of serum into the subdural space to replace the withdrawn blood. The fluid is thick and dark red at first and gradually becomes chocolate, xanthochromic and finally clear. If there are more than 20 ml. of fluid to be withdrawn daily after 10 days then a membrane has probably formed around the collection. Once this tough, inelastic membrane has formed a formal craniotomy is necessary for its removal. Before the craniotomy is undertaken the dry side should be aspirated once, lest a collection has silently been re-gathering there. Burrholes are made to confirm the position of the membrane. A wide craniotomy is then necessary to remove the membrane completely. *Persistence with aspiration is tempting but useless once the membrane has formed. Delay or failure to evacuate the fluid and eradicate the membrane may cause cortical atrophy.*

Subdural hæmatoma, or subdural hygroma, is a condition which is found in direct proportion to the persistence with which it is sought. The secret of diagnosis is suspicion, and suspicion should be followed by tapping. Negative taps, properly carried out, are completely safe. If the number of patients with subdural hæmatoma could be reduced, or if the condition were treated promptly and properly, the incidence of cerebral palsy might decline considerably. However anoxia, cerebral hæmorrhage and subdural hæmatoma are not the only causes of cerebral palsy. There is also a group apparently caused by genetic factors and with no evidence of perinatal trauma.

LIMBS

Birth injuries involving the limbs cause either *fractures* or *nerve lesions.*

Birth fractures are often of the greenstick type. The fibrillary elements of the bones are so strong that the bone cracks across without complete loss of continuity. Disability may be slight and discomfort seems minimal. A fracture of the clavicle may be recognized only later as a profuse mass of callus grows. The large mass will resolve spontaneously after several months. Fractured ribs may also be recognized only as the swelling of callus appears, and again no treatment is required. Fracture of the humerus, or displacement of the upper epiphysis may result from traction on the arm. It may be recognized when failure to use the arm freely leads to observation that the limb is angulated. Remodelling of the bones is highly effective at this young age, and healing with gross angulation may be accepted in the expectation of spontaneous correction over the next year or two. Treatment consists of simple protection. Strapping or bandaging to the side for two weeks is adequate.

Fracture of the shaft of the femur is of some importance. If left unsupported it will heal with 90° angulation, due to the flexed position in which the muscles hold the proximal fragment. Even this deformity will be corrected with growth over several years, but a degree of shortening may result. It is therefore wise to support the limb in 90° flexion for about two weeks. A felt-padded Cramer wire splint can be specially made to support the limb, or the neat traction device of Watson-Jones used. Either method allows for toilet management, which is a big consideration. Plaster of Paris is of little value, owing to the difficulty of achieving a good fit on a chubby baby without enveloping it in a mass of plaster, which makes toilet impractical and soon becomes a stinking mess.

Nerve lesions are a well-recognized result of traction during delivery. They usually affect the brachial plexus. Occasionally similar lesions occur in the lumbar plexus or spinal cord.

Traction affecting the upper cords of the brachial plexus produces the internally rotated arm hanging by the side typical of an Erb's palsy. The main paralysis affects the deltoid, supraspinatus, coracobrachialis and brachioradialis. While the nerves are given time to recover, overstretching of the muscles must be avoided and thus the development of fixed joint contractures prevented. Most of these injuries are at least in part recoverable. A bandage to the wrist from the top of the cot is a convenient way of maintaining the shoulder in abduction and external rotation in the early stages. Two or three times a day the mother should put the limb through a full range of passive movements.

A less common form of palsy affects the whole arm, or occasionally only the lower roots are affected resulting in paralysis of the small muscles of the hand. The damage to the nerves is more severe and recovery is uncommon.

VISCERAL INJURIES

Visceral injuries are rare. Sudden collapse of the newborn baby due to intraperitoneal hæmorrhage from intrapartum rupture of the liver can occur. The tear is usually adjacent to the falciform ligament, a relatively fixed part. The bleeding may thus be amenable to surgical arrest with transfusion.

Patches of cutaneous gangrene may arise in the newborn, usually affecting the lower limbs. Certain cases have been traced to the unintentional injection of stimulants into the umbilical artery instead of the vein. Vascular spasm then occurs. This does not explain all the cases. Areas of necrosis have also occasionally been seen in the bowel of premature babies and elsewhere, with no evident cause for the vasospasm. The stress of delivery may possibly play some part.

REFERENCES

Johnson, E. W. (1960) Brachial palsy at birth. Collective review, *Surg. Gynec. Obstet. Internat. Absts. Surg.*, **111**, 409.

Russell, P. A. (1965) Subdural Hæmatoma in Infancy. *Brit. med. J.*, *ii*. 446 (includes cases due to birth trauma).

CHAPTER 3

VOMITING IN THE FIRST WEEK OF LIFE

ABOUT a quarter of babies vomit during the first week of life. In the great majority the cause is not serious and treatment, if necessary, is simple and symptomatic. A presumptive diagnosis can usually be made from the timing and character of the vomit.

When did the vomiting begin? If it occurred in the first twelve hours of life it may be due to swallowed liquor amnii and secretions setting up a gastritis. If there is much mucus, gastric lavage with normal saline will help. *Is the vomiting persistent?* Unimportant types of vomiting are usually occasional and intermittent, and the vomitus is gastric juice and curdled milk. In most cases some simple cause of the vomiting will be found. For example, poor feeding technique allowing the baby to swallow too much wind, or failure to give the baby a rest and encouragement to bring up wind during the feed. Human milk virtually never "disagrees with" the baby, but an artificially fed baby may be having too concentrated a formula to start with. Sedatives and powerful anti-emetics or antispasmodics should not be given at this stage. They may mask symptoms of the uncommon serious lesions or may cause a drowsy baby to aspirate a vomit. There is never any need to force feeds on a reluctant baby in its first days of life and the attempt may be dangerous. The nature of the vomitus is of even greater importance.

Was the Vomit Green? This is the most important question. *Bilious vomiting in the first seven days of life of a full-term infant should be considered as due to mechanical intestinal obstruction until proved otherwise.* Yellow vomits are not uncommon. The pigment is not bile but is carotene from the colostrum milk, and is of no special significance.

Was the vomit bloodstained? In œsophageal hiatus hernia and chalasia of the œsophagus, there is usually a history of vomiting during the first few days of life and this is frequently bloodstained. The vomiting is typically regurgitant, effortless and responds to management by propping up the baby.

What was the nature of the stools? Meconium will be passed unless there is an imperforate anus, meconium ileus, or a severe form of Hirschsprung's disease. It is important to see whether the stools show milk curds in a case seen later, in which feeding has been attempted.

NOTE :

(1) Babies with œsophageal atresia present with respiratory distress due to unswallowed mucus. Attempts at feeding would make it

worse. These babies do not really vomit. They splutter frothy mucus and become intermittently cyanotic. (See page 32.)

(2) If no vomitus is available, aspirate the stomach and note the quantity and quality of the aspirate. If empty:—

(3) Test feed the baby with 5 per cent glucose *when* sure the feed is reaching the stomach.

(4) Inspect the anus and do a digital examination. A full-term infant's anus will accommodate an average doctor's little finger.

At least the nurses should realize the extreme danger of attempting to force feeds on a reluctant baby.

There are three serious causes of vomiting in this period. *They all produce green vomits.*

Mechanical Intestinal Obstruction
Cerebral Birth Injuries
Infections

Intestinal obstruction may occur anywhere along the tract from the beginning of the duodenum to the anus. It is usually complete. The vomiting is persistent and becomes copious. It is bilestained, *except* in those cases of duodenal obstruction proximal to the ampulla of Vater including the rare case of hypertrophic pyloric stenosis of precocious onset. Distension may be completely absent in duodenal obstructions whereas it may be marked in large bowel obstructions before vomiting is manifest. The individual causes of obstruction are described in the next chapter.

Cerebral birth injuries may cause repeated bilious vomiting. There is usually a suggestive history of difficult or precipitate delivery. Abdominal distension may be considerable, and accompanied by increased peristalsis. Clinically, the appearance of intestinal obstruction may be closely simulated. Indeed, the condition is one of obstruction, although the cause is neurogenic and not mechanical. Irregular pulse and respiration, bouts of peripheral circulatory failure, unusual flaccidity or irritability, or even frank fits may lead one to the diagnosis. The fontanelle is often tense. There is often increased but disordered peristalsis. These injuries are discussed in Chapter 2.

Infections may cause vomiting during the first week, but they are not common until later. Septicæmia can cause adynamic ileus. A dirty umbilicus may be the forerunner of a portal pyæmia, septicæmia or peritonitis. Meningitis may be present even without neck stiffness or a bulging fontanelle. External signs of infection may be slight or absent. The urinary tract should not be forgotten as a possible site of infection.

At this age infection may not cause pyrexia. The temperature may even be subnormal—a serious sign. The baby is typically hypotonic and looks more ill in the early stages than one suffering from mechanical obstruction.

Every baby who is even suspected of having an intestinal obstruction, the usual reason being green vomits, should have an upright radiograph of the abdomen. This can be carried out with minimal disturbance to the baby, even in the home if necessary. It will diagnose every case of complete obstruction. Further observation or investigation may be needed to exclude the less common incomplete or intermittent obstructions.

REFERENCES

Craig, W. S. (1961) Vomiting in the early days of life, *Arch. Dis. Childh.*, **36**, 451.

Dunn, P. M. (1963) Intestinal Obstruction in the Newborn with special reference to transient functional ileus associated with Respiratory Distress Syndrome *Arch. Dis. Childh.*, **38**, 459.

Editorial (1962) Vomiting in the newborn, *Brit. med. J. i*, 995.

CHAPTER 4

INTESTINAL OBSTRUCTION IN THE NEWBORN

ABOUT one in every fifteen hundred babies develops intestinal obstruction in the newborn period. Most causes of the obstruction are remediable, and in the majority it is an isolated abnormality.

The cardinal signs of intestinal obstruction are:

Vomiting
Distension
Absolute Constipation

The important symptom of mechanical obstruction is colic. Clearly in this age group this symptom is unlikely to be of much value. Of the three signs vomiting is the most important. Distension may be entirely absent in a high obstruction of the duodenum. Furthermore, it is difficult to assess in the early stages in the protuberant belly of the newborn. Constipation is not manifest until the bowel below the obstruction has emptied itself of meconium. This takes two or three days. One is left with *vomiting as the usual presenting symptom.* Obvious distension may, however, precede vomiting in large bowel obstruction. Visible peristalsis is fairly common in all types but is not a reliable sign of mechanical obstruction at this age.

The vomiting of intestinal obstruction is typically persistent and copious and is green except in obstruction of the duodenum above the ampulla of Vater. It persists even though feeds are withheld.

A new-born baby who is vomiting is in grave danger of aspirating vomitus. This may cause death rapidly from asphyxia or more gradually as a result of pneumonia or lung abscess. If obstruction is suspected a 12 F.G. catheter should be passed orally and the stomach aspirated. The quality and quantity may help in the diagnosis. This should be done *before the baby is transferred* to hospital. If the stomach is kept empty by quarter-hourly aspiration of the indwelling tube the distance to hospital is of little importance. The child's head should be kept low and the pharynx sucked out frequently.

The diagnosis will usually be pretty certain on the clinical grounds described. It can be confirmed by taking a plain radiograph of the abdomen in the upright position. The chest is usually included on the same film for it will be useful to see if there have been any ill effects of pulmonary aspiration. This is the only special investigation likely to be needed. If the stomach has already been aspirated 50 ml. of air should be put down the tube to provide a gaseous contrast before radiography.

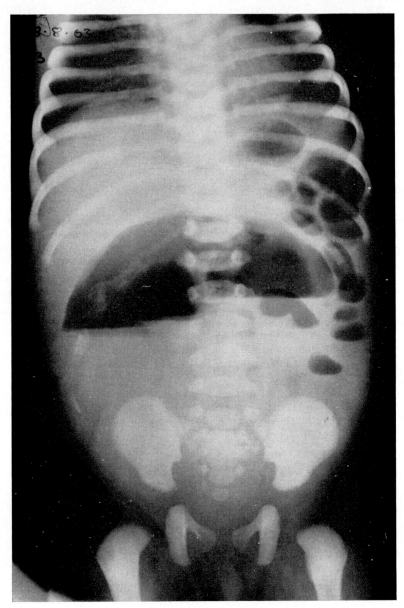

FIG. 4. Erect radiograph of ileal atresia
(with calcified meconium peritonitis).

Air is the safest contrast medium and the only one that should be used, except in the further investigation of those patients known not to be completely obstructed but thought possibly to have an incomplete or intermittent obstruction.

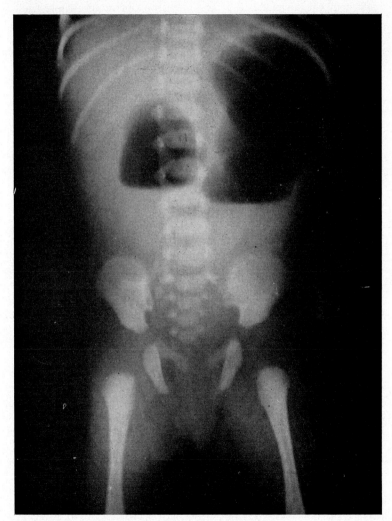

FIG. 5. Erect X-ray of duodenal atresia.

The small bowel of the newborn normally contains enough air to show fluid levels throughout. In the presence of mechanical obstruction the levels will be seen to be in progressively distending loops of bowel down to the level of the lesion. Below this there will be an opaque area.

In functional obstruction due to infections or neurogenic causes the distension is diffuse and affects the whole of the bowel equally. In peritonitis the loops may be seen to be separated by the fluid in the peritoneal cavity. Vigorous crying can also produce an impressive gas pattern in the normal baby's abdomen, but again the whole tract is equally affected.

When organic obstruction has been diagnosed then operation is indicated. Modern anæsthesia and supportive therapy have made a wide laparotomy the procedure of choice in virtually every case. Preparation for surgery is not prolonged as fluid and electrolyte disturbances are generally slight unless there has been serious delay in diagnosis into the third or fourth day of life. Blood must be available and a safe intravenous infusion which can be accelerated if need arises should be set up before operation.

A 7-lb. baby has a blood volume of about 250 ml. A loss of 50 ml. is hence the equivalent of a loss of a litre to an adult. Prompt and accurate replacement is essential.

CAUSES OF INTESTINAL OBSTRUCTION

We will now consider the individual causes of obstruction. None of them are common, yet they add up to about 500 infants each year in England and Wales. The four main groups are:

Atresia and stenosis
Malrotation
Meconium ileus
Hirschsprung's disease

ATRESIA

Atresia literally means no lumen. In *stenosis* the lumen is narrowed. Either may occur anywhere in the alimentary tract, but atresia is much more common than stenosis except in the duodenum. There may be a blind enlarged end to the bowel with a gap before the collapsed distal bowel is reached; or the ends may be joined by a cord of varying development from a fibrous thread up to a narrow but normally formed segment of the bowel (stenosis). Less commonly the bowel may look normal from the outside but be blocked by a complete or incomplete mucosal septum. Twenty-five per cent occur in the duodenum, fifty per cent in the ileum and most of the remainder are in the jejunum. The colon and stomach are very rarely affected. Varying lengths of bowel may be affected or lost in the formation of the lesion and there may be multiple atresias but there is almost always enough bowel left for reconstruction.

Associated disturbances of rotation are common in midgut loop atresias (jejunum and ileum) and there is some evidence that these atresias arise as a result of a vascular accident to the loop after it has formed. Outside the alimentary system the baby is usually normal.

Duodenal atresia, however, is associated with Down's syndrome in about a third of cases. It may be that these atresias result from persistence of the solid stage of the formation of the bowel though this is only hypothesis.

Jejuno-ileal atresia. Treatment of jejunal or ileal atresia is particularly urgent, for with delay the enlarged blind end of bowel proximal to the atresia will undergo tension gangrene. The abdomen is usually opened by a wide transverse muscle-cutting incision. The bowel is delivered out of the wound to elucidate the cause or causes of the obstruction. The few inches of bowel immediately above the block are greatly enlarged, for the acute postnatal obstruction is superimposed on a chronic prenatal obstruction to the passage of meconium. This bowel is inefficient in propulsion so it is resected and an end to oblique end anastomosis is carried out. One carefully placed row of fine silk invaginating mattress sutures may be used, so as to produce an accurate apposition of the serosa without obstructing the narrow lumen of the distal bowel, or an inner layer of continuous 50 catgut with an outer layer of interrupted 50 silk is probably more reliable. (One of us (B.O'D.) prefers en Y anastomosis with ileostomy as described below for meconium ileus.)

Duodenal atresia is commonly treated by duodeno-duodenostomy.

If the peritoneum is cut around the convexity of the proximal duodenum, it can be mobilized to reach the distal duodenum, allowing anastomosis to short circuit the obstruction without leaving a blind loop.

A gastrostomy is made in duodenal obstructions and in all obstructions in small premature babies—i.e. those in which postoperative vomiting is a particular risk—for nasogastric tubes have to be so small that blockage is common. In duodenal obstruction a tiny PVC tube can be passed through the same gastrostomy and on through the anastomosis to allow early milk drip feeding.

MALROTATION

Disturbances of rotation are often grouped together as malrotation. This is inaccurate although convenient. The common error is *failure to complete the normal process of rotation and fixation* of the bowel rather than an aberration of these processes. The cæcum remains high and near the midline of the abdomen. As a result the bands which pass to the posterior abdominal wall to fix it take a course across the duodenum and obstruct it. Furthermore the failure of descent of the cæcum and terminal ileum leaves the midgut loop suspended from a narrow stalk containing the superior mesenteric vessels instead of from the broad base of the normal root of the mesentery. This narrow pedicle renders the midgut loop liable to volvulus. When this occurs it obstructs the bowel first at its upper end. "Malrotation" can thus cause extrinsic obstruction of the duodenum in two ways. If the condition is neglected the bowel may also obstruct at the lower end of the volvulus forming a closed loop obstruction with rapid distension of the abdomen. This progresses to strangulation, and early death if unrelieved.

Malrotation usually presents from birth, but the obstruction by bands or volvulus may occasionally be delayed even into adult life. Clinically it may present as a complete or incomplete or intermittent duodenal obstruction. Blood may be passed per rectum. This, in association with the vomiting, can lead to a dangerous misdiagnosis of dysentery.

Treatment is by laparotomy, and unwinding of the volvulus if present. Then the transduodenal bands of Ladd are divided and the cæcum and colon brushed over to the left side of the abdomen. The duodeno-jejunal flexure is freed and coaxed to the right. This leaves all the small bowel on

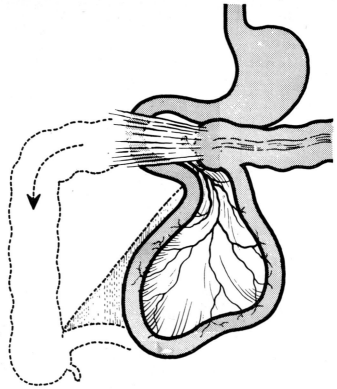

FIG. 6. The mechanism of intestinal obstruction due to incomplete rotation of the midgut (malrotation). The dotted lines show the course the cæcum should have taken. Failure has left bands across the duodenum, and a narrow pedicle for the midgut loop making it prone to volvulus.

the right side and the large bowel on the left, i.e. the bowel has been completely unrotated. This is an abnormal position, but a stable one compatible with a normal life and freedom from recurrence. It is technically much more satisfactory than attempts to produce a normal anatomy. Appendicectomy should be performed if the infant's condition permits.

It is to be hoped that the above account of the basis of the management of atresias and malrotations will not give an impression of simplicity or that a set procedure can be applied to every case. The patients present endless variations and combinations of disorders. The key to successful handling of the problems is an understanding of the underlying embryology so that the significance of variations can be assessed and the procedures modified to suit the individual case.

MECONIUM ILEUS

Meconium ileus is a mechanical obstruction of the bowel due to inspissated abnormal meconium. The meconium becomes solidified to a chewing gum consistency, and forms a complete barrier. The abnormality results from the generalized disorder of the mucous glands of the body called cystic fibrosis or mucoviscidosis.

All degrees of the condition occur from meconium retention with delayed but spontaneous passage of the material to complete obstruction with an abdomen distended at birth and green vomits within an hour or two. Masses of meconium in hypertrophied loops of bowel may be palpable through the abdominal wall. Little more than a mucus plug will be passed from the rectum even with the aid of a gentle washout. Radiography often shows a characteristic pattern of mottled meconium shadows, without even the normal fluid levels in the bowel as the meconium is so thick that it is not sufficiently fluid to form these levels.

Once a case has presented with the clinical picture of obstruction it is futile to hope for spontaneous relief. Operation is urgently required.

Bishop and Koop's 'en Y' operation has been most reliable in our hands. The maximally enlarged loop of bowel is resected and the proximal end anastomosed into the side of the distal bowel. The open end of the distal bowel is drawn out through a stab wound as an ileostomy. This acts as a safety valve until the inspissated meconium beyond is cleared. The natural colonization by *Escherichia coli* will do this, but postoperative instillation of pancreatin may expedite it. Any solid meconium proximal to the resection should be milked out with the help of injection of 1 per cent hydrogen peroxide before making the anastomosis. Either N-acetyl cysteine or Tween 80 may well prove a better substance to inject.

Half of these patients have complications in the shape of prenatal volvulus with or without the development of atresias or perforation or both. Nevertheless, it has proved possible to correct the intestinal obstruction in most cases.

The tragedy is that these patients are not saved for a normal life.

They still suffer from mucoviscidosis with its more usual presenting syndromes of pancreatic achylia with steatorrhœa, and persistent respiratory infections secondary to bronchial obstruction by the tenacious mucus. Many die in the early months of staphylococcal lung infections. But the medical management of these conditions is improving rapidly and the outlook is no longer one of unrelieved gloom. Methicillin should be given from the time of admission and a high humidity atmosphere maintained. Neomycin inhalations and mucolytic agents are used. N-acetyl cysteine shows promise.

Mucoviscidosis is a genetically determined condition. When it has occurred in a family there is one chance in four of subsequent siblings being affected though only 15 per cent of the affected babies will have meconium ileus.

HIRSCHSPRUNG'S DISEASE

Hirschsprung's disease usually presents symptoms from the first month of life. It is a condition in which the terminal bowel has no parasympathetic ganglia within its walls. The result is a functional obstruction due to inability to produce a co-ordinated wave. Most cases involve the rectum and the lower part of the sigmoid colon. Less commonly the segment involved may be shorter or it may be longer, even extending up into the small intestine.

A common story is that the baby passes little or no meconium during the first few days of life; develops tense abdominal distension, and then begins to vomit bile-stained fluid. Rectal examination may produce a dramatic passage of stool and flatus with prompt reduction of the distension. The baby may then remain well for days, weeks, or months before symptoms recur. Alternatively the baby may require saline rectal washouts to relieve the obstruction. In longer segment cases even this may fail to relieve the obstruction. If expert facilities are available an urgent barium enema will usually confirm the diagnosis.

Laparotomy will then be required. It will reveal a distended colon above the aganglionic segment coning down to a normal calibre at this level. A colostomy above the cone will relieve the obstruction. Biopsy of the rectal wall will allow histological confirmation of the aganglionosis but is usually more conveniently carried out later. Biopsy from the colostomy orifice will confirm that this is correctly placed above the affected bowel. The definitive treatment of the condition, usually by resection of the abnormal bowel right down to the anal canal with colo-anal anastomosis, is carried out later.

Hirschsprung's disease has classically been looked on as a type of chronic constipation with megacolon. But it is now realized that the true aganglionic condition is a distinct entity with a high infant mortality from obstruction. Now that pædiatricians are alerted to the clinical picture of complete, partial or recurrent obstruction in early infancy we are seeing more of these babies who would have succumbed in the past before reaching the later stage of the disease with chronic constipation and vast megacolon. At present about a third of patients with neonatal intestinal obstruction have Hirschsprung's disease.

It is still not widely recognized that the disease may present paradoxically with diarrhœa. For these babies may have fulminating attacks of enterocolitis (so-called putrefactive diarrhœa) in which the passage of liquid stools and prostration may detract attention from the underlying obstruction. They may die labelled as severe gastro-enteritis. Abdominal distension occurs in gastro-enteritis with hypokalæmia, but it is a feature which should alert the physician to the possibility of underlying Hirschsprung's disease. The passage of a flatus tube, repeated as necessary and perhaps with the addition of careful washouts, will usually bring the crisis under control. Intravenous infusions may be needed to combat dehydration or collapse. Colostomy should follow without delay.

Hirschsprung's disease is a genetically determined congenital lesion and it is considered further in Chapter 22.

RARE FORMS

There are several rarer forms of neonatal intestinal obstruction, but one must remember the possibility of incarcerated or strangulated inguinal hernia at this, as at every other age. Annular pancreas, duplication of the intestine and intussusception may all cause obstruction in the neonatal period.

REFERENCES

Louw, J. H. (1959) Congenital intestinal atresia and stenosis in the newborn, *Ann. roy. Coll. Surg. Engl.*, **25**, 4, 209–234.

Nixon, H. H. (1960) Experimental study of propulsion in isolated bowel and applications in intestinal obstruction in the newborn, *Ann. roy. Coll. Surg. Engl.*, **27**, 106.

Santalli, T. V. and Blanc, W. A. (1961). Congenital atresia of the intestine. *Ann. Surg.*, **154**, 939.

Bishop, H. C. and Koop, C. E. (1957). Management of Meconium Ileus, *Ann. Surg.*, **145**, 410.

Holsclaw, D. S., Eckstein, H. B. and Nixon, H. H. (1965). Meconium Ileus: a 20 year review of 109 cases, *Amer. J. Dis. Child.* **109**, 101.

CHAPTER 5

IMPERFORATE ANUS

IMPERFORATE ANUS is the name usually given to the group of congenital anomalies which may arise in the formation of the terminal gut. It is a convenient name but an inaccurate one. In the great majority there is a small though abnormal outlet for the bowel, either on the surface of the perineum or vulva or internally as a "fistula" into the prostatic urethra of the male or the vagina in the female. These anomalies occur in about 1 in 3,000 babies.

Prompt diagnosis of the type is important because there is a large group in which simple, though painstaking, management will produce normal continence, and another large group in which management is much more difficult, control is less complete and associated defects are more common. Inadequate or delayed treatment of the former can make their childhood miserable and mar their chances of fæcal control.

CLASSIFICATION

The most important practical subdivision of ano-rectal anomalies is into the *Low* and *High* types. In the former the bowel extends down through the levator ani and its puborectalis sling before becoming abnormal. In the High type the bowel ends on (or occasionally some way above) the pelvic floor. It usually has a small orifice into the posterior urethra in the male or into the intervening vagina in the female.

The Low types should virtually all achieve normal continence. The High types rarely achieve normal continence though the majority develop, through voluntary effort, a socially acceptable form of abnormal continence by the age of 5 to 7 years or even later. In this High group there is a considerable mortality from associated serious abnormalities particularly common in the urinary system and the heart.

Development. The usual causative embryological processes are excessive fusion of the anal tubercles and genital folds, and failure of migration of the anus from its primitive intra-cloacal position. The latter process can alternatively be stated as a failure to complete the separation of the primitive cloaca into urogenital and rectal portion. Some of the apparent differences of opinion on these embryological processes are little more than a play on words. The two invaluable concepts of *Excessive Fusion* and *Failure of Migration* were brought into clinical use by Denis Browne and Douglas Stephens.

The three main anomalies, covered anus, ectopic anus and anorectal agenesis are about equal in frequency.

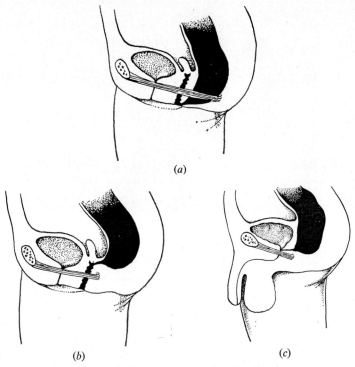

(*a*)

(*b*)   (*c*)

FIG. 7. Certain malformations of anus and rectum.

(*a*) Vulval ectopic anus. The small opening remains in the vulva, but the bowel passes through the puborectalis sling before it becomes abnormal.

(*b*) Rectal agenesis with vaginal fistula. A more primitive condition in which separation of the lower rectum from the urogenital sinus has failed to occur. A primitive cloacal termination in the posterior vaginal fornix usually persists. The abnormality occurs above the puborectalis.

(*c*) Rectal agenesis with urethral fistula. The male condition corresponding to (*b*) in which the primitive bowel termination is in the prostatic urethra (interposition of the Müllerian cords in the female transfers it to the vaginal fornix). Again the abnormality lies above the puborectalis.

Low Anomalies

Covered Anus. This anomaly usually occurs in the male. As the genital folds or the anal tubercles develop their posterior ends fuse excessively so as to cover the normal anal site. A median bar may thus extend over the anus leaving a small opening to one side of it. More commonly the orifice is covered completely leaving a subcutaneous track under the perineal raphe which runs forward towards the scrotum and opens at the front of the perineum as the so-called perineal fistula. Occasionally the orifice is carried even further forward along the ventral surface of the penis.

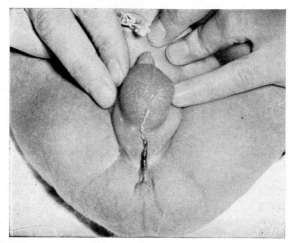

FIG. 8. This covered anus shows meconium tracking forward in the perineal and scrotal raphe.

It is important to realize that there is a complete and normal anus underlying the epithelial excrescence in these cases.

Ectopic Anus. This type usually occurs in the female. The usual site is in the vestibule or vulva. The suggestion is that the anus fails to migrate from its primitive site back to the surface of the perineum. The bowel extends through the normal pelvic floor and the pubo-rectalis sling before taking its abnormal course. Like all ectopic orifices the anus is usually stenosed. The external sphincter does not usually surround it. (This sphincter is at the normal anal site and may be poorly developed). Yet full continence is regularly achieved with management as described below. This fact is difficult to explain on normal concepts of defæcation control and suggests that the pubo-rectalis portion of levator ani is very important in continence.

A less severe failure of migration may produce a perineal ectopic anus in either sex. The opening is on the perineal surface but farther forward than normal.

High Anomalies

High anomalies are commoner in the male. The basic error is a developmental arrest. One may say that the uro-rectal septum has failed to develop or that the primitive anus has failed to migrate down

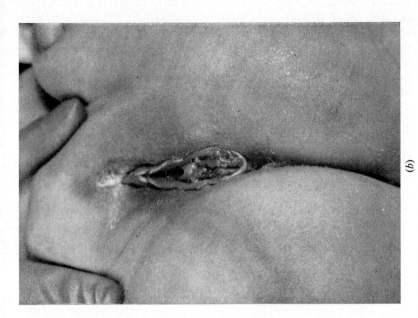

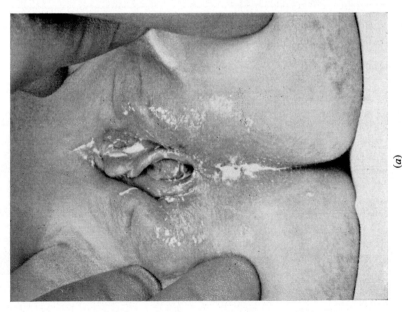

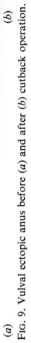

(a)

(b)

Fig. 9. Vulval ectopic anus before (*a*) and after (*b*) cutback operation.

the cloaca and across the perineum, depending on the interpretation of the differential growth pattern one prefers. The result is that the bowel stops above the levator ani with a small terminal orifice (or occasionally a fibrous cord) entering the prostatic urethra. If the anomaly arises in the female its presentation is modified by the interposition of the Müllerian ducts so that the orifice usually enters the posterior fornix of the vagina. The perineum shows no orifice; the natal cleft is usually shallow, and the anal site is marked by a slight dimple or more commonly a raised ridge of epithelium in the raphe. *Anorectal agenesis* with urethral or vaginal fistula is one of the names which have been given to this type.

Rectal atresia occurs rarely. The anal canal is normal, but ends as a blind pouch at the level of the upper border of levator ani. The rectum ends as a pouch above this and there is no attachment to the urethra or vagina. There may be a wider gap with a cord between the patent rectum and the anal canal, i.e. the findings are similar to those of small intestinal atresia. Of course in these cases the sphincter mechanism is intact around the normal anal canal and it is unfortunate that they are so rare compared with the anorectal agenesis or persistent cloaca type.

INTERMEDIATE ANOMALIES (uncommon)

Anorectal stenosis occurs due to a fibrous ring stricture inside the anal canal where the proctodæum joins the rectum and may be associated with incomplete development of the anal sphincters.

Anorectal septum, due to failure of the anal membrane to break down is rare. Most so-called septa are at the lower end of the anal canal in cases of covered anus.

Diagnosis

This can almost always be made on inspection, according to the descriptions given above. Passage of meconium *per urethram* or *vaginam* may signalize a fistula in anorectal agenesis. Radiography of the inverted baby will confirm the findings if necessary. A lateral view centred on the greater trochanter (Stephens) will enable one to relate the level of the air bubble outlining the end of the bowel to the "pubococcygeal line" which marks the level of the levator floor of the pelvis. It also allows one to assess the development of the sacrum. Incomplete sacral development is not uncommon particularly in the high anomalies. A sacrum with three segments or less is likely to be associated with a neurological defect which will not only render levator control of the bowel deficient but also lead to a neurogenic bladder lesion.

TREATMENT

Almost every case needs prompt neonatal treatment for its best management. This may be of a minor nature—perhaps only dilatation—

but delay can cause much misery and can rarely achieve any benefit. There is nothing gained by tiding a baby over with aperients and enemas before referring to surgery. Most of the bad results are due to rectal inertia with overflow incontinence. The lack of control is due to constipation (and consequent overflow of liquid fæces) and not as might be expected to inadequate sphincter ability. The tedious treatment of rectal inertia is described in the chapter on constipation, but the condition is better avoided by correct early management.

It must be emphasized that the operation is only the beginning of the treatment. The anus produced will require daily dilatation (mother's fifth finger or Hegar's dilator size 12) for three months after which the frequency is reduced over the next three months. Follow-up examination and advice on management follow at least to school age. The anomalies should be tackled only by someone prepared to carry out this prolonged supervision and management. The results of such care are most rewarding.

Primary treatment of the low varieties is by enlarging the opening so as to enable it to work where it lies (Denis Browne). A perineal ectopic anus may need only dilatation. The commoner vulval ectopic anus is better treated by a cutback. This consists of a simple midline episiotomy enlarging the opening backwards to make it big enough. It is followed by dilatations. The end result is a shotgun perineum with both barrels alongside without the usual bridge of intervening skin (Denis Browne). Functionally this arrangement is fully adequate. In a few cases the anus may be difficult to keep clean and later troubles may arise which justify transplantation to the normal site. This can be done easily at say four years of age in the minority who need it. It is carried out from the perineum, dissecting only below the competent levator floor. Whenever possible the toddler period should be avoided for the operation because after-care with dilatations are particularly likely to be upsetting at this age and co-operation in training will not be obtained.

The covered anus only needs enlarging by cutting back from the minute opening, following the track to the underlying anus, and removing the epithelial cover. Dilatations for three months to prevent contraction and constipation will result in a normal anus.

The high anomalies (rectal agenesis) are usually treated by abdomino-anal operation. The end of the bowel has to be freed from its attachment or fistula to the urethra or vagina; it is mobilized and then brought through the pelvic floor in front of the puborectalis sling to an opening made at the anal site. The unpredictable degree of continence obtained has led to modifications and to the development of an alternative sacro-coccygeal approach. Others believe that the sensory side of control has had inadequate consideration.

In the absence of full facilities for major neonatal surgery or in a grossly distended baby, a transverse colostomy may be a wise primary procedure which will save life and leave the pelvis and sigmoid colon free for later surgery. Many believe it is always wise in the "high" anomalies so that the perineum can be dissected later with less risk of injury to muscles and nerves.

The urinary system should be investigated in every case as at least a third are abnormal.

The three main anomalies—covered anus, ectopic anus and rectal agenesis (or persistent cloaca) are about equal in frequency.

REFERENCES

Bill, A. H. Jr. and Johnson, R. J. (1958) Failure of migration as the cause for most cases of imperforate anus, *Surg. Gynec. Obstet.*, **106**, 643.

Browne, Denis (1955) Congenital deformities of the anus and the rectum, *Arch. Dis. Childh.*, **30**, 149, 42.

Kiesewetter, W. B. and Turner, C. R. (1963) Continence after surgery for imperforate anus, *Ann. Surg.*, **158**, 498.

Nixon, H. H. (1961) Imperforate Anus. British Surgical Practice. Surgical Progress. Butterworth's, London.

Nixon, H. H. and Callaghan, R. P. (1964) Ano-rectal Anomalies: Physiological Considerations, *Arch. Dis. Childh.*, **39**, 158.

Scott, J. E. S. and Swenson, O. (1959) Imperforate anus, *Ann. Surg.*, **150**, 477.

Stephens, F. D. (1963) Congenital Malformation of the Rectum, Anus and Genito-urinary Tracts. E. & S. Livingstone Ltd., London.

CHAPTER 6

RESPIRATORY DIFFICULTIES IN THE NEWBORN

Breathing and Swallowing Difficulties

THESE two problems are frequently associated in the neonatal infant. The first sign of respiratory distress may be a rise in the respiratory rate (tachypnœa) or dyspnœa. The dyspnœic infant often holds its head back in a typical manner. If the condition is really severe there will also be cyanosis.

Difficulty in swallowing in infancy is usually a consequence of difficulty in breathing. The baby is unable to afford the delay in respiration necessary for deglutition. Difficulty in swallowing may also arise from incoordination resulting from a cerebral lesion, or less commonly from a congenital palatal palsy. Even unfed babies have to swallow their own saliva, and inability to do so may be the first sign of trouble.

Most of the difficulties encountered are due to conditions requiring management rather than operation, but it is not easy to give figures of the relative incidence.

The conditions fall into three main groups:

1. RESPIRATORY DISTRESS SYNDROME OF THE NEW-BORN
2. RESPIRATORY DIFFICULTY DUE TO OBSTRUCTION OF THE UPPER AIR PASSAGES
3. INTRATHORACIC SURGICAL CONDITIONS

Respiratory Distress Syndrome of the Newborn

This is perhaps the commonest single condition causing respiratory distress. It is associated with a variety of conditions including prematurity, atelectasis and hyaline membrane. Hyaline membrane is particularly common in premature infants. The membrane forms on the wall of the alveoli and prevents normal gaseous exchange, resulting in cyanosis and possibly death. The origin of the membrane is still disputed, and the descriptive term hyaline is from the histological appearance. The infant is kept in an incubator and disturbed as little as possible. The oxygen pressure is only raised enough to relieve any cyanosis, and the humidity kept high. The acidosis is treated by THAM. However, active treatment is not very effective, and the object is to bring the infant through the first vital 48 hours. If they survive to that stage they usually thrive from then on.

Inhalation of liquor amnii occurs frequently and indeed it may well be a normal condition. However, it upsets some infants more than others, and it may cause respiratory distress and the secretion of copious mucus. The treatment is frequent pharyngeal aspiration.

Obstruction of the Upper Air Passages
Micrognathia
Choanal Atresia
Congenital Laryngeal Stridor
Subglottic Stenosis

Micrognathia. In this condition of underdevelopment of the lower jaw the relatively large tongue has inadequate room in the mouth. The tongue can fall back and choke the baby. This tendency is exaggerated

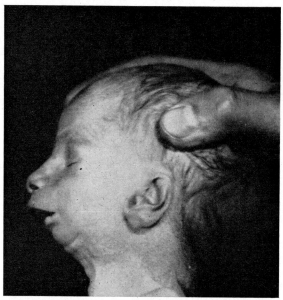

Fig. 10. Micrognathia. Note the emaciated appearance, the result of feeding difficulty.

when micrognathia is associated with a cleft of the soft palate (the Pierre Robin syndrome). Respiratory distress is due to the narrow airway, and feeding difficulties occur owing to the increased respiratory obstruction resulting from attempted swallowing.

Posture is the prime factor in treatment. These babies should never be allowed to lie on their backs, or the tongue may fall back and sudden fatal asphyxia may occur. Feeding may be helped by holding the angle of the jaw forwards. A more severe case may require feeding through an indwelling naso-gastric tube to avoid exhaustion. Oxygen may be required at first. A crisis of asphyxia may be resolved by a tongue-stitch to hold the tongue forward. This is a purely temporary measure and in a few cases it may be necessary to do a tracheostomy. Failure of tracheostomy is usually due to doing the correct operation too late. Nevertheless, with skilled nursing care, it should rarely be needed.

Micrognathia tends to improve with age. As the baby grows the air passages widen and the relative narrowing becomes less significant. The infant gains more control over his tongue by the third month. The jaw also improves relative to the baby. An unsightly tiny jaw at birth may become an attractive small chin in a pleasant-featured baby with a small "rosebud" mouth. After the first three months of life the difficulties are usually over. If the palate is cleft this may be repaired at the usual time. *There is no urgency about the palate repair* as the technical difficulties of early surgery may prejudice the speech results without helping the problem of the respiratory passages.

CHOANAL ATRESIA. In this condition the openings of the nose into the nasopharynx are closed by a septum containing bone. The nasal channel is often also diminished in size. A unilateral case may escape recognition for years, until a chronic nasal discharge leads to investigation. A bilateral case will usually present as an urgent problem of respiration. The baby will go blue, making violent inspiratory efforts. If the mouth is opened and the tongue drawn forward air can be inhaled easily. But mouth-breathing is an unnatural habit which a new-born baby has to learn. Meanwhile some form of tube over the back of the tongue may be used to allow mouth-breathing until the choanæ can be opened by operation. If the posterior end of the septum is nibbled away as well as the offending diaphragms it seems that less postoperative bouginage is likely to be necessary.

CONGENITAL LARYNGEAL STRIDOR. This is a label given to a condition characterized by a harsh inspiratory stridor. It may be accompanied by intercostal recession, due to the difficulty of getting air into the lungs. It tends to be outgrown, and no active measures are necessary. Some cases have an inter-arytenoid cleft allowing the cords to be sucked-in on inspiration. A few have a delicate laryngeal web. A small proportion later show cerebral damage.

SUBGLOTTIC STENOSIS. Congenital subglottic stenosis will give rise to respiratory distress, and may require tracheotomy. It is important not to over-investigate such patients. A little œdema of the larynx after laryngoscopy means a relatively severe encroachment in the narrow air passages of the newborn, and may tip the scales against the baby. Tracheostomy should be performed early, before the baby becomes exhausted by his efforts.

INTRATHORACIC SURGICAL CONDITIONS

In addition to the abnormalities described above, there are several important surgically remediable intrathoracic lesions which can mimic these conditions so closely that it is vital always to bear them in mind. In many instances clinical examination of the infant will allow the doctor to go no further than realizing that there is something gravely the matter with the respiratory system. There are serious limitations to clinical methods in the examination of an infant's chest. An X-ray is essential.

The X-ray must have good definition and, because the infant's respiratory rate is so rapid, a short film exposure of not more than one-thirtieth of a second is necessary. It may well be that the mobile or portable X-ray unit does not give this short exposure, in which case the patient should be moved to the X-ray department, in oxygen if necessary, to give him the benefit of a clear, definitive picture. Surgery within the chest of an infant should never be contemplated without an X-ray.

The following conditions, all usually surgically remediable, should be borne in mind in any infant with respiratory distress.

1. **Œsophageal atresia with tracheo-œsophageal fistula**
2. **Congenital diaphragmatic hernia**
3. **The tension syndrome, to include staphylococcal lung-cysts, congenital lobar emphysema, and congenital lung-cysts**
4. **Congenital heart disease**
5. **Vascular rings**

Œsophageal Atresia

This is a congenital interruption of the œsophagus. The usual type (85 per cent) has a blind upper pouch and a fistula from the lower segment of the œsophagus to the trachea at or about its bifurcation. An

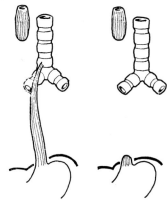

FIG. 11. Œsophageal atresia. 1. The usual type with fistula from lower segment to trachea. 2. The type next in frequency. Atresia without fistula and with a wide gap between the ends.

infant with this condition will be found to have much mucus in its throat, and this rapidly collects again after aspiration. The mucus tends to be inhaled, causing respiratory distress. Air tends to be drawn into the stomach through the tracheal fistula, and distension of the abdomen may interfere with diaphragmatic movements and exacerbate this distress. A new-born baby's breathing is almost entirely diaphragmatic. Gastric juice regurgitating through the fistula is another factor contributing to the respiratory distress, and it may be responsible for a chemical pneumonia which sometimes becomes serious after operation although it has arisen some time before any treatment is undertaken.

The recurrent collection of mucus in the baby's throat should give rise to immediate suspicion of atresia. Classically the mucus overflows at the mouth and the baby blows it out in little bubbles.

If the condition is unrecognized and feeding is attempted, the milk soon fills the œsophageal pouch and spills over into the trachea, choking the baby and causing acute cyanosis. This phenomenon should rarely be seen for the suspicion of atresia can be confirmed simply at the bedside if the significance of persistent frothing is realized. A rubber catheter, French gauge 10, is boiled up and passed through the mouth down the gullet. It is advisable to pass it through the mouth, as in this way there is less possibility of it passing through the vocal cords. Fine catheters have passed down the trachea through the fistula into the stomach or have coiled in the upper pouch and given the false impression of a normal œsophagus, but this will not happen if a catheter of this size is passed through the mouth. If atresia is present the catheter will stick about four inches from the gums. If not, the catheter will pass on into the stomach.

If the catheter will not pass then the patient is treated as having œsophageal atresia until proved otherwise, and no time should be lost in transfer to a unit where the diagnostic X-ray can be carried out. A radio-opaque catheter is passed into the gullet and on X-ray will be seen in the air shadow of the upper pouch of the œsophagus. *No dye of any kind in any quantity should be used*, as diagnosis can always be definitely established without it. If a few cubic centimetres of air are blown through the catheter just before the film is taken it will often outline the upper pouch of the œsophagus.

If the infant is to be transferred, then it is important that repeated pharyngeal suction be made during the journey so as to minimize pulmonary inhalation complications. The infant should be nursed in a head up position and virtually continuous suction of the mucus maintained. We have seen a baby arrive in a surgical centre three hours after birth when a shrewd midwife suspected atresia and passed a catheter in the home. Such promptitude, resulting in diagnosis before feeding is attempted, is clearly of great value in avoiding pulmonary collapse and its possible sequelæ. Once the lesion is diagnosed pharyngeal suction must be persistent. The operation to repair the defect will follow later.

The usual procedure is a right thoracotomy with division of the fistula and primary anastomosis of the upper and lower segments of the œsophagus. A gastrostomy can also be performed to allow early feeding. This should certainly be done if the anastomosis has been

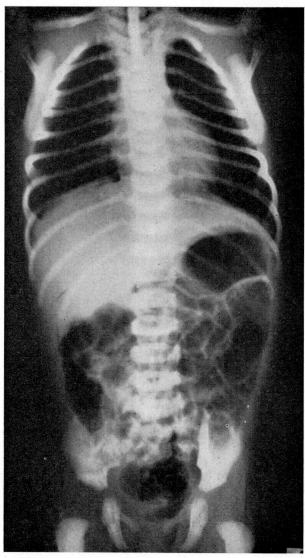

FIG. 12. Œsophageal atresia of the usual type with fistula. Tube stops at lower end of upper pouch which is outlined by the contained air. Normal gas pattern in the abdomen confirms presence of fistula and absence of associated obstruction in the abdomen.

performed under tension. If the anastomosis has been performed without tension then the infant may be fed through a fine-bore polythene tube which goes through the anastomosis and enters the stomach. The results of treatment in a mature baby with no other deformity are good. Break-down is rare. A tendency to stricture at the anastomosis may necessitate later œsophagoscopic dilatation in some cases. This narrowing is particularly liable to show itself when mixed feeding begins, but it almost always responds to bouginage.

Many of the babies have a harsh raspy cough which may cause undue alarm. This tends to be outgrown. It is probably due to vibration of the mucosal fold which is present at the tracheal end of the fistula, though occasionally the vagus nerve is damaged at operation and this may be the cause.

A large proportion of these babies are premature or have other abnormalities (about 40 per cent), and in particular there is a definite association with imperforate anus, duodenal atresia and congenital heart lesions. If any of these conditions is present the outlook is much less favourable. There is such a close relation between birth-weight and prognosis that it is usual to restrict primary operation in premature babies under 4 lb. weight to a division of the fistula and gastrostomy with continued pharyngeal suction or cervical œsophagostomy to drain the upper pouch. When the baby has established itself and gained weight the definitive repair follows.

A less common type (10 per cent) of atresia occurs without a fistula to the trachea. In these cases the lower segment is usually only represented by a nubbin of tissue above the diaphragm and there is a long gap between the two segments of the œsophagus, so that primary anastomosis is impossible. This type can often be recognized clinically because the abdomen is dull to percussion since there is no fistula. (In the usual type of atresia with a fistula air soon enters the stomach and the abdomen becomes resonant.) The outlook in this type is not so good. At primary operation the upper pouch is brought out into the neck (cervical œsophagostomy) so that the saliva can drain away, and a gastrostomy is performed for feeding. The stomach is small and considerable nursing skill may be required to enable adequate feeding to be maintained.

When the infant is a few months old a substitute œsophagus must be made. A technique used at the present time is to isolate the transverse colon and bring it up through the chest, anastomosing it to the upper pouch of the œsophagus and to the distal œsophagus. Good results have been obtained in this manner.

Rare variants occur in which both upper and lower segments of the œsophagus communicate with the trachea, or in which there is a common tube or œsophago-trachea, or in which a fistula may be present without atresia. This latter (H fistula) is a cause of respiratory distress which is difficult to diagnose. In our experience the fistula is high up, at the root of the neck, where it is extremely awkward to demonstrate even when the lesion is suspected. In this condition a small foroblique cystoscope may be a more useful instrument in searching for the fistula's opening than the conventional bronchoscope or œsophagoscope. A little methylene blue blown down the endotracheal tube may enable the fistula to be visualized from the œsophagus. A cine barium swallow in the prone position may also reveal the fistula.

Congenital Diaphragmatic Hernia

This is one of the few "fire brigade" emergencies where minutes may count. Once the diagnosis has been established, the patient should be taken to the theatre straight away and the operation started as soon as possible.

There are several types of diaphragmatic hernia, but a defect in the left dome of the muscle accounts for at least 80 per cent of cases, and defects of the right dome account for 15 per cent. The small bowel, the spleen and a portion of the large bowel are usually within the chest cavity. The mobility and shape of the mesentery usually found makes it clear that a large proportion of the small intestine has been developing in the chest before birth. The lung on the side affected is completely collapsed. The other lung may not yet be fully expanded, or at least may not be adequately aerated because of mediastinal displacement by the bowel in the chest. Because of this symptoms are usually early and dramatic.

Cyanosis and dyspnœa occur spontaneously and are exacerbated by attempted feeding. If there has been time for gaseous distension of the intestines to occur then the symptoms will be further exacerbated. The chest is usually resonant to percussion on the affected side, though fluid in the intestine may sometimes render it dull. The heart is pushed over, away from the affected side, and may frequently give the impression of a dextrocardia in the common defect of the left dome of the diaphragm. It is the combination of severe, sometimes intermittent cyanosis with displacement of the heart, and consequently the heart sounds, which make one suspect the diagnosis:

TRIAD: Cyanosis

Dyspnœa

Apparent dextrocardia.

The abdomen is suspiciously empty when palpated. Auscultation of the affected side may reveal bowel sounds in the chest, but this is one of those classical signs which is better not waited for. Once the diagnosis is suspected, these patients should always have a doctor who is capable of passing an endotracheal tube watching them until the anæsthesia is induced, and nasogastric suction to prevent swallowed air from distending the intestine. Asphyxial death may occur rapidly and unexpectedly. Even if the distress seems to have settled completely, this condition remains one of the utmost urgency for operation. An erect chest X-ray is taken immediately. It will confirm the presence of intestinal gas shadows in the chest and their rarity in the abdomen. Cysts of staphylococcal pneumonia can give similar shadows in the chest X-ray and a similar clinical story. But infection will not be a cause in the first few days of life and a normal gut pattern will still be visible in the abdomen. Asphyxia may be so severe as to need endotracheal intubation and positive pressure respiration before and during transfer to a surgical unit. *Face mask insufflation, or worse still, intragastric oxygen may kill the baby by filling the misplaced intestine with gas.*

Operation is usually undertaken from the abdomen in the neonatal period, so that any concomitant bowel condition, e.g. malrotation, can be inspected and treated at the same time. The bowel is first withdrawn from the chest and this part of the operation has sometimes to be carried out with the urgency which used to be associated with the performance of tracheostomy in the past. There may or may not be a sac of peritoneum extending into the chest. If present, it is so closely applied to the pleura as to be easily missed. A nick allows air between the layers and clarifies the situation. When the viscera have been withdrawn from the chest, the lungs can be inflated and the defect closed at leisure. The affected lung is usually slow to expand, but one must be careful not to exert too much pressure on the endotracheal tube for fear of damaging the lung on the opposite side. There is no need to attempt to expand the collapsed lung, which will gradually come to fill the chest cavity over the suc-

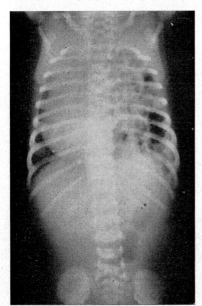 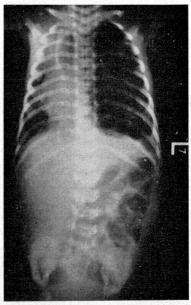

FIG. 13. Diaphragmatic hernia. The left chest contains most of the bowel and the abdomen is seen to be almost free of bowel shadows.

FIG. 14. Staphylococcal lung cysts. The left lung contains many large cysts which have pushed the mediastinum across and collapsed the right lung.

ceeding few days. There is usually ample tissue for the repair of the diaphragmatic defect, and pericostal sutures should be used if there is any doubt about the safety of the closure due to a poor posterior rim of the defect. At the end of the operation the chest should be aspirated, to avoid any possibility of tension pneumothorax from trapped air delaying the expansion of the lung. Closure of the abdomen is rarely difficult with relaxant anæsthesia. However, tension limiting diaphragmatic movement after operation may lead to acidosis causing unexpected collapse, so there is still a place for closure of skin only, particularly in prematures. The peritoneum should be sutured to the anterior layer of fascia to avoid adhesions to the cut muscle ends. Then formal closure in layers can be performed a week later. Gastrostomy also helps by diminishing gaseous distension of the abdomen.

It is particularly important to avoid excessive administration of intravenous fluids in these cases, as the brain may have suffered considerably from anoxia before operation, and excess fluid would exacerbate postoperative cerebral œdema.

Results are good in mature infants seen before 24 hours old unless anoxia has caused irreversible brain damage. A group of patients with hypoplastic lungs and other severe associated anomalies, which used to die within 24 hours, may now reach the surgeon, but the results of treatment are poor.

The Tension Syndrome

This name is given to the picture of cyanotic collapse resulting from an expanding lesion in the chest causing collapse of the lungs. The neonatal mediastinum is so freely mobile that the effects are soon felt by both lungs.

Diaphragmatic hernia presents thus. Other expanding lesions may be the cysts of staphylococcal pneumonia, or a tension pneumothorax or pyopneumothorax of the same disease, congenital lobar emphysema, or congenital lung cysts. The physical signs of all may be similar. Cyanosis, rapid respiration and pulse rate, a hyper-resonant chest and a displaced heart are common to all. Any clinical distinction between these problems and congenital diaphragmatic hernia is largely a chronological one, as the diaphragmatic hernia often causes serious trouble during the first few hours of life, whereas these conditions tend to occur later in the first week or two. Evidence of sepsis elsewhere may lead to suspicion of staphylococcal pneumonia as the underlying cause. Radiology distinguishes the conditions. In addition to an anteroposterior picture of the chest, a good true lateral view is essential for accurate localization.

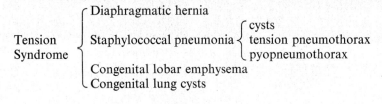

Staphylococcal cysts or pneumothorax, or pyopneumothorax all respond well to an intercostal drain with low-pressure motor suction. This method of suction is essential to deal with the amount of air which may leak through the damaged bronchus. The organism's sensitivity to various antibiotics should be established as early as possible, but full doses of antibiotics (at present cloxacillin) should be given immediately. These staphylococcal lung cysts tend to resolve spontaneously so that residual cysts may be watched by occasional chest-X-rays once the tension phenomenon has been controlled. Despite the dramatic appearance and extensive distortion of the lung, staphylococcal cysts normally resolve completely without dilated bronchi and subsequent lobectomy is rarely necessary.

Congenital lobar emphysema occurs as the result of a congenital deficiency of the bronchial cartilages causing valvular obstruction to expiration. The affected lobe expands enormously and compresses the remaining lobe on the same side as well as moving the mediastinum to the opposite side and compressing the opposite lung. The marked translucency of the affected lobe is seen clearly on X-ray, and the other lobe of the lung may be compressed into a tiny space. Despite its dramatic X-ray picture, really urgent treatment is rarely necessary, and while eventual lobectomy is essential the diagnosis can be firmly established before thoracotomy.

Congenital lung cysts may also occur, and they are frequently taken for staphylococcal cysts because of the relative frequency of this latter variety. However, congenital lung cysts are a definite entity and may occasionally be accurately diagnosed. Unlike staphylococcal lung cysts, congenital lung cysts often develop bronchiectatic changes and may spill over pus to the opposite lung. Lobectomy is necessary for this condition.

Congenital Heart Disease

This may present in the neonatal period as cardiac failure, or acute cardiac illness. There is dyspnœa, tachypnœa, increased pulse rate, hepatomegaly, possibly cyanosis and failure to thrive. Many of the conditions encountered are complex and indeed the outlook is poor no matter what is done. A special look-out should be kept for remediable conditions such as patent ductus arteriosus, coarctation of the aorta and Fallot's tetralogy. The subject is discussed in Chapter 26. *It must be stressed that cardiac illness in the neonatal period may be due to a remediable defect.*

Vascular Ring

"Dysphagia Lusoria': Cyanosis on feeding
Inspiratory stridor

This is a composite group of anomalies of the aortic arch or its branches, which cause compression of the trachea and the œsophagus.

There is usually no cyanosis except on feeding, but there is a constant inspiratory stridor. The aorta bifurcates in its ascending part and the two limbs enclose the trachea and œsophagus. The two limbs join at the beginning of the descending aorta. The ring formed is a tight one and a bolus of food in the œsophagus presses on the posterior part of the trachea and occludes the airway, causing cyanosis. Some believe that a little of the food regurgitates onto the glottis and causes the cyanosis. Tube feeds are well tolerated and the infant thrives on them. A barium swallow shows a posterior indentation of the œsophagus and a tracheogram will show a narrowed air passage. Œsophagoscopy shows a pulsating vessel behind the œsophagus. Aortograms are unnecessary for diagnosis. The treatment is a left thoracotomy, early division of the narrower limb of the ring, whichever that may be, and freeing of local connective tissue.

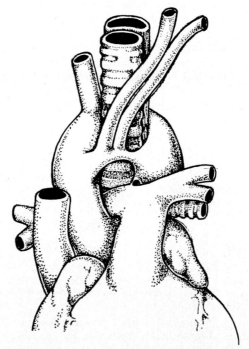

Fig. 15. A congenital vascular ring constricting trachea and œsophagus. Persistence of the posterior aortic arch.

After operation the swallowing is dramatically improved, but the stridor persists perhaps for a year due to a hypoplastic tracheal cartilage at the site of compression.

Vascular anomalies other than double aortic arch may cause the same symptoms. An anomalous vessel from a right-sided aortic arch from which the left subclavian arises; or an aberrant right subclavian from the descending aorta (the classical cause of dysphagia lusoria), or an aberrant right common carotid artery may all cause the same symptoms. It is the local connective tissue which causes the compression in these latter conditions, and if the vessel is not itself divided at operation the connective tissue must be thoroughly freed so that it can be displaced to obtain a satisfactory result.

REFERENCES

Bonham Carter, R. E., Waterston, D. J., Aberdeen, E. (1962) Hernia and eventration of the diaphragm in childhood, *Lancet, i,* 656.
Butler, N., Claireaux, A. E. (1962). Congenital diaphragmatic hernia as a cause of perinatal mortality, *Lancet, i,* 659.
Haight, C. (1961) The management of congenital esophageal atresia and tracheoesophageal fistula, *Surg. Clin. N. Amer.* **41**, 1281.
Potts, W. J. (1958) Respiratory emergencies in the newborn, *Ann. roy. Coll. Surg. Engl.,* **23**, 275.
Waterston, D. J., Bonham Carter, R. E., Aberdeen, E. (1962) Œsophageal atresia; tracheo-œsophageal fistula. A study of survival in 218 infants, *Lancet, i,* 819.

CHAPTER 7

INFECTIONS IN THE NEONATAL PERIOD

THE fall in neonatal mortality has focused attention on *infection* as still the most important single cause of neonatal death after the first week of life. Infections at this time of life have not been controlled by the widespread use of antibiotics and the problem remains serious. Severe infection is uncommon in babies born at home, but the modern trend to have more confinements in hospital exposes the babies to the resistant staphylococcal organisms which are so much more common there and which are now spreading outside the hospital environment.

The streptococcus used to be the scourge of the obstetric wards. Puerperal fever, erysipelas, pemphigus and septicæmia killed mothers and babies. The introduction of sulphonamides dramatically changed the picture. But the price paid for the control of the streptococcus is the emergence of virulent, drug-resistant strains of staphylococci. The staphylococcus, which used to be looked on mainly as a cause of annoying local lesions like boils, is now a serious cause of severe or fatal illness in mothers and babies. Its ability to acquire resistance to a drug kept ahead of the discovery of new antibiotics and necessitated a return to the older hygienic methods of control of infection. Now, whilst the newer penicillins (e.g. cloxacillin) are maintaining their powers against the staphylococci, *Pseudomonas pyocyanea* is emerging as a new source of danger.

The great problem in cross-infection, as hospital infection is commonly called, is that the organisms are everywhere, They are plentiful on the floors, blankets, walls, utensils and fixtures. *The noses and perineum of the medical and nursing staff, and the patients' own infections are the most serious sources of organisms.* The unfortunate infant may acquire the infection from passage through the genital tract of his mother, while the mother in turn may have acquired the organism since her entry to hospital. Thus the infant's entire environment is often contaminated, and the majority of infants themselves may be carriers of resistant organisms at the time of their discharge from hospital.

The control of cross-infection in maternity wards and nurseries is a huge problem. The antibiotic umbrella is not the answer. The organisms quickly become resistant to any antibiotic or combination of antibiotics which are used as a routine in a hospital. A return to the older mechanical methods of antisepsis has helped the position, and a Listerian approach to the problem has paid dividends. Thorough mechanical cleansing of utensils, more care in sweeping and bed-making to avoid raising dust, together with the reduction of resistant carriers by local applications to the anterior nares have all contributed to a great reduction of infection in those units where the measures have been carried out. Finger nails should be kept short and cleaned frequently. Even small skin lesions in the staff should be cleaned with an antiseptic such as hexachlorophene and kept covered with zinc oxide strapping.

Staphylococcal infection in the new-born infant often presents in a trivial form. Little pustules on the face, conjunctivitis (sticky eye) paronychia or eponychia, or a moist umbilicus are the common ones. Each must be treated with great respect. A swab should be taken and wide spectrum antibiotics given until sensitivities are obtained. Not only may the organism spread to produce a serious lesion, but it may be transferred to other babies.

Neonatal mastitis is not uncommon. At birth the breasts may be enlarged and secrete "witches milk". This is a response to maternal œstrogens and requires no treatment. Staphylococcal infection may occur in the engorged breasts. Injudicious handling or expression of the milk will encourage such infection. The correct treatment is early incision, and antibiotics are required to prevent severe spreading cellulitis of the chest wall. The incision into the abscess is made on the under-surface of the nipple and as far from it as possible, so that there will not be a disfiguring scar later in life.

SEPTICÆMIA

The great danger of staphylococcal infection is that it may cause a septicæmia. This in itself may rapidly overwhelm a baby. If it is less fulminating the infection may settle in the lungs, causing *pneumonia;* in the brain causing *meningitis* or *brain abscess;* in the peritoneum causing staphylococcal *peritonitis;* or in the bones and joints causing *osteitis* or *septic arthritis.*

The diagnosis of septicæmia in the new-born infant is quite a difficult one. The responses at this age are different from those of an older child. Pyrexia may be absent and the infant is frequently *hypothermic.* It is essential to use a thermometer reading down to 85°F routinely for these sick infants. There is circulatory collapse and usually vomiting, possibly diarrhœa. The spleen is enlarged. The generalized infection may produce abdominal distension with paralytic ileus and bile-stained vomiting. This may imitate the picture of mechanical intestinal obstruction. Bowel sounds may be diminished, but as this also occurs in the late stages of many organic obstructions it is unreliable in differentiation. White cell counts are also unreliable in making the distinction between a functional and mechanical obstruction. However, a plain radiograph of the abdomen, one supine and one erect, will differentiate these conditions. Infection produces an even distension of the intestines with similar sized fluid levels throughout. Mechanical obstruction produces a picture of progressively dilating loops of bowel down to the site of the obstruction, and an area without gas shadows below this. The treatment of septicæmia is by the use of wide spectrum antibiotics singly or in combination. The combination used at the outset should be that one which has been found to be most effective against the particular strain of organisms predominant in the institution where the infection occurred. A blood culture should be taken at the outset and therapy adjusted according to the sensitivities found. But commencement of treatment cannot await these findings.

Hæmorrhages may occur into the skin as petechiæ, or into the alimentary tract, causing hæmatemesis and melæna. The septicæmia in itself causes blood destruction and the infant should have frequent hæmoglobin estimations. Repeated small blood transfusions may be of great value. In the early stages, a shock-like state in the presence of a normal hæmoglobin may require plasma infusions. The suprarenal glands may be destroyed by hæmorrhages. This produces the Water-house-Friderichsen syndrome of peripheral vascular collapse. Hydrocortisone has been life-saving when used promptly in this fulminating condition.

If paralytic ileus develops, continuous gastric suction and intravenous fluids will be required. Vomiting is dangerous because of the risk of a weakened baby inhaling his own vomitus. Distension restricts diaphragmatic breathing, which is the principal mode of breathing in an infant.

Sclerema Neonatorum. This is an ill-understood condition in which the limbs, face and trunk may be progressively involved in a diffuse hardening of the subcutaneous tissues. It occurs in debilitated infants and often affects infected infants who have become hypothermic. Intracellular œdema and physical changes in the fat have been described, and probably a number of different conditions are present in different types of cold injury.

Sclerema is usually a fatal condition. The use of hydrocortisone 5 to 10 mg., intravenously, followed by cortisone 5 to 10 mg. thrice daily, along with a suitable antibiotic has probably reversed the lesion in some apparently hopeless postoperative cases. The treatment has not had the expected deleterious effects on wound healing in such cases.

Metastatic Lesions

In other cases the immediate toxæmia may be less intense and then metastatic lesions may develop before the baby is overwhelmed or treatment begun. *Staphylococcal pneumonia* may be found and is discussed below. *Staphylococcal peritonitis* occurs, causing paralytic ileus. It is difficult to distinguish this entity from a septicæmia with paralytic ileus, but an X-ray of the abdomen may show a quantity of fluid within the abdomen separating the coils of bowel. If one is certain that there is no mechanical cause for the peritonitis, then it should be treated conservatively with gastric suction, intravenous fluids and antibiotics.

A *brain abscess* may arise in which general signs of intracranial pressure usually overshadow localizing neurological signs. *Meningitis* may coexist, or occur alone.

Hæmatogenous osteitis and suppurative arthritis neonatorum is an increasingly important condition and is considered more fully in Chapter 30. It may occur in a clinically mild form or with a severe illness. Though the mortality of the former is low, the results of inadequate treatment may be crippling. Any bone may be affected, but the region of the hip is an important site. Because it is deep and covered by muscle, swelling of the joint is not immediately obvious but movements, including abduction, are limited and painful. The maxilla is also frequently attacked, from a focus in a tooth germ.

Early diagnosis is vital. Any swelling of soft tissues, irritability, immobility of a part or a superficial lesion associated with signs of a generalized infection must raise suspicions. Localized tenderness over bone is the important sign. X-rays do not show the true extent of destruction, as the cartilage destroyed is radio-translucent and demineralization of affected bone is not evident for two weeks.

The treatment is intensive, uninterrupted and long-continued chemotherapy. Pus should be aspirated, using a very wide bore needle or trochar, and repeated needling may be necessary. If needling fails, the abscess should be incised, the pus evacuated and the incision closed. Drilling of the bone is unnecessary. Early arthrotomy is advisable in infections of the hip joint, however. The chemotherapy should continue until the lesion is completely quiescent, and the minimum course of treatment should be three weeks, but much longer may be required.

Even with full treatment some children will develop a deformity in one or more joints. Late diagnosis, inadequate length of treatment and failure to evacuate pus are all causes of failure, but in septic arthritis of the hip results may be bad despite all possible care. On the other hand, regeneration of bone at other sites can be astonishing. Early diagnosis is the key to good results and this means suspecting osteitis when the signs are still slight.

RESPIRATORY INFECTIONS

Respiratory infections are the commonest cause of morbidity and mortality later in the first year of life. Occasionally they may affect the new born.

Staphylococcal pneumonia in the newly born has already been mentioned as a cause of respiratory distress. Again it must be remembered that the generalized effects of the infection may overshadow the local signs. Physical examination of the chest may mislead at this age and prompt resort to a chest X-ray is fully justified in a baby with a persistently rapid respiratory rate. Treatment is primarily with antibiotics, and oxygen may be needed. The tendency to form air-containing retention cysts in the lung and to complication by pneumothorax has already been mentioned. The tension syndrome which can result needs urgent decompression by the insertion of a needle between the ribs, followed by continuous suction through an intercostal catheter. Lobectomy may occasionally be required later.

It is now realized that the *Escherichia coli* may be a pathogenic organism in this age group, and may also cause pneumonia. Indeed the treatment of sensitive infections by penicillin at this age is sufficiently frequently followed by reinfection by *Escherichia coli* to justify a general rule that streptomycin is always given along with cloxacillin or penicillin during the first month of life.

MENINGITIS

Coliform meningitis may be the precursor of hydrocephalus. The picture of the initial infection may be simply that of a baby who refuses his feeds, becomes hypotonic, has cyanotic attacks and perhaps a low, irregular pyrexia or hypothermia. Vomiting may occur, but the specific meningeal signs like neck stiffness are frequently absent. Only the performance of a lumbar puncture on suspicion reveals the site of the infection. Even without treatment the lesion may recover, but the residual adhesions in the subarachnoid space are one of the causes of so-called congenital hydrocephalus.

Meningitis may also present with more typical signs and be caused by other organisms, such as the staphylococcus. Raised intracranial pressure may also be due to brain abscess.

GASTRO-ENTERITIS

Gastro-enteritis due to specific organisms such as Salmonella or Shigella, pathogenic strains of *Escherichia coli* or undetermined organisms, including viruses, is usually seen later in the first year of life. But this is usually because the newly born is more carefully guarded and more likely to be breast-fed. The newly born must be carefully protected against gathering infection in hospital by cross-infection. The disease is more likely to be serious or fatal, the younger the patient.

Familial infection will frequently be found in the background of the baby's illness. The organism which causes the father to have a whitlow or a sore throat may cause osteitis in one of the children, and may overwhelm the unresistant baby with a meningitis or septicæmia. The immunity responses of the baby are undeveloped, so that infection may be catastrophic. It is important that parents should realize the need for care to avoid transferring to the baby an apparently trivial infection. Infections are common in the neonatal period. They are serious because tissue and general responses may be slight. There is often no pyrexia. Chemotherapy must be prompt, accurate and long continued in full dosage.

REFERENCES

Williams, R. E. O., Blowers, R., Garrod, L. P. and Shooter, R. A. (1960) *Hospital Infection: Causes and Prevention.* London: Lloyd-Luke.

CHAPTER 8

SPINA BIFIDA AND HYDROCEPHALUS

SPINA BIFIDA

THIS common and usually serious malformation occurs about once in every three hundred births in these islands and it has a tendency to recur in families. When one affected child has been born the risk of a second child being affected is about one in twenty-five.

Development

The spinal cord develops by invagination and tubulation of the dorsal ectoderm and it is then enveloped in mesoderm which subsequently differentiates into the spinal column. Spina bifida results from failure in varying degrees of these processes (Fig. 16). The most serious problems arise from failure of development involving the neural tissue itself—meningomyelocele. This is by far the most common form presenting clinically, and only 5 per cent of spina bifida aperta are pure meningoceles with a normal cord. Minor failures only involving incomplete fusion of the bony arch (spina bifida occulta) are common and symptomless and often unnoticed.

In virtually all cases of spina bifida aperta there is an associated Arnold-Chiari malformation. This consists of a small posterior cranial fossa with displacement of parts of the medulla and cerebellum into the cervical region. Arachnoid adhesions around this abnormality may obstruct the flow of cerebrospinal fluid causing hydrocephalus. This hydrocephalus is present in about 85 per cent of meningomyeloceles although it is only progressive in about 60 per cent.

Meningomyelocele

This is far the commonest type to reach the surgeon (Figs. 17 and 18). The neural tissue remains exposed on the surface looking like granulation tissue. At the upper end the central canal may be recognized as a fistula discharging cerebrospinal fluid. This tissue is surrounded by a thin translucent membrane representing the meninges and circumferentially an area of ill-formed skin may be present. Left untreated the sac fills with cerebrospinal fluid and distends to a cystic appearance. The base of the lesion is broad and the separated bony pedicles of the spine can be felt down either side. These cases always show some degree of paralysis below the lesion, varying from minor sphincter or foot weakness to complete paralysis of the lower limbs, bladder and anal sphincters. There is also a variable degree of anæsthesia. The extent of the paralysis does not necessarily relate accurately to the level of the lesion

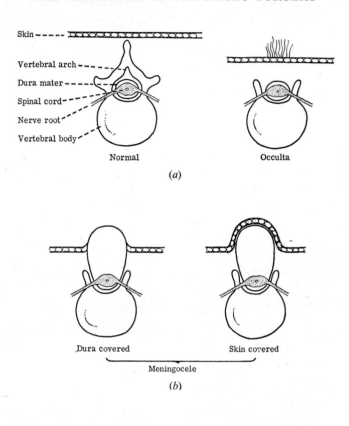

Skin
Vertebral arch
Dura mater
Spinal cord
Nerve root
Vertebral body

Normal Occulta

(a)

Dura covered Skin covered

Meningocele

(b)

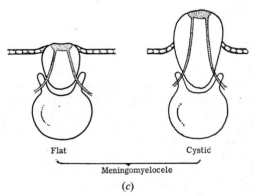

Flat Cystic

Meningomyelocele

(c)

FIG. 16. The varieties of spina bifida.

because dysplasia in the spinal cord may be more extensive than the overt lesion. Bizarre deformities of the lower limbs, and particularly the feet, occur. These seem to result from muscle imbalance and from the effects of uterine pressure on the limb. Recently it has been realized that within a few hours of birth extensive function of the legs may be present but this may soon be lost as the exposed neurones become dry or infected, or are destroyed by spirit or other antiseptics. Swelling of the sac may also cause traction injury on the nerve roots.

The Arnold-Chiari malformation, as has been said, is present in virtually every case and causes hydrocephalus in the great majority. However, this may not be clinically obvious at birth and may only be revealed by ventriculography. In about 60 per cent of cases arachnoid

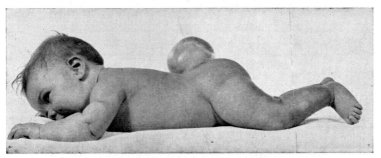

FIG. 17. Lumbo-sacral myelomeningocoele.

adhesions around the displaced brain cause progressive hydrocephalus and this can be expected to be clinically obvious within the first two months.

These conditions are commonest in the lumbar region but can occur anywhere along the neuraxis including the brain itself (encephalocele). Even grosser forms may occur in which the entire cord lies open and untubed on the surface. Such babies usually have other gross defects. They are commonly stillborn and few reach a surgical clinic.

Meningocele

Here there is a failure of the vertebral arch to form and a protrusion of the meninges through the gap. A cystic swelling is thus formed on the back which is usually covered by thin modified skin. The coat may, however, vary from a thin translucent membrane to normal skin. In the great majority the cord is normally formed and there is no neurological defect but each case must be watched with care because there may be an associated dysplasia of the spinal cord. The cyst may be large reaching several inches in diameter but the neck is narrow. A lipoma round the base of the sac may give the false impression that it is wide. Radiology will show that the interpeduncular gap is not so extensive. Unfortunately this type of spina bifida aperta is uncommon—certainly not more than 5 per cent.

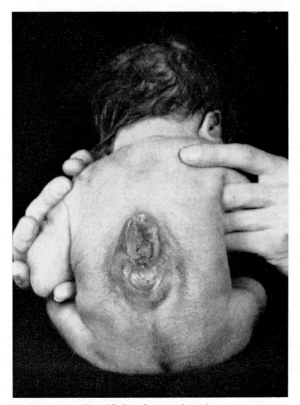

FIG. 18. Lumbar myelocoele.

Spina Bifida Occulta

The spinal cord forms normally in these cases but the arch of mesoderm which should cover it dorsally fails to form completely. On examination there will be an absence of the spinous processes in the midline at the level of the lesion. There may be simply a gap in the series, or the remnants of the vertebral arch may be palpable on either side of the midline—spina bifida. The defect is purely vertebral and there is no neurological defect. It is not an uncommon incidental finding and has been blamed for various neurological conditions such as enuresis. But the evidence that it has been more than a chance association is unconvincing.

The lesion is called occulta because it is hidden below the intact skin. But there is often a superficial clue to its presence. The skin may bear a scar or dimple or it may have an angioma or a hairfield. There may be a subcutaneous lipoma.

Dysraphism

Disraphism is a cord which has abnormal tethering fibres usually at its lower end around the lumbar enlargement or conus. The cord itself may be dysplastic and often reaches a lower level than the usual. The results of tethering may become evident as the child grows. Often the condition is recognized at the age of three or four when the child develops, say, a varus foot or evidence of bladder dysfunction. Diastematomyelia is a type of dysraphism in which the cord is split down the midline around a midline spur of cartilage or bone which also tethers the cord, traction with growth of the child being more likely the lower down the cord it occurs.

Dysraphism may occur in isolation or in association with spina bifida occulta or aperta.

The New-born Baby with Spina Bifida

The new-born baby with spina bifida is a social and surgical emergency. There is a wide spectrum of neurological involvement, and hydrocephalus although not always manifest is present in all but the most minor of lesions.

EXAMINATION. The majority of overt lesions have a raw looking area of varying size over part of the spine, the lumbar region being most commonly affected. This looks somewhat like granulation tissue but is in fact the exposed spinal cord. If it is left there is the danger of infection and dehydration destroying its function as well as the risk of infection ascending to cause meningitis and precipitating progressive hydrocephalus.

Careful examination with stimulation and with changing postures of the baby will enable one to make a reasonable assessment of the function of the lower limbs and in higher lesions that of the abdominal muscles. A patulous anus may give evidence of sphincter paralysis. The perineum may be flat due to absence of tone in the pelvic floor allowing the floor to bulge down between the buttocks obliterating the natal cleft. Dribbling of urine or a firm enlarged bladder may give indication of damage to the nerve supply of the lower urinary tract.

In a minority of infants there is a cystic swelling on the back which has a complete epithelial cover. In these meningoceles the outlook is better and there will usually be no neurological defects. A few of them have a covering of normal skin and, since in these there is no risk of infection entering, treatment is not so urgent.

Prognosis at Birth

It is important not to be too dogmatic in prognosis as the effects of faulty advice to the parents in the first few days of life may never be entirely eradicated. The degree of spinal paralysis is difficult to assess in the early days and no assessment of mentality at that time can be reliable, though the outlook is bad if hydrocephalus is clinically evident at birth. Upper thoracic lesions appear to be less likely to have neurological involvement than the common lumbar and lumbosacral lesions.

Management

Survival must be anticipated in all but the most severe anomalies. It is very unwise to tell the parents that the infant is likely to die in a few days or weeks and that, since nothing can be done to cure him, this will really be a good thing. It is all but impossible to predict which infants treated or untreated will die and this must be borne in mind in all counselling. It is necessary to explain that this is a serious lesion but that the exact outcome cannot be predicted so early. The fact that treatment can and will be given as problems may arise is stressed. An attitude of living from day to day rather than attempting to work out a comprehensive prognosis needs to be encouraged. Now that it is realized that myelomeningoceles may have extensive function which can be lost within a few hours of birth, treatment becomes no longer a matter of appearance and convenience but one of function and makes immediate treatment difficult to deny. There are some cases so severe and who have other gross abnormalities in whom active treatment does not appear justified. For the majority in whom active treatment is the correct course it should be given within twenty-four hours. In the meantime the cord must be kept moist with saline soaks or with a bland non-adherent, non-greasy dressing such as Nusan B.

A wide defect can be tubed with dural closure but a narrow defect is better simply covered with skin. Attempts to mobilize and tube it may produce pressure which itself damages the nervous tissue. The peripheral meningeal area may be sacrificed and the skin is drawn over the lesion by wide undermining—even out to the rectus sheath if necessary. The use of elaborate rotation flaps is more effective on paper than on patients. Suction drainage under the flaps minimizes seroma formation and contributes to primary healing. Partial breakdown may occur but the use of adhesive strapping from flank to flank to take pressure from the widest possible area minimizes this. Local interference is unwise as it breaks down the protective surface barrier of the granulation tissue and increases the risk of meningitis. A cerebrospinal leak from the wound is not, in the authors' opinion, a sign of poor closure but rather of raised spinal pressure and is an indication for the insertion of a Holter valve.

Progressive hydrocephalus will be a problem in about 60 per cent of the infants whether or not operation is performed. It is wise to see that at least one of the parents appreciates this and appreciates the likelihood of some sphincter involvement so that the operation is not blamed for the complications which may arise.

In the rarer form of pure meningocele the epithelial cover is complete but rather thin so that there is still a danger of infection entering and causing meningitis. Early closure is therefore advisable here too.

In those even less common types in which the swelling is covered with normal skin it used to be considered that there was no important indication for operation because infection could not enter. The swelling below the skin is largely lipoma but it is now realized that in a proportion of these cases there is an underlying dysraphism which may produce a progressive traction lesion with growth. There is therefore a case to be made out for operation to free the tethering of the cord lest such symptoms should occur, if myelography confirms the presence of dysraphism with or without diastematomyelia. However, such prophylactic surgery has at least a 10 per cent risk of causing some neurological defect and opinions remain divided as to whether it is wiser to wait for the first signs of neurological involvement before recommending operation.

MANAGEMENT OF THE RETAINED SAC

In those few cases where it seems wise not to operate urgently on the spina bifida epithelialization can be expected within several weeks. There is a real danger of meningitis but this is not as common as might be expected. The most useful protection is a thick ring of cotton wool wrapped in a bandage and fitted around the sac like a doughnut. It should be deep enough to prevent pressure on the sac when the infant is rolled on his back. The sac is dressed with a suitable non-adherent dressing until healed and the ring kept in place with a crêpe binder. Whatever their effectiveness in protecting the sac these rings are a great comfort to the mother when the baby is being discharged and enable her to handle the infant more easily. Some of the sacs are acutely tender though the majority are not. Management is also more difficult because the baby cannot be nursed on the back. If the baby is nursed on the side flexion contractures of the hips develop easily so part of the time should be spent in the prone position (this applies to all cases of spina bifida with neurological involvement of the legs whether or not the sac is retained). Those in whom the sac has been left untreated are usually those who are expected to succumb to associated abnormalities or to extensive paralysis, for example that involving the respiratory muscles. However, should this baby survive, the difficulties of nursing and the difficulties of later fitting calipers to teach walking may justify the more difficult operation of later excision of the sac with its scarred apex.

The Disabilities of the Survivors

Disabilities of the survivors arise in the following four groups:

1. Associated hydrocephalus
2. Orthopædic defects
3. Urinary problems
4. Bowel control

Associated Hydrocephalus. Obstruction to the flow of cerebrospinal fluid causes distension of the ventricles and damages the stretched brain around them. The result is mental retardation and enlargement of the head. A balance may eventually be struck and the condition arrest itself. If it continues to progress, intracranial pressure eventually leads to death by pressure effects on the vital centres of the hind brain. The hydrocephalus may be evident at birth, or it may become so at any time during the first year of life, usually during the first months.

It has been widely taught that the spina bifida sac acts as a safety valve against the development of hydrocephalus and that it should be preserved as an absorptive surface. Dye studies and clinical experience have now amply shown that this is not the case. Indeed, overt or clinically silent infection in the sac may cause ascending arachnoiditis and precipitate hydrocephalus. Recent pathological studies have shown this to be so common that this is now considered an added reason for removal of the sac as a neonatal emergency. Again, ventriculography when the baby is first seen may show some degree of hydrocephalus even though it is not clinically obvious. The treatment of hydrocephalus is discussed in a later section. Early use of the Holter valve has achieved 85 per cent educability in survivors.

The Orthopædic Defects. The hip joints may be flail in a gross paralysis. With lesser degrees of paralysis, the muscle imbalance may deform or dislocate the joint. Such cases are commoner with early repair of the lesion on the back. These changes may begin before birth. Strong and unopposed adductors will tend to force the head of the femur out of the joint. Abduction exercises carried out by the mother and the use of a home applied "H splint" can counteract this tendency, and later on an adduction osteotomy of the femur may enable a stable joint to be maintained. Prone nursing with adhesive felt knee pads avoids flexion contracture of the hips.

The psoas major and the sartorius receive an innervation from higher segments of the cord than the other muscles of the hip. They may frequently remain active alone and cause a typical deformity. The hip is grossly externally rotated—so much so that the foot may point backwards—and a flexion contracture is present. It has been shown by Sharrard that the early application of the principles of muscle transplantation learnt in the management of poliomyelitis (also a lower motor neurone paralysis) can help these children. Transplantation of the lower end of the sartorius to the outer side of the knee removes its external rotating effect. Transplantation of the psoas muscle through a hole in the blade of the ileum removes its flexor effect and allows it to support the joint in the manner of a gluteus maximus.

Training, manipulation, transplants and splinting can all help also in the management of the knee and foot deformities. Infantile paralysis victims with flail lower limbs can be taught to walk with callipers, and the same methods can be applied to children with spina bifida. The problem may be more difficult because the baby may be born with contractures already developed, and anæsthesia of the limbs may make them unduly sensitive to pressure effects and trophic sores. Associated hydrocephalus may result in a temperamental inability to persevere sufficiently to learn to walk even in the absence of gross mental retardation. However, the great majority should be able to walk, with or without appliances.

Urinary Problems. The innervation of the bladder and its sphincters is deficient. A mild weakness may lead to a stress incontinence. This increases the risks of urinary infections and supervision is needed. But there is often a spontaneous improvement in control at about 7 or 8 years of age, so that radical surgical measures should be delayed. Improvement is apparently much less common in boys, but at least they can avoid accidents by the use of a sponge rubber penile clamp, or a light urinal with replaceable plastic bags. Plication of the bulbous urethra, though not reliable, may help some of the milder cases who are improving, as a later measure.

A more severe weakness will produce a complete incontinence. Nursing to avoid the miseries of a sore perineum is difficult in the early years. Orthopædic attention to the hips may at least make this problem more manageable. A plastic operation narrowing the muscle of the bladder neck may also help, but in many diversion of the urinary stream will have to be considered. Transplantation of the ureters into an isolated loop of ileum brought out on the surface of the abdomen is often required. The disposable bags designed for ileostomy use can be fitted. If the ureters are elongated and dilated they can be brought out through one opening as a double-barrelled cutaneous ureterostomy avoiding the risks of reabsorption, especially with kidneys already damaged.

A less common problem, but one more serious for the child, is the development of an enlarged bladder secondary to a tight bladder neck, the result of unbalanced muscle power between detrusor and sphincter. A large residual urine and overflow incontinence arises with all the dangers of back-pressure effects on the kidneys and infection of stagnant urine. It may be thought that bladder neck resection would always convert these children to a similar problem to those with a lax bladder neck described above. But the results are not as good as one might expect because there is often an associated weakness of the muscle of the bladder itself and emptying remains inefficient. Furthermore weakness of the ureterovesical junctions may allow persistent reflux, increasing the effective residual urine and the tendency to infection. In infancy a regular routine is instituted of expression of urine by suprapubic manual pressure each time the napkins are changed. This, with chemotherapy if necessary, helps to control infection. Urinary diversion by uretero-ileostomy usually becomes necessary and should not be left until pyelonephritic changes are irreversible.

Urine examination, blood urea, blood pressure estimation and intravenous pyelography are essential investigations. Bladder and emptying views may give a good idea of the lower urinary tract as well as the upper. But voiding cystography and cysto-urethroscopy will usually be needed as well.

Bowel Control. This is often a happier facet of the disability. These children can almost always be trained to bowel cleanliness when they have reached a co-operative age. The usual measures are the use of a constipating diet with enemas, say twice a week, to evacuate the bowel. Many can learn voluntary control of defæcation by making a habit of straining hard at some regular time after a meal with a hot drink.

In the earlier stages the important point in management, paradoxical as it may seem, is the avoidance of constipation. For these children have no normal urge and may become loaded with fæces so as to overstretch the rectum. It then becomes an inert sac with the constant liquid soiling of overflow incontinence. Many of these children are looked on as hopelessly dirty because the difference between involuntary defæcation and overflow incontinence is not appreciated.

There remains an occasional case of completely uncontrollable automatic defæcation in which a terminal iliac colostomy may be considered after thorough trial of training regimes has failed.

General Management

In some hopeless cases, especially those with multiple deformities, it may be kinder to keep the child from the mother. But in cases with a reasonable hope of survival it must be remembered that early separation is likely to lead to rejection from the family. The child is then condemned to an institutional life in addition to its deformities. In general, therefore, treatment should be planned so that the baby can go home soon. At this age all babies are incontinent and none can walk so that the parents have time to adapt to the situation. Furthermore the mother who may at first seem glad to have the problem taken out of her hands will sometimes later feel guilty about the abandoned child. In the long run the mother will usually be less upset by this tragedy in the family if she has made some attempt to cope with it even though institutional care may later become inevitable. For some will be so handicapped as not to be reasonably manageable at home. Attempts to do so may lead to neglect of the other children, and even disrupt the family.

Clearly, decisions as to treatment cannot be made on purely medical grounds. The social circumstances and ethical considerations are quite as important.

To start treatment early will mean a lot of "wasted" work on babies who succumb to progressive hydrocephalus, meningitis or urinary infections. Yet it will give the favourable cases their best chance. However, indiscriminate use of surgery may unnecessarily prolong the existence of hopelessly retarded and handicapped babies.

At present "management" often means neglect until the baby has proved its viability by prolonged survival and then attempts at "salvage surgery" for contractures, dislocations, sores and chronic urinary infections in children retarded by late arrest of hydrocephalus. The application of similar principles of training and physiotherapy and "prophylactic" surgery, such as muscle transplants, can achieve in many cases as much as they have in poliomyelitis and spastics.

HYDROCEPHALUS OF INFANCY

Hydrocephalus is an excessive accumulation of cerebrospinal fluid in the dilated ventricles. It occurs in about 4 per 1,000 births and 3 out of 4 are associated with myelomeningocele. It is usually caused by obstruction at some point along the circulation—e.g. stenosis of the aqueduct

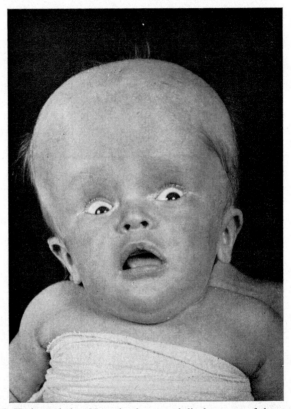

Fig. 19. Hydrocephalus. Note the downward displacement of the eyes due to raised intracranial pressure—"the setting sun" appearance.

of Sylvius, or arachnoidal adhesions around the outlet foramina of the fourth ventricle or in the basal cisterns. Increase in pressure is usual, but in the young baby the skull may expand so easily that this remains normal. The condition may progress until "coning" of the medulla causes death by damage to the vital centres; or an equilibrium between secretion and absorption may arise with "arrest" at varying degrees of cerebral damage. An occasional case is due to oversecretion of c.s.f. without any obstruction (e.g. papilloma of the choroid plexus). CLINICAL FEATURES. The clinical features are obvious. There is a gradual increase in the size of the head. This is best measured as a maximum circumference. The eyes become downcast with sclera showing above the pupil—the so-called "setting-sun" appearance. Their prominence may be masked by the overhanging forehead. The veins of the scalp stand out. It may be obvious at birth but usually becomes clinically recognizable during the first three or four months of life. (Occasionally a similar condition arises later in life, due to injury, infection or tumour in a previously normal person. If the bones of the vault have already united, enlargement of the head will not be obvious.)

Causation. The condition may result from:

(1) Congenital defects.
   i.   Arnold-Chiari malformation, the commonest, usually associated with spina bifida.
   ii. Stenosis of the aqueduct.
   iii. Absence of the foramina of Magendie or Lushka.

(2) Infections.
   i.   Perinatal meningitis (which may itself be almost asymptomatic).
   ii. Ascending arachnoiditis causing posterior fossa block (often associated with Arnold-Chiari malformation and spina bifida).
   iii. Meningitis later in life.

(3) Trauma.
   i.   Birth trauma, causing e.g. 'forking' of the aqueduct.
   ii. Sequel to head injury later in life.

(4) Tumour.
   i.   Causing obstruction, usually after infancy.
   ii. Choroid plexus papilloma causing oversecretion (a non-obstructive cause).

It will be seen, therefore, that there is no one cause of hydrocephalus. The condition was often called congenital hydrocephalus because the cause was assumed to be *some congenital defect*. This, indeed is one of the important causes—for example the Arnold-Chiari deformity often associated with spina bifida or aqueduct stenosis. It is now realized that many of the cases arising in early infancy are due to *perinatal accidents*. *Neonatal meningitis*, often coliform, may present few clinical signs and be self limiting. It may leave behind obstructive adhesions. *Intracranial birth trauma* may cause bleeding into the cerebrospinal pathways and leave a block, for example in the aqueduct ('forking of the aqueduct'). The importance of this is that it means that many of the babies who present with hydrocephalus began with normal brains, and should at least theoretically be amenable to treatment. *Tumours* are extremely rare and in any case usually incurable.

Division into communicating and non-communicating types depending on the freedom of flow from lumbar to ventricular levels is of little value, except in relation to certain forms of treatment which have been used less recently. Communication is a relative matter and many cases have more than one site of blockage.

Treatment

The key question in treatment is "Is this lesion still progressive?" If the head is progressively enlarging then steps may be taken to halt it. If it is stationary in an infant with its unfused sutures then nothing should be done.

Serial measurements of the head circumference will demonstrate the rate of progression. If these are recorded on a percentile chart the progress can be more readily assessed. As long as the head is enlarging the fontanelle may be kept open. An open anterior fontanelle at 18 months is definitely abnormal. In some unfortunate infants the head goes on enlarging for years, and to wait for a spontaneous arrest once a circumference of 20 inches has been reached is the ultimate in Micawberism. Arrest does occur spontaneously in many infants, but it will often happen too late to prevent a secondary cortical atrophy with severe mental retardation and a hideous cranial deformity which cannot be disguised.

Investigation

The most important investigation which should be carried out in every case of hydrocephalus is needling of the subdural space as far laterally as can be managed in the angle of the enlarged anterior fontanelle or if necessary through the suture line high in the temporal region. A narrow lumbar puncture needle may be used, but a shorter needle is more convenient. The finding of more than a drop or two of fluid will demonstrate the presence of a subdural collection— usually a subdural hæmatoma draining bloodstained or yellow fluid, and occasionally a subdural hygroma draining relatively clear c.s.f. Subdural collections (see Chapter 2), which usually follow birth trauma, are the other important cause of intracranial pressure and enlargement of the head. It is important not to miss them because they are amenable to treatment.

It is then usual to proceed to ventriculography. In babies the ventricle can be tapped from the angle of the fontanelle. About 20 ml. of c.s.f. are removed in 5-ml. stages, being replaced by air. By tilting the baby and taking X-rays a "bubble study" can be carried out which will show the degree of dilatation of the ventricles and the site of the block. In older children it may be necessary to make burr holes in the skull to allow tapping of the ventricles. It is important never to attempt to empty the ventricles as is done for a standard ventriculogram. The

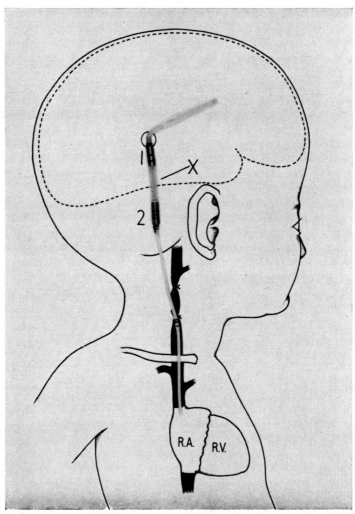

FIG. 20. The principle of ventriculo-atrial shunt with the Holter valve. 1 and 2 are slit valves. X marks the pump.

reaction to the pressure changes induced by even a bubble study can be considerable, and removal of more fluid will produce dangerous collapse. In very young babies with an easily distended cranium, the head size may increase progressively with a normal cerebrospinal fluid pressure. The use of percentile charts of head size are invaluable in assessing the significance of serial measurements.

The thickness of the cerebral mantle can be estimated from the radiographs, but this bears little relation to the mental state of the baby. More can be learned from playing with the baby and putting it through the manœuvres designed to test its developmental staging in relation to the chronological age. The opinion of the sister who nurses and feeds the baby can be invaluable. The affect of the baby can be assessed in a rough way, and crude as it is, this method is more valuable than radiography in deciding which babies will respond to treatment designed to relieve the block. The baby who does not respond to attention and who feeds badly is likely to be severely retarded. It must be remembered that irritation may obscure the picture and that the baby may presumably be suffering from severe headaches from the raised pressure. This may produce an appearance of greater defect than is actually present.

Surgery

The most widely used operation at present is a ventriculo-atriel shunt using the low pressure Holter valve. The device consists of two one-way silicone slit valves opening at a pressure of 25 mm. cerebrospinal fluid and joined by a silastic tube. Pressure on this tube allows 'pumping' to test the function of the system. It is placed subcutaneously over the mastoid region. A catheter leads from the lateral ventricle to the valve and a tube leads down from it into the jugular vein, whence it is threaded down the superior vena cava so that its end lies in the atrium. The fluid is thus discharged at a controlled rate back into the blood stream, but reflux of blood cannot take place. Results have been gratifying, though complications are not uncommon. In perhaps 15 per cent fibrin depositions in the venous system blocks the system necessitating reoperation. Obstruction of the ventricular catheter is easily dealt with by replacement. In about 10 per cent hydrocephalus slowly progresses in spite of a functioning valve. The dreaded complication is low grade septicæmia, usually with *Staphylococcus albus*, which occurs in about 10 per cent. It cannot be controlled until the valve is removed, and later it may be impossible to insert another. Despite these drawbacks, the shunt is successful in about 70 per cent—far better than any other procedure.

REFERENCES

Lawrence, K. M. (1958) The natural history of hydrocephalus, *Lancet*, ii, 1152.
(—) (1964) "The natural history of spina bifida," *ibid* **39**, 41.
Macnab, G. H. (1965) Chapters "Hydrocephalus in Infancy" and "Spina Bifida Cystica" in *Recent Advances in Pædiatrics* (ed. Gairdner), Churchill, London.
Nash, D. F. E. (1963) Meningomyelocele, *Proc. roy. Soc. Med.*, **56**, 506.

CHAPTER 9

INFANTILE HYPERTROPHIC PYLORIC STENOSIS

THIS is one of the common conditions requiring surgery in infancy. It affects one in every 200 male children and one in every 1,000 girls. This gives a male preponderance of 5 to 1. First-born infants do not now appear to be so much more susceptible as was described in the past.

Hypertrophic pyloric stenosis has been recognized for over 80 years and has had a specific treatment for almost 50 years. Yet the ætiology is still obscure. There is a proven genetic factor, and an uncertain environmental factor. It may be transmitted by either parent to male or female offspring but an affected mother is more likely than an affected father to produce an affected infant. The pathology is apparently a postnatal work hypertrophy of the pylorus following on a congenital slowness of the pyloric sphincter to open. It can thus be appreciated that maternal inexperience in baby-handling could account for an increased tendency for symptoms to arise from the hereditary factor in first-born babies. Conversely, skill in feeding the baby may postpone the onset of symptoms. There is some evidence that constitutional muscularity may be the environmental factor.

CLINICAL PICTURE

Symptoms usually begin in a well-developed infant during the third or fourth week of life, but the condition may show itself earlier, and it can occur in premature infants. For practical purposes the disease does not occur after the third month and rarely begins after the second month. *Vomiting* is the presenting symptom. At the onset it is occasional and little more than regurgitation. Soon it becomes regular, copious and projectile, sometimes occurring with the first gulp of milk. The distended stomach is usually emptied in one or two large vomits. The infant is characteristically eager to feed again immediately after a vomit. The stomach becomes enlarged so that it can retain large volumes of milk and vomiting is therefore infrequent, though regular, and does not occur with every feed.

The vomitus consists of curdled milk and gastric juice containing a lot of mucus. There is always some degree of gastritis as a result of the gastric stasis. The vomitus is sometimes bloodstained or coffee ground if the gastritis is severe. Occasionally it is stained yellow but the pigment is not bile.

The baby will usually have been taken from the breast and had various brands of artificial milk in the mistaken belief that vomiting is due to failure of the milk to agree with the baby.

With *projectile vomiting, visible gastric peristalsis* is a characteristic feature. It may be seen particularly well towards the end of a feed. Waves pass across the upper abdomen from left to right "like a golf ball under the skin". But visible peristalsis is not a specific finding of this condition and may be seen in any wasted baby who has active peristalsis.

The general appearance of the baby is rather typical. There is always a failure to gain weight satisfactorily and in the more severe cases there

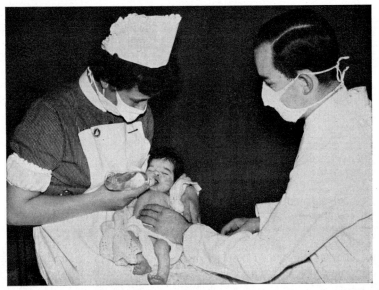

Fig. 21. The method of palpating a pyloric tumour.

will already have been *loss of weight* before the baby is seen. The baby has an anxious expression and with his wrinkled brow has been said to look like a little old man. He is restless and remains *hungry*. Dehydration results in loss of the normal tissue turgor when a fold of skin is picked up, and malnourishment is revealed by its laxity.

The baby is usually *constipated* although he may pass frequent green hunger stools consisting largely of mucus and bilestained intestinal secretions. The urine becomes scanty and darkly coloured.

The onset of hypotonicity and disinterest in feeding is of serious import and suggests a severe electrolyte upset or superadded infection of the weakened baby. A subnormal temperature is another sign of severe illness.

The most important feature, because it is absolutely pathognomonic is the palpation of the *pyloric tumour*. In size, shape, edge and consistency it feels like an olive in the right upper abdomen. It may be difficult to feel. It is easiest to do so during a feed when the baby is relaxed. The mother or nurse should feed the baby on her left arm so that the doctor can sit opposite on a low stool and lay his left hand across the baby's upper abdomen with the finger tips on the upper right quadrant. As the baby feeds the tumour will be felt coming up against the fingers as the baby relaxes. Once felt the firm sensation is so typical that there is little doubt.

It has been said that satisfactory palpation needs three comfortable people. Mother or nurse on a suitable chair; baby (by feeding him); and the doctor on a low stool so that his left hand rests easily across the baby's abdomen. Kneading with the fingers merely annoys the baby and prevents the relaxation which is essential to allow the fingers to sink back and feel the tumour. It may be necessary to palpate during a whole feed. If unsucessful then the procedure is repeated at the next feed. Immediately after a large vomit there is a moment of great relaxation of the abdominal wall; the stomach is empty and it is then that the tumour is most easily felt.

Projectile vomiting and palpation of the tumour are the characteristics of the disease. Other signs and symptoms are less constant and less specific.

The Differential Diagnosis

The two important conditions in differential diagnosis are gastro-enteritis and feeding problems. Other obstructive conditions are much less common, and would require operation in any case. The distinction should be made however, because the operation of pyloromyotomy for pyloric stenosis can be performed conveniently, if desired, under a local anæsthetic and with a limited access whilst most other operations cannot.

Gastro-enteritis is considered first. It is distinguished by fever; unformed, offensive smelling frequent stools; bilestained vomiting, and a sick looking baby who is unwilling to feed.

In contrast the baby with the mechanical obstruction of pyloric stenosis remains hungry and alert and has few but copious and projectile vomits, and is constipated. It should be reiterated that in the late stages of pyloric stenosis the baby may have the hypotonicity and illness of electrolyte imbalance and show "dehydration fever". Furthermore a true gastro-enteritis may complicate the picture, for the baby, weakened by starvation, is particularly prone to catch infections such as gastro-enteritis or pneumonia. Palpation of a typical tumour remains as the crucial sign.

When the vomiting is accompanied by a less typical history and findings it is important to enquire into the feeding methods and the nature of the feeds. Correction of technique or quality or quantity of feeds may be all that is required. This is not the place for a full discussion of *feeding management* but too small a hole in the teat is a frequent cause of that common problem, the windy baby.

Pylorospasm merits individual mention. It seems to be a definite entity and the differences between it and pyloric stenosis are probably more of degree than of kind. All the signs except for a palpable tumour may be similar, but the condition is essentially transitory, and the diagnosis often rests on this factor alone. Vomiting tends to be more frequent but less copious and forceful. The pylorus may be palpable but has not the typical hard discrete feel. Onset is often earlier. Gastric lavage, perhaps repeated once or twice seems to hasten recovery.

Œsophageal hiatus hernia also merits individual mention. It is not an uncommon condition and the symptoms almost always begin in the first 6 weeks of life. Vomiting may be projectile as in pyloric stenosis. The history is important in that vomiting more often dates from the first days of life and early *hæmatemesis* is more frequent.

RADIOLOGY. A barium meal is helpful in a doubtful case. A large stomach and delay in emptying are found in many conditions, but the significant sign of pyloric stenosis is the elongated and narrow pyloric canal. The meal will also reveal œsophageal reflux and any hiatus hernia. It will also show the other rare causes of a similar clinical picture, such as high duodenal obstruction by stenosis, or malrotation.

TREATMENT

Surgery is the treatment of choice in the vast majority of cases. Medical treatment has for a long time been popular, particularly in Scandinavia, but it carries a mortality of its own, a fact sometimes forgotten. Medical measures consist of gastric lavage, small frequent feeds and resuming feeding the infant after a vomit. An antispasmodic is given before feeds. Atropine methyl nitrate (Eumydrine) has been the most popular of these since its introduction in 1926. A dose of about 8 drops of a 1 in 10,000 alcoholic solution is given before feeds five times a day. Conservative measures are usually successful, but treatment may be prolonged. In severe cases prolonged skilled nursing care may be needed and the baby is at risk of complicating infections whilst it remains in a debilitated state. The more obvious risk of an operation is avoided at the cost of other less obvious risks. In milder cases of late onset medical treatment may safely avoid hospitalization but clinically apparent dehydration is a complete bar to medical treatment other than as a preparation for surgery. Any comparison of statistics showing the results of surgical and medical treatment must ensure that both are treating the same condition. The difficulty arises that cases of pylorospasm are often included in the medical, but not in the surgical series.

Recent surveys of adults who had been treated for pyloric stenosis in infancy showed that a proportion still have interference with the mobility of the pyloric canal and that the incidence of peptic ulcer was above the normal. The changes and the ulcers were significantly more frequent after medical treatment than after operation. This led to a revival of interest in surgical treatment in Denmark.

PREPARATION

If the patient is to be treated surgically the operation itself is not urgent, although the treatment is. It must be emphasized that adequate preparation for operation is as important as the skill of the surgeon. There are many régimes which have proved their value. More important is the management of the baby by nurses and an operator who are accustomed to the method. Cases do not fare so well in the unit which treats only an occasional case. Adequate barrier nursing is all-important.

Many patients are nowadays brought to hospital at an early stage of the disease, and once the diagnosis is confirmed they are ready for operation. There are still some infants who have had severe and prolonged vomiting, and arrive seriously dehydrated and starved. The chloride, potassium and sodium concentrations in the serum should be measured. The serum chloride is usually low, but the potassium is normal in all but the most severe cases. Losses have been by gastric secretion and hence there is a tendency to alkalosis. The chloride level is sometimes reduced from the normal level of about 100 M.eq/l. (360 mg. per cent) to say 60 M.eq/l. (215 mg. per cent). Such a baby will show obvious clinical signs of dehydration, but the estimation is a valuable check on clinical judgment and a base line for evaluation of treatment.

The malnutrition is not so easily estimated, for the plasma protein concentrations usually remain normal. Such information as is obtainable about the child's fluctuations in weight, and the weight change after rehydration, will give some guidance. A baby admitted weighing less than its birth-weight must be considered as seriously dehydrated and malnourished.

In the moderately ill infant the mainstay of treatment is intravenous infusion of normal saline. Oral intake of milk should be stopped *completely*. The stomach is washed out with normal saline (to avoid removing further chloride as may occur if water is used) and this is repeated if necessary. Clear fluids are given by mouth and it will be found that there is always a temporary cessation of vomiting. This gives time for preparation and the oral fluid and electrolyte intake will supplement the parenteral. Attempts to get the starved baby to absorb some protein by using milk feeds, however dilute, only lead to persistence of vomiting and further losses.

Some of the very ill babies with circulatory collapse will require expansion of the blood volume by plasma or blood before further fluid and electrolytes are given. 200 ml. of half strength plasma or 100 ml. of whole blood given over 8 to 12 hours may suffice. The fluid requirements can be roughly estimated from the usual weight formulæ, i.e. 40–60 ml. per pound body weight. A moderately dehydrated baby can be given 50 per cent more than its maintenance needs over the first 24 hours and a really seriously ill one double the requirements (some of which will be a protein containing solution, plasma or blood). The maintenance salt requirement is about 1 g. per day and 1 ml. per pound of normal saline should raise the plasma chloride 1 M.eq/l. in theory. Clinical examination, weighings and biochemical estimations will guide further therapy.

Potassium replacement may be needed in the baby who has been ill a long time and it is always best given by mouth to avoid the danger of toxic levels arising in the blood; 0·5 g. potassium chloride by mouth three times a day will allow the baby to correct his deficit.

For parenteral therapy we use the intravenous route exclusively. Scalp vein needles attached to polythene tubing are used, but a cut-down infusion may be necessary and is fully justified. The subcutaneous and particularly the rectal routes are much less certain and have their quota of complications.

Probably the most reliable sign that treatment is effective is a weight gain without œdema. It is our practice not to operate until the serum chloride level reaches 90 M.eq/l (about 320 mg. per cent). This will usually be achieved in one day, sometimes two may be needed. A peristently subnormal temperature is of serious portent and contra-indicates operation at that time. Ideally one tries to have the baby at such a stage that the infusion can be taken down before he goes to the operating table in the certainty that he will be feeding normally shortly after surgery.

After all this discussion of the preparation of the sick baby to make him safe for surgery it is important to stress that *nowadays the majority are seen when only mildly dehydrated and not seriously starved. They do not need any parenteral preparation.* Gastric lavage with saline, repeated twice daily if necessary, until the washings are almost free of mucus enables the baby to take his fluid and electrolytes by mouth as sweetened half or fifth normal saline. Attempts to persist with modified milk formulæ only lead to persistence of vomiting and may move the baby into the class needing parenteral therapy.

THE IMMEDIATE PREPARATION FOR OPERATION

If a Local Anæsthetic is to be Used. The stomach is washed out 1½ hours before operation. (If the washings contain much mucus the procedure is postponed until the stomach is cleaner. This avoids troublesome postoperative vomiting from mucous gastritis which may otherwise interfere with the prompt establishment of oral feeding.)

Chloral hydrate is put down the tube before it is withdrawn in a dosage of $\frac{1}{2}$ gr. (30 mg.) per pound body weight. The child is then bandaged on to a padded crucifix and left to go to sleep. The gastric tube accompanies the baby to the theatre so that it can be passed again during operation if acute distension of the stomach with gas makes delivery of the organ difficult. It is not left down or it irritates the baby and prevents sleep. When the child is brought into theatre small points such as the avoidance of shining the operating light in his eyes and the use of warm solution to clean the skin minimize irritation and hence crying and air swallowing. This is a great help to the surgeon.

If a General Anæsthetic is to be Used. The stomach will be washed out in the same way and a nasogastric tube may be left down at this time. Atropine will be required ($\frac{1}{200}$ gr.) (0·3 mg.), but the anæsthetist will probably prefer to avoid sedatives.

Modern endotracheal anæsthesia for infants is very safe. The indication for local anæsthesia has become largely the unavailability of a practised anæsthetist—which must be rare in clinics which have the other facilities to justify embarking on the management of these babies. It should be stressed that a sick baby is no longer an indication for local anæsthesia. If special circumstances require operation on a sick baby, he will be maintained in better oxygenation by the correct general anæsthetic than by breathing by his own efforts with the handicap of an open abdomen and depressant drugs can now be avoided. Furthermore, in this condition there must be few reasons for not making such a patient fit before operation.

The Operation

Ramstedt's operation (1912) for which the originator suggested the name pyloromyotomy, has replaced all others. It is an almost perfect procedure.

The peritoneal cavity is opened through a high incision over the liver. This makes it easier to retain the small bowel within the abdomen, but more important, it protects the wound after operation. These babies are malnourished and special care is needed to avoid wound dehiscence. For this reason many use a right subcostal muscle splitting incision instead of the usual paramedian rectus splitting incision. The delivery of the tumour is rather more awkward, but the benefits may offset this disadvantage. The operation is carried out systematically and as the baby is well prepared there is neither necessity nor value in hurried smash and grab surgery. Rough handling will always cause shock. Gentle surgery can be prolonged as may be required without any anxiety. Speed will come of practice.

The pylorus is firm when palpated at operation. The less vascular anterosuperior aspect of the peritoneum and muscle overlying the pylorus are split down to the mucous membrane throughout the whole extent of the elongated canal. A superficial incision is made with the knife and it is deepened through the muscle by stroking this with a semi-blunt instrument such as a small periosteal elevator of the type used in cleft palate surgery. The muscle is then spread widely so that the mucosa pouts out above the level of the visceral peritoneum. It splits with a characteristic grating feel and slides easily over the mucous membrane so that the latter is safe from perforation except at the zone of adhesion in the fornix at the duodenal end, where care is needed to complete the

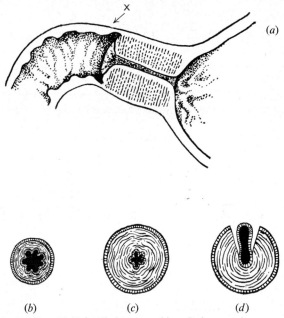

FIG. 22. Infantile hypertrophic pyloric stenosis.

(*a*) Section through the pyloric region. X marks the dangerous zone of adhesion in the fornix at the duodenal end where the reflected mucosa is adherent and is easily torn close to the surface.

(*b*) Transverse section of normal pylorus.

(*c*) Showing obstruction of the lumen by infolded mucosa when the circular muscle hypertrophies.

(*d*) Showing how the lumen is re-established by division of the muscle in Ramstedt's operation, allowing the mucosa to unfold and pout to the surface.

freeing. Perforation is no tragedy *provided* it is noticed. A single stitch will close it and a pad of omentum is tied over the area.

Once in a while there may be difficulty, especially if local anæsthesia is unsatisfactory and the baby heaves. The assistant holds a moist gauze in his hand and is ready to thrust any protruding coils of bowel back into the abdomen without waiting to be asked. If bowel is allowed out it blows up with gas and is more difficult to replace. In these circumstances the following manœuvre will keep matters under control. All intestine is replaced. A narrow gauze is then pushed down into the abdomen and withdrawn. It will bring up adherent omentum. This guides one to the transverse colon which is withdrawn and held down over the lower end of the wound. Thus the small bowel is prevented from leaving the abdomen and the colon leads one in turn to the stomach. The stomach is grasped near the greater curve and traction delivers the pylorus. The assistant can control the field by holding the stomach out to the left and caudally whilst the surgeon is free to carry out the pyloromyotomy.

POST-OPERATIVE CARE

After the operation the temperature is checked with a thermometer which reads down to 85°F and the baby returned to his cubicle. Feeds can begin 4 hours after the operation. A start is made with a drachm of 5 per cent glucose every hour. After 4 hours this quantity is doubled and after 8 hours half an ounce is given. If there is no vomiting by 12 hours after the operation then half-strength milk is given. The feeds and the intervals between them are increased step by step until the baby is back on full feeds within 48 hours.

An occasional vomit is not uncommon after operation. This is due to a combination of habit and gastritis. Troublesome persistence of vomiting is most likely to be due to the gastritis not having had time to settle. Gastric lavage is more helpful than fiddling with the feeds. It must be remembered that although the obstruction is immediately relieved there will be some delay in the establishment of normal gastric peristalsis and settling of the concomitant gastritis. The medically oriented staff who are so often caring for these babies after operation do not always appreciate this.

If the baby should still be breast feeding when admitted, then of course every effort is made to keep the milk supply going by expression. The baby is given expressed breast milk in his schedule and should return to the breast within 48 hours of operation.

The patient is ready for discharge when he has been taking full feeds for a day. It is unwise to retain a thriving infant in hospital longer than is essential because of the inevitable risks of cross-infection even with the greatest care.

The results of treatment are excellent. About 15 years ago at a discussion of this subject several régimes were supported and mortalities of under 4 per cent quoted. Yet the registrar-general's figures still showed a mortality of 15 per cent for the country as a whole. The inference is that it is more important that these babies be cared for in a unit experienced in a technique than to follow one particular régime. Mortalities of less than 1 per cent have been achieved in many clinics.

REFERENCES

Benson, C. D. and Warden, M. J. (1957) Seven hundred and seven cases of congenital hypertrophic pyloric stenosis. *Surg. Gynec. and Obstet.*, **105**, 348.

Hayes, M. A. and Goldenberg, Ira S. (1957) Collective review, *Surg. Gynæc. Obstet. Internat. Absts.*, **104**, 105–138.

Proc. roy. Soc. Med. (1951), Discussion on the treatment of congenital hypertrophic pyloric stenosis, **44**, 1055.

Jacoby, N. M. (1962) Pyloric stenosis: selective medica and surgical treatment *Lancet, i*, 119–121.

$\frac{\sigma}{\varphi} = \frac{3}{1}.$

CHAPTER 10

INTUSSUSCEPTION

INTUSSUSCEPTION (intus = within, suscipere = to take up) is the invagination of one portion of the intestine into another. The invagination almost always occurs in the direction of peristalsis and is most common at the ileocæcal region. It is a form of strangulation (interference with the blood supply of the bowel) as well as obstruction. Treatment is therefore even more urgent than in a simple intestinal obstruction. The results vary inversely with the duration of the condition.

Intussusception is the commonest cause of intestinal obstruction between the ages of 2 months and 5 years. It may occur earlier or later than these times but its maximum incidence is between 3 and 18 months with a peak at 6 months. The cause is unknown in the majority of cases, but there is sometimes a history of diarrhœa suggesting that inflammatory enlargement of the Peyer's patches in the terminal ileum

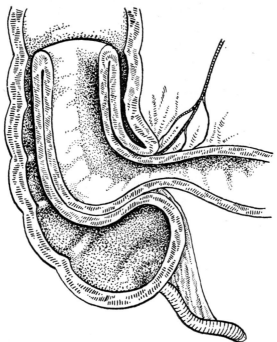

FIG. 23. Diagram of origin of ileocolic intussusception.

76

together with the resultant hyperperistalsis may be factors. Weaning frequently used to be incriminated, and a change of diet may be a precipitating factor. A definite local cause such as a polyp, Meckel's diverticulum, or intestinal duplication at the head of the intussusception is found in under 3 per cent. Henoch-Schönlein purpura causing hæmorrhage into the bowel wall so that the lumen may be almost totally occluded, may imitate the picture of intussusception or may, less commonly, cause a true one.

There appears to be a seasonal incidence varying from place to place, and it is certainly a "cropping" disease. Adenovirus infection is a common aetiological factor.

The intussusception consists of three layers or cylinders of bowel and an included portion of the mesentery. The outer layer of bowel is called the intussuscipiens and the middle and inner layers are called the intussusceptum. The advancing point is called the apex whilst the reflection of the middle layer to the outer is called the neck. Intus-susceptions are usually ileocæcal or ileocolic. In the former the apex is in the cæcum and in the latter in the ileum. But they may be ileo-ileal or colo-colic, whilst combinations of these may occur. Occasionally there may be more than one present. (In severe gastro-enteritis there may be multiple small transient intussusceptions. If the abdomen is opened through a diagnostic error they can be seen to form and reduce as one watches the bowel.)

SIGNS AND SYMPTOMS

The disease classically presents in a fat, previously healthy, infant. The first symptom is *intermittent colicky pain*. The spasms make the baby cry and usually draw the knees up to the abdomen as babies will do with abdominal discomfort. The infant goes pale with the pain. The spasms, though severe, are fairly short. Because of the pain-free intervals which may last 15 to 20 minutes the parents will often temporize before sending for advice. The infant goes off his food and the majority *vomit*. Early vomiting is of reflex origin and the vomitus is gastric content. Later bilestained obstructive vomits occur if the diagnosis is delayed. There is usually a history of *constipation*, but blood and mucus may be passed from the anus. This really does quite often have the appearance of *red-currant jelly*. It is unusual in the first day of the disease when diagnosis should be made. Often the first observation of blood follows a rectal examination, and this is an essential part of the examination of a baby suspected of intussusception. Rarely the intussusception may present per anum. It cannot really be mistaken for a prolapse on more than the most casual inspection, though the differential diagnosis is laboured in many texts.

Many babies suffer from colics caused by wind, indigestion, gastro-enteritis, respiratory infections and so on. But these babies tend to be persistently irritable and grizzly. They won't lie still to be examined. They go red in the face during their screaming bouts. This contrasts with the periodicity of the symptoms in intussusception—severe pains causing *pallor*, not flushing of the facies—with exhaustion soon becoming evident between the pains; the baby lies limp and still.

On examination there is usually moderate *pyrexia* and a tachycardia. The infant is exhausted and lies quiet or sleeps between attacks of pain. The abdomen is usually *moderately distended* and on auscultation the heart sounds may be heard clearly between spasms of peristalsis—a sign of distension of the gut. There are then almost no bowel sounds. When a spasm comes on the sounds are loud, turbulent, splashy and high pitched. Auscultation should be performed before palpation, and should continue for at least 3 minutes in suspicious circumstances. Palpation of the abdomen should begin gently in the left iliac fossa and continue slowly anticlockwise. Under the bedclothes may be the most successful method, to avoid disturbing the baby. The left hypochondrium should be carefully palpated as it is here that the typical *mass* is often missed. The mass is nearer the centre of the abdomen than might be expected, because the mesentery is shortened by its invagination. The mass is less likely to be missed in the epigastrium, though it may underlie the firm liver edge and make examination difficult. On the other hand, the liver edge, rolled under the fingers has been mistaken for an intussusception.

If the infant is really difficult to examine then he should be sedated with 1 ml. of intramuscular paraldehyde, or 25 mg. of intramuscular pethidine, and the examination repeated half an hour later. Although the intussusception varies in length with the distance it has progressed the mass of bowel palpated is usually about 3 inches long and 2 inches wide. It is a distinctly tender mass. It may be felt to harden under the hand, as palpation often stimulates peristalsis and precipitates a painful spasm.

Rectal examination should never be omitted and a fresh normal stool after the first few hours is against the diagnosis.

It is important to remember that although severe colics are the most frequent symptoms, there are about 10 per cent of intussusceptions in which there is no evidence of pain. Blood and mucus in a motion or on an examining finger are very reliable signs and should not be ignored.

If after physical examination under good conditions there is still genuine doubt about the diagnosis, then one should proceed to radiology. There is *no place for observation* because this is a strangulating condition and delay may mean all the hazards of resection of the bowel instead of simple reduction of the invagination. As has already been said, *the mortality varies directly with the duration of the disease.*

Plain radiography in the prone and erect positions is performed. If it shows fluid levels in progressively dilating loops of bowel then obstruction is confirmed. Laparotomy is indicated and intussusception is the likely lesion. (It must be remembered that fluid levels may be seen in the small bowel of normal babies under the age of 2 years, and that they may be marked in the presence of gastro-enteritis, or with the air-swallowing of persistent crying. It is the progressive dilatation down to the level of the lesion that is characteristic of organic obstruction.) If the plain films are inconclusive then a barium enema will give a definite diagnosis in virtually every remaining case. (It may not penetrate far enough to show an ileo-ileal intussusception, but such a small bowel lesion will almost certainly have caused sufficient obstruction even in the early stages to show obstruction on the plain films.) *The obstruction may be incomplete* especially in an older patient and this may lead to delay in diagnosis. The urgency is no less because there may still be strangulation of the intussuscepted bowel.

Differential Diagnosis

The common imitators of intussusception are *gastro-enteritis* and *upper respiratory infections with colic*, as has been mentioned. *Sonne* dysentery in particular may present with pain, fever and blood from the rectum without diarrhœa. Indigestion, wind and irritability also cause colic in the same age group. The differences in the picture have already been described

TREATMENT

SURGERY. In our experience the treatment of choice has been operative reduction. This can be achieved through a high McBurney incision. It is a reliable procedure.

The preparation of the patient for operation is important. Early diagnosis and careful preparation and postoperative management have reduced the mortality from almost 25 per cent before 1940 to 1 or 2 per cent in the last 15 years. Operation should not be performed until the circulatory volume has been restored by blood or plasma. The shocked condition of the child is due to blood and plasma loss at the site of the strangulation; 200 ml. to a 16-lb. infant is the equivalent of a 3-pint transfusion to an adult, and is just as dramatic in its effect. Again, it is impossible to be sure before operation whether the reduction will be easy or whether resection will be necessary—and if resection is unavoidable blood or plasma replacement is essential. If a Meckel's diverticulum, polyp or duplication is the cause of the trouble it may have to be excised, and this is another reason for being prepared in every case. If the bowel cannot be reduced or if reduction reveals non-viable bowel then resection is necessary. An end-to-end anastomosis is performed. Resection should be wide, reaching back to really healthy bowel, so that healing will be sound. An end-to-end anastomosis is always possible and preferable.

HYDROSTATIC REDUCTION. There is a trend, particularly in parts of the U.S.A. and Scandinavia, towards non-operative reduction of intussusception by hydrostatic pressure. The refinement of using a barium enema instead of water, and controlling the reduction by radiological screening is usual. This method is most successful in cases with a history of less than 24 hours and in babies over 6 months of age. Even then a laparotomy is necessary in about a quarter of the cases to confirm or complete the reduction. Objections are uncertain control of ileo-ileal intussusception, possible reduction of gangrenous bowel, perforation of weakened bowel, increased frequency of recurrences, and loss of valuable time if the method fails. Finally, it must not be forgotten that the procedure itself may be a shocking one, and this may not always be appreciated in the darkness of the X-ray room. In our practice hydrostatic reduction is not used as a deliberate policy. However, if a barium enema is required to diagnose a case it seems reasonable to make a limited trial of the method by raising the enema can to about 3 ft. and waiting 5 to 10 minutes and watching for reduction. This will avoid some operations and facilitate others by moving the intussusception back to the right side. There is no risk of trouble if prolonged or forceful efforts are avoided.

Spontaneous reduction. Spontaneous reduction of intussusception probably occurs more often than is realized. There is a classical history of colic, pallor and passage of blood. Later, the mass which was felt on diagnosis is found to have gone. But it must be stressed that such an outcome must never be awaited in a doubtful case. *Diagnostic doubt after examination is an indication for further investigation, and not for observation.*

Operation

A cut-down infusion in the left antecubital fossa is usually necessary, as the fat infant is a difficult subject for an intravenous needle. This should be put up in the ward as the patient normally requires preparation for surgery—200 ml. of half-strength plasma over about 3 hours before operation on a 4-month-old baby would be a typical requirement. A naso-gastric tube is passed to keep the stomach empty. Antibiotics, for example penicillin and streptomycin, should be given because of the risk of septicæmia beginning in the devitalized bowel.

The anæsthetic agent employed will depend on the anæsthetist. Controlled respiration with an endotracheal tube and small increments of muscle relaxants seems ideal.

The abdomen is palpated before the incision is made. A high McBurney incision is adequate for the vast majority and has the advantage of easy sound repair. It can be extended for the occasional awkward case by a rectus-displacing or a muscle-cutting medial extension.

When the abdomen is opened two fingers are inserted and the mass palpated within the abdomen. Pressure beyond the apex will usually reduce the intussusception easily as far as the right side of the abdomen. The mass can then be lifted gently out of the wound, because there is almost always a mobile mesentery in these babies. When the mass is controlled by both hands reduction may be completed under vision. This is done by squeezing gently on the distal portion (the apex) and massaging it out of its sheath. It may become progressively more difficult. The last inches are the most difficult. Rather than use heavy pressure the intussusception should be wrapped in warm packs and the œdema slowly reduced by even pressure before squeezing out the last piece of bowel like tooth-paste from a tube. Traction must never be used to reduce an intussusception. There is a grave risk of tearing the bowel. In reducing the last portion the œdematous peritoneal coat may split. It should be repaired with fine sutures.

It may be that the mass cannot be reduced, or that the reduced bowel is not viable. There are two courses of action. The mass may be resected with primary anastomosis, or it may be exteriorized. If it is exteriorized it may be amputated at the end of the operation and anastomosis is carried out later at a second operation three to five days later. If the baby is well prepared the first course is to be preferred. If its condition is poor or blood is not available, then the second course may be wiser.

An occasional case is still seen in a desperately ill toxic condition. Abdominal distension is gross and the baby is not only dehydrated but shows peripheral circulatory failure. Reduction of the bowel in such a case often produces a fatal exacerbation of the shock. Urgent blood transfusion followed by a rapid exteriorization and excision of the mass without any attempt at reduction will save some of these cases.

Appendicectomy in passing is safe in most cases. It is particularly advisable if the McBurney incision is used. No attempt to prevent recurrence should be made. Most plication operations designed to prevent recurrence seem to precipitate it. Cæcostomy or resection seem the only reliable ways of prevention. Either may be required to deal with a chronic intussusception or with a third recurrence.

Recurrence is rare—about 3 per cent. Mortality is negligible with treatment in the first 24 hours of the disease. It rises to 5 or 10 per cent by the third day. Thereafter it comes down again as one begins to include the less common cases of subacute intussusception in which strangulation is not a feature.

The series of papers from the Newcastle school on this subject show how such a clinical problem can be studied and the effect of such attention—the 1950 paper quotes a consecutive hundred cases without mortality.

REFERENCES

Morrison, B. and Court, D. (1948) Acute intussusception in childhood, *Brit. med. J.*, *i*, 776.

Spence, J. and Court D. (1950) Acute intuss usception in childhood, *Brit. med. J.*, *ii*, 921.

Jones, J. D. T. (1953) Treatment of irreducible intussusception, *Brit. Med. J.*, *ii*, 1304.

Knox, E. G., Court, S. D. M., and Gardner, P. S. (1962) Ætiology of intussusception in children, *Brit. med. J.*, *ii*, 692–697.

Ravitch, M. M. (1959) *Intussusception in Infants and Children*, Charles C. Thomas, Springfield, U.S.A.

CHAPTER 11

CIRCUMCISION

CIRCUMCISION is the most widely practised surgical procedure in the world. One-sixth of the male population have a ritual circumcision, the Jews in infancy and the Moslems at three years of age or later. It would appear that it is mainly in these islands and North America that the merits or otherwise of the procedure are still open to debate. Circumcision is uncommon in France, Germany, Italy and Scandinavia.

The procedure was a purely religious rite up to the 1880s, but it is now a common operation. Every male in the English-speaking world comes under scrutiny at some time or other as a possible candidate for circumcision. There are various medical indications but the firmly held beliefs of parents, grandparents, nurses, midwives and many doctors are the commonest reasons for operation.

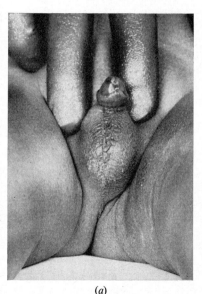
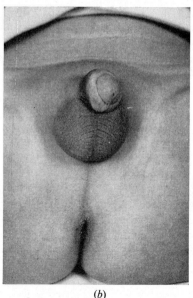

(a)   (b)

FIG. 24. (a) Meatal ulceration after circumcision.
(b) Meatal stenosis following healing of meatal ulcer.

The prepuce has a protective role for an infant in napkins. If the operation were postponed until the patients were out of napkins then fewer operations would be requested. The prepuce is normally non-retractile for the first 9 to 15 months of life. It is non-retractile in four

83

out of five males at the age of 6 months; in 50 per cent at the age of 1 year, and 10 per cent at 2 years. The prepuce protects the glans from meatal ulceration. There is at birth a layer of squamous cells present between the glans and the prepuce. These cells usually begin to degenerate sometime between 6 and 18 months and then the prepuce becomes fully retractile. Previous to that the glans is muzzled (Greek—phimosis) and that is as it should be. The small preputial orifice and the adhesions between the prepuce and glans are physiological. If the infant has been observed to pass a stream of urine and there is no ballooning then no intervention is necessary. If at the age of 4 years the layer of cells has not degenerated, then a gentle probing will often suffice to prove that everything is in order. In a few boys the prepuce will still not retract owing to a real narrowing of its outlet. To circumcise then will avoid the risk of paraphimosis when erections occur.

Ammoniacal Dermatitis

The commonest reason given for circumcision is balanitis. Balanitis strictly should mean an inflammation of the glans and posthitis an inflammation of the prepuce. The term balanitis is loosely used, and in the majority of cases so described there is no inflammation in the subpreputial pocket which indeed is usually still closed by the persistent squamous layer in infancy. *There is inflammation of the prepuce resulting from external irritation by ammonia in the urine.* This ammonia burning of the prepuce is usually associated with ammonia dermatitis in other parts of the napkin area. The distribution is typically on the prepuce, scrotum and in severe cases also on the upper thighs and lower abdominal wall. The depths of the skin creases which are protected from contact with the urine escape the dermatitis in an unmistakable fashion. *Where there is active ammoniacal dermatitis circumcision is contra-indicated.* If the circumcision is performed in these circumstances preputial ulceration is likely to be exchanged for meatal ulceration when the glans is exposed. The ulcerated meatus causes excruciating pain on micturition and there is typically a speck of blood at the beginning of each act of micturition. If meatal ulceration persists for long enough scarring may produce meatal stenosis and even require eventual meatotomy.

Ammoniacal dermatitis is extremely common even in the social groups where hygienic standards are high. It is caused by urea splitting organisms in the infant's fæces acting on the urea in the urine and decomposing it into ammonia. The napkin area has many patches of red, raised and sore skin, with ulceration in the more severe cases. It is the prepuce which suffers first and most, however. It is tender, œdematous and boggy. Any attempt at retraction is painful and may cause bleeding, while the external urinary meatus may be completely concealed. Naturally the passage of urine further irritates the lesion.

Treatment. The basis of the treatment is simple hygiene. It must be said that powders, lotions and ointments have a small place in keeping the skin clear. There are two common causes of the trouble: (1) *The child wears waterproof pants for most of the 24 hours.* These pants, whether plastic or rubber, keep the child wet and warm when he has passed urine, and give the bacteria a greater chance to decompose the urine. They are particularly apt to be worn through the night, and this is the time when the rash is most likely to develop, in warm surroundings. Waterproof pants should be worn only on important social occasions. (2) *Failure to boil the napkins is a frequent source of trouble.* If the child has ammoniacal dermatitis the napkins require to be boiled after each wearing whether they are soiled or merely wet. Many mothers only boil

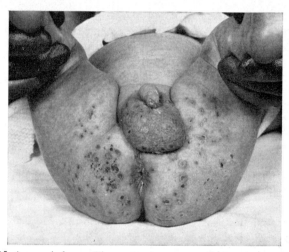

FIG. 25. Ammonia burns. The prepuce, scrotum and buttocks are affected. The flexures are spared. (Case of Dr. R. T. Brain.)

the napkins when they have been soiled. Ideally they should be boiled for 20 minutes in a soft detergent to destroy the bacteria. Washing machines with a boiling action do not usually produce adequate temperatures to *sterilize* napkins. These rules must be rigidly adhered to if the skin is to heal. Some mothers will say that none of her previous boys had the trouble and that she adopted the same standards of hygiene with them. The explanation for this is that skin textures vary and that some children are abnormally prone to this condition. Ammoniacal dermatitis is quite common in little girls also, but it is not such an important problem for the surgeon because the question of the operation does not arise.

The boracic régime has been in use for many years for the treatment of ammonia dermatitis and is of undoubted value. Boracic is a poor antiseptic but in these conditions it is being used not as an anti-septic but as a non-irritant weak acid to neutralize the ammonia. The kind of routine usually described is to use boracic ointment 5 per cent on the sore parts and to rinse the napkins after boiling in a solution of a tablespoon of boracic crystals in half a pint of hot water, allowing them to dry with the boracic impregnating them. It is possible to produce boracic poisoning by means of injudicious use of boracic powder applied directly to large raw areas denuded of epithelium. However, this has been a greatly over-emphasized danger, and the use of 5 per cent ointment on the kind of lesion seen in these children is completely safe. There is certainly little reason to turn to more expensive proprietory quaternary alkyl ammonium compounds in its place. Indeed as has already been said *these local measures are of secondary importance to the matter of hygiene and regular boiling of the napkins.*

Ammonia dermatitis is one of the commonest conditions seen in infants presented for circumcision. It is a contra-indication at that time, but the infection may cause fibrosis of the prepuce and result in an acquired phimosis. This acquired phimosis may require circumcision when the infant is out of napkins.

Surgical Indications for Circumcision

Balanitis. If separation of the prepuce is delayed into the second year of life a few cases will be seen in which separation is associated with infection under the prepuce. The organism is usually a staphylococcus. The story is that a previously well boy complains of a sore penis and on examination the prepuce is seen to be swollen and a few purulent drops of discharge can be expressed from the orifice. There is naturally dis-comfort on micturition. This acute balanoposthitis is readily treated by baths and local sponging and application of penicillin cream. Within a few days it settles completely. At this stage the child is often referred to hospital for an opinion on circumcision. The more fortunate child may have completely stripped his remaining subpreputial ad-hesions with this attack of balanitis. It is an unpleasant manner of completion of the natural process, but results in a completely retractile prepuce and the mother can be reassured that with ordinary standards of hygiene he will have no more trouble. In a number of these children, however, the separation of the glans will have been incomplete so that it can be only partially retracted. If these children are left for a natural separation to continue they may have recurrences of this unpleasant infection. Attempts to separate the adhesions without anæsthesia at this age can be extremely frightening as well as painful. It is therefore usually preferable after such an attack to proceed to circumcision to avoid the risk of further recurrent attacks of balanoposthitis. At this age the children will be developing control of their micturition and getting out of their napkins so that the danger of meatal ulceration is no longer an important one.

True Phimosis. This is uncommon as a primary condition. Often the diagnosis is made when the prepuce is merely long. If an attempt is made to demonstrate the meatus, it can usually be shown to be unobstructed. Genuine phimosis does occur and the possibility should not be ignored. Ballooning of the prepuce may occur on micturition. This usually follows much meddlesome stretching in infancy and makes circumcision advisable.

Paraphimosis. This is a definite indication for circumcision. It is the result of the leading edge of the prepuce being retracted behind the corona of the glans, and becoming too tight to be pulled forward again into its normal position. Engorgement and œdema of the prepuce set up a vicious circle and the penis is a sore and sorry sight. The prepuce forms a swollen ring behind the penis eventually ulcerating if untreated. Paraphimosis should be reduced as soon as possible. A general anæsthetic will usually be necessary. The first and second fingers of each hand are placed behind the swollen ring of the prepuce and the thumbs are placed on the glans. Firm pressure will reduce the glans through the prepuce and relieve the venous pressure. A nick in the dorsum of the most constricted ring of the prepuce will ease reduction in a neglected case. Early circumcision should be performed. This can be done as part of the emergency treatment under a general anæsthetic if the tissues are not too grossly œdematous.

Redundant Prepuce. A long prepuce may lead to recurrent irritation and discomfort from retention of urine inside the sac and justify circumcision.

PSEUDO INDICATIONS. An argument frequently put forward in favour of circumcision is the mother's statement that he cries when he wets. What happens in fact is that he wets when he cries. For crying increases the intra-abdominal pressure, and anything which increases the intra-abdominal pressure of an infant whose bladder happens to be full will stimulate the automatic emptying of that bladder.

One of the commonest medical arguments constantly heard in favour of circumcision is that carcinoma of the penis is almost unknown in those who have the procedure in infancy. The incidence of this condition varies tremendously in various countries and races, and it is an uncommon form of cancer amongst the English-speaking peoples. It accounts for perhaps 1 in 500 cancers. It appears almost always to occur in the dull and the dirty. If one considers the protection from this cancer worth while then the rational outcome is universal infant circumcision. Carcinoma of the penis has been recorded in patients circumcised in infancy, but it is undoubtedly much less common in these patients.

Conclusions

There is no doubt that there are many genuine indications for circumcision and that many parents are happier when the procedure has been completed. If any procedure is to be performed it should be a full circumcision. The dorsal slit has lost favour on cosmetic grounds. *Stretching with an artery forceps is only asking for further stricture formation at the prepuce as the resultant fissures heal by fibrosis.* Furthermore it is a painful procedure and its repetition is distressing to the mother as well as the child.

The reason for the development of various minor procedures instead of circumcision is the desire to preserve a protection for the glans while making the opening big enough. However, if the policy of deferring circumcision beyond the napkin wearing age is carried out wherever the danger of meatal ulceration is high, the risk of baring the glans is negligible.

In uncircumcised infants with retractile prepuces one should not be too insistent on "pushing it back" and "frequent powdering". Such advice often causes anxiety and doubt.

UNDER TWO YEARS

DO NOT STRETCH:

EITHER CIRCUMCISE OR LEAVE

OVER TWO YEARS

GENTLE PUSH BACK MAY HELP.

FORCEFUL RETRACTION AT ANY AGE

NEVER HELPS BUT MAY HARM

Few uncircumcised males have cause to regret their condition.

OPERATION

The operation itself is basically an easy one but has an uncommonly long list of common faults or complications. Bleeding (it has been called a diagnostic test for hæmophilia!), removal of too much skin (causing painful tension at the frænum on erection), removal of too much mucosa (so that the sutures are inadequate and the skin slips forward to heal in front of the glans with recurrent phimosis requiring further operation), removing too little mucosa, untidy tags, circumcision in hypospadias (removing valuable and irreplaceable repair material), fistula of the urethra (by placing the frænal stitch too deeply) and accidental amputation of the glans. Meatal ulceration with meatal stenosis often follows either trauma at operation or ill-advised operation in the presence of ammonia dermatitis.

It is best to use a technique which requires no special instruments. In the neonatal period the operation is often performed using a bone forceps without an anæsthetic. The trouble with this method is that it may leave too much mucosa so that the prepuce is able to slip forward during healing and a recurrent acquired phimosis may result. It is perhaps a convenient trick for one who practices frequent circumcision but it is not very satisfactory for the occasional operator. All resection methods require general anæsthesia. The first step is to retract the prepuce completely, even if a dorsal slit is necessary to allow this to be done. The adhesions are completely separated back to the coronal sulcus, the surfaces are cleaned and the foreskin pulled forward again. Artery forceps are put on the skin and mucosa at 2 o'clock, 6 o'clock and

10 o'clock of the prepuce. The prepuce is drawn forward over the glans and a heavy artery clip put across the excess skin at an angle parallel to the corona, just distal to the glans. The amount of skin removed is such that it is judged that the remaining skin will lie just beyond the coronal sulcus. It is particularly important in fat babies with a short looking penis partly buried in the pubic fat to make sure that some preputial shaft skin is left all round. It is much easier than one might think to draw too firmly on these foreskins and remove too much. (This type has been described by the Americans as toad-in-the-hole penis, and the result of removing too much skin so that the glans lies flush with the pubic skin is to produce a buried penis.) The excess skin is amputated by a scalpel running along the distal edge of the forceps. The artery forceps is left in position for a few minutes after the actual cut to give the vessels time to thrombose. When the artery forceps is removed there is usually some bleeding which need not be attended to immediately. The skin is once more pushed back beyond the corona and the mucosa inspected. If, as is usually the case, enough mucosa has not been removed then it must be trimmed until between one-quarter and one-eighth of an inch ring of mucosa remains. Hæmostasis is now secured by catching the bleeding points with forceps and ligaturing with the finest catgut. Only performing hæmostasis in this way, as would be carried out in any other surgical operation, can the risks of post-operative hæmatoma formation and bleeding be reduced to proper proportions. The ring of mucosa is then stitched to the skin. On the ventral surface the frænum and frænal artery are secured by single mattress suture. Elsewhere a number of single interrupted sutures of catgut are used. It is important to be careful of hæmostasis to avoid the risk of hæmatoma formation. If a large hæmatoma occurs it may disrupt the stitches and cause a raw area greatly retarding healing and it is also a cause of considerable post-operative discomfort.

No dressing is required in a formal circumcision. If one is preferred, a roll of gauze impregnated with compound ointment of benzoin may be applied, or a few of the catgut sutures can be left long and tied over a piece of tulle gras.

It is important that the suture line should be allowed to heal in the retracted position behind the glans. If an inadequate amount of mucosa is removed and the prepuce slips forward in front of the glans it will almost always heal with a tight cartilaginous scar producing a severe recurrent phimosis. Yet if the same skin is made to heal behind the corona any thickening which may occur proves temporary and settles within a few months. This curious re-action of the penile skin was pointed out by Denis Browne. It is unexplained but it is undoubtedly a fact. It is for this reason that minor procedures such as modifications of the dorsal slit with transverse suture are to be looked on with caution because they give an opportunity for such forward healing. The standard circumcision with a small fringe of mucosa, properly performed, is such an operation that this kind of forward displacement of the suture line is impossible.

REFERENCES

Gairdner, D. (1949) The fate of the foreskin, *Brit. med. J.*, *ii*, 1433.

CHAPTER 12

BIRTHMARKS

BIRTHMARKS may actually be present at birth but the majority are first noticed a few days or even weeks later. The two main groups are the *angiomas* and the *benign pigmented melanomas*. They are common and advice on treatment is frequently sought. This must be based on a knowledge of the natural history of the various types.

ANGIOMAS (VASCULAR NÆVUS)

The usual types are:

NEONATAL STAINING. Milk spots, salmon patch, erythema nuchæ.

CAPILLARY ANGIOMA. Stellate angioma (spider nævus) and port-wine stains.

CAPILLARY-CAVERNOUS ANGIOMA. Strawberry mark.

CAVERNOUS ANGIOMA.

HÆMANGIOMATOUS VARICOSITIES Diffuse hæmangiomatosis and hæmangiomatous gigantism.

Neonatal Staining

Neonatal staining is so common as to be considered a variation of the normal. It is flat, dull pink patch of skin often seen on the forehead, upper eyelids and most frequently at the back of the neck. It is present at birth and almost always fades within a few months. No treatment is needed. The common association of a patch on the occiput with one on the glabella has given rise to the popular name of storkbites.

Capillary Angioma

SPIDER NÆVUS

The spider nævus is another innocent capillary lesion. It consists of tiny vessels radiating from a central venule. Cosmetic treatment by diathermy of the central venule may be applied if the appearance seems to justify it.

PORT-WINE STAIN

The port-wine stain is a much more unfortunate lesion. It is a flat diffuse intradermal capillary angioma which commonly affects the greater part of one side of the face. Its extent sometimes follows the distribution of the cutaneous nerves. The usual colour is a mauve tint though some are paler and pinker and others a more dusky and dirty

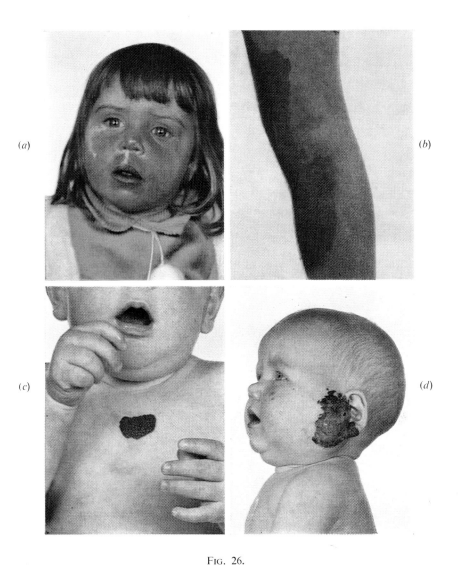

FIG. 26.

(a) Portwine Stain (flat capillary angioma, Nævus Flammeus). (b) Hairy Mole (intradermal nævus). (c) Strawberry Mark (raised capillary angioma). (d) Cavernous angioma.

[*facing page 90*

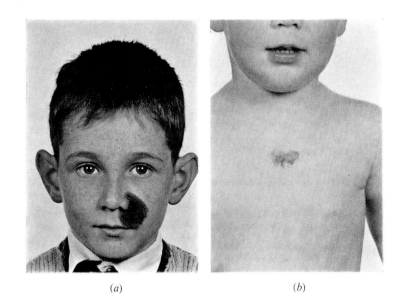

(a)   (b)

FIG. 27.

(a) Brown Mole on Face (intradermal nævus).
(b) The Strawberry Mark shown in Fig. 26 (c)
fading spontaneously two years later.

looking hue. The angioma blanches on pressure. This lesion grows with the child. It does not spread to other areas but shows no tendency to regression. Attempts may be made to improve the unsightly blemish by punctate diathermy or the application of the radioactive substance thorium X. These may help some of the paler lesions but an uneven response may leave a blotchy lesion that looks worse than its original state. Extensive grafts are also cosmetically inadequate. The treatment of choice is the use of make-up. Special cosmetics are available to disguise these blemishes, e.g. Covermark.

Capillary-Cavernous Angioma (Strawberry Mark)

The *strawberry mark* is the commonest birthmark seen by surgeons. It is a raised dull red angioma with well-defined margins. It looks full and shiny. The mark may be present at birth or more commonly appears during the first few days or weeks of life, and occasionally later. It is a mainly capillary angioma, but at least microscopically there are larger spaces in most of them justifying the description of capillary-cavernous angioma. It is an essentially benign lesion. It does not require biopsy despite the rapid growth which is common in the first few months of life.

Angiomas are hamartomas rather than true tumours. The enlargement is due to postnatal expansion of the spaces rather than real spread.

This lesion will *always* regress spontaneously though it will take an average of about 4 years to do so. At about 9 months of age the growing stage ceases. The condition then hangs fire and little change may be seen for a year or so. Regression then begins. The colour may become a duller red and the lesion less tense. Pale grey or whitish spots appear centrally and join together so that a peripheral ring of red is left. As healing progresses this ring gradually narrows and disappears. The remaining skin is usually quite normal. It may be thin or pale or redundant. The healing process is one of spontaneous thrombosis in the vessels. It may be associated with ulceration. Then there may be a more noticeable residual skin blemish. Hæmorrhage may be brisk if ulceration occurs, or following trauma—such as scratching or catching a comb in an angioma on the scalp. Although alarming to the mother it responds to a simple pressure dressing. Spontaneous healing of the lesion is often accelerated after such an occurrence.

Treatment by carbon dioxide snow or diathermy hastens healing but causes a permanent patch of pale, shiny skin. Carbon dioxide snow has the advantage of convenience in the surgery, but it is difficult to control precisely the extent and depth of treatment and a blotched appearance may result. It is applied direct to the lesion for not more than 20 seconds at any one application. The diathermy needle produces a more easily controlled effect. But it may cause a pock-marked appearance if it is used over a wide area and is probably better used only in regions where the cosmetic result is not important, such as the perineum. A radium plaque hastens resolution but radiotherapy is unjustified in such a benign condition. The best results (usually no trace) are obtained by natural cure.

Cavernous Angioma

Cavernous angioma is a lesion which is subcutaneous rather than dermal. A blue discoloration may show through the overlying skin. It can be emptied easily by pressure but rapidly fills again. It may enlarge quite quickly in the early months of infancy.

Many angiomas combine surface capillary and deeper cavernous elements.

In treatment it must be emphasized that the majority disappear with little trace by the time the child is ready for school. The best cosmetic results (complete disappearance) again result from natural cure without interference. A problem which often arises, however, is the angioma seen at an early stage when it is obviously spreading and on a conspicuous place such as the face. It is sometimes difficult to advise expectancy under these circumstances. Cavernous lesions, in particular, go through a phase of quite rapid growth early in life, especially those combined with the capillary type. Although we know that these will later involute, growth should usually be stopped and the skin changes following involution will be less widespread. In certain situations there may be distortion or destruction of tissues, e.g. a lip or the cartilage of the ear. In some extensive cavernous hæmangiomata their development may even cause cardiac failure as a result of the arteriovenous shunt through them.

There is a less common type of angioma in which the skin surface is abnormal and "warty". It seems more likely to persist into adult life.

Denis Browne draws attention to a type which begins as a small bright red smooth-surfaced spot at birth. It does not grow in the early stages like the strawberry mark. Later it may begin to spread producing a progressive and grossly disfiguring lesion. It usually arises on the face. Although it is pathologically benign he calls it the malignant facial angioma to stress the unpleasant course it may take and to distinguish it from the much commoner strawberry mark. In the early stage it can be simply obliterated by the application of surface diathermy.

Management of Cavernous Angiomas. Expectancy is usual. The principal active treatments which have been employed are X-ray therapy, radon seeds, injections of sclerosants including saturated saline solution and boiling water, carbon dioxide snow, diathermy needle and surgical excision.

All forms of radiation have their hazards. Despite what is said by enthusiasts damage to normal growing tissue sometimes occurs and the scar may become more noticeable later, as the patient grows around the irradiated tissue. The result may at first appear perfect but later growth of the part may fail to occur (e.g. a case in which an angioma of the chest was treated with apparently perfect cure until puberty. The breast on the affected side failed to develop).

In the rapidly growing cavernous angioma with or without an overlying capillary element the treatment of choice is the *injection of a saturated solution of saline* into the lesion. The solution is injected a minim at a time throughout the lesion and is never injected so close to the skin as to cause complete blanching of the surface capillary portion, or into the normal skin. If this precaution is neglected necrosis may occur and scarring follow. A small lesion may only need ½ ml., but as much as 10 or even 20 ml. may be required to fill and make tense a large angioma. A series of injections at monthly intervals may be required. The injection is always followed by a reactionary swelling before the shrinkage begins and the effect cannot be judged under 3 weeks. The parents should always be forewarned that the phase of swelling is expected.

Surgical excision is reserved for lesions in important positions (e.g. the eyelid, when the swelling is causing the baby to squint); very exposed positions where they may be subject to trauma; for lesions in which hæmorrhage has occurred without subsequent regression, and for cases in which the parents flatly refuse conservative treatment. Cosmetic surgical excision of redundant tissue is sometimes required after spontaneous or treatment induced healing.

On the trunk and limbs in particular an angioma may be combined with a lipomatous element. If this is so then treatment other than excision is irrational.

Hæmangiomatous Varicosities

This is a deep cavernous lesion which may only be demonstrable with the limb dependent. It usually affects the lower limbs or buttocks. There is a port-wine stain on the surface and there may be raised capillary elements also. These lesions bleed easily and the bleeding may be severe. The skin may ulcerate and healing be unsatisfactory. Sclerosant injections are of limited value and usually the only treatment of value is staged surgical excision and skin grafting. Hypotensive anæsthesia may be of considerable assistance. Recurrences are frequent and may need treatment in the same way as the original lesion.

Diffuse angiomatosis of a limb may be restricted to the skin and subcutaneous tissues. In some cases the deep tissues are also affected, including the bones. There may be considerable arteriovenous shunts through the lesions and in some there is gigantism of the limb. Amputation may be called for in the worst cases.

BENIGN PIGMENTED MELANOMA ("MOLES")

These are the brown birthmarks and different types are recognizable: *The Intradermal Nævus or Common Mole*. It is flat or slightly raised and the surface may be smooth or papillary, warty or hairy. The nævus cells are mature and it is a stable lesion. It may be removed for cosmetic reasons. They do not become malignant and local excision is adequate. Serial excisions of an extensive lesion are often useful. The end result is a linear scar, cosmetically much preferable to a skin graft. On the face large advancement flaps from the neck and even pedicle flaps may be justified to remove an ugly dark brown stain, especially if it has a profuse growth of hair.

The Junctional Nævus. The nævus cells are in the basal layer of the epidermis at its junction with the dermis. It is light or dark brown and occurs on the palm of the hand, the sole of the foot and on the external genitalia. It may "mature" to the intradermal type, but it may undergo malignant change in adult life. It is quiescent before puberty and local excision is advisable.

The Compound Nævus. This is clinically indistinguishable from the intradermal variety. It consists of intradermal and junctional elements and 98 per cent of children's moles are of this type. Because of the danger in the junctional area excision is advisable when practicable.

The Juvenile Melanoma. This looks like the other pigmented moles but is usually small and occurs on the face, trunk or limbs. Its rapid growth leads to a histological picture with many which may arouse suspicion of malignancy. However, their course is benign and local excision is adequate. True malignant melanoma is exceedingly rare in children.

The Blue Nævus. This is a dark blue black, smooth, hairless lesion. It is entirely intradermal and heavily pigmented.

"Mongolian Spot". This is a flat blue black lesion over the sacral area seen in babies of the Mongolian races and sometimes in others. It is of no importance.

REFERENCES

Cade, S. (1961) Malignant melanoma, *Ann. roy. Coll. Surg. Engl.*, **28,** 331.
Simpson, J. R. (1959) Natural history of cavernous hæmangiomata. *Lancet, ii,* 1057.
N.B. This paper refers to the lesions usually called "strawberry marks" or capillary cavernous angiomas.

CHAPTER 13

HARE LIP AND CLEFT PALATE

CLEFTS of the lip and palate may occur together or separately. In about half the lip and palate are involved. In a quarter the lip alone is cleft and in a quarter the palate alone is affected. Most probably result from failure of the mesenchyme to penetrate the junctions between the primary processes which fuse to form the nose, lip and palate. In the absence of such penetration the gaps between these processes reappear in part or throughout. It is thus possible to have incomplete or complete clefts of the lip or palate. Fusion seems to occur earliest at a point just behind the alveolus so that the clefts begin at the vermilion of the lip and the uvula respectively and extend a varying distance towards this postalveolar point. It is also possible to have clefts on either or both sides of the midline. The photographs (Fig. 26) show cases of unilateral and bilateral hare lip with cleft palate. They illustrate the fact that the entire skeleton of the middle third of the face is distorted. Good repair of a hare lip requires attention to the twisted nose, which is a more difficult problem than the closure of the lip. The twist is due to the congenital division of the orbicularis oris allowing growth free from the moulding influence of the oral sphincter. Repair of this muscle brings the nasal tip near the midline and the alveoli into juxtaposition within a few weeks. Secondary distortion of the cartilages of the nose and of the pyriform fossa may necessitate secondary operations. Postalveolar cleft of the palate alone is probably due to simple failure of fusion of the embryonic secondary palate.

Inheritance. These disorders occur in about 1 per 800 births. There is a strong genetic factor in the tendency to develop hare lip with or without a cleft palate. Isolated clefts of the palate form a separate though heterogeneous group, in some of which a genetic factor is important whilst others appear to be due to different factors. If one child in a family has hare lip the chance of a subsequent sibling being involved is about 1 : 20. The degree of the defect as manifest in the individual may be anything from a complete bilateral hare lip and cleft palate down to a mere notch on the red margin of the lip. If one child of the family has a cleft palate the chance of a subsequent sibling having the defect is about 1 : 50. But there is no increase in the risk for hare lip. If one parent is affected the risks rise to 1 : 7 and 1 : 5 respectively. This kind of information is valuable in counselling the parents. It is not the doctor's place to tell them whether they should attempt to have further children. But he should be able to tell them the risks entailed and perhaps advise further if he is asked to do so.

The Disability

The hare lip is a severe cosmetic blemish. It does not interfere with sucking unless it is so gross that the baby cannot make an airtight seal between the lips and breast or teat. Sucking is performed by the muscles of cheeks and tongue together with the palate, and not with the lips.

Cleft palate will usually prevent sucking for the cleft prevents oronasal closure. This inefficiency of the sphincter is the serious result of the cleft. Later it will prevent normal speech. Nasal escape of air causes honking. There is an articulatory inability to make plosive consonants and other sounds which need a raised pressure in the oral cavity or contact of tongue with hard palate for their performance, and there is an increased nasal resonance and nasal escape of air.

Inability to create pressure and clear the nose by sneezing and the free communication from the mouth makes the child prone to respiratory infections and otitis media.

Some cases of isolated cleft of the palate are associated with a very small lower jaw and hence a tendency to tongue swallowing (Pierre Robin syndrome). This puts them in danger of asphyxial death during the first months of life. The baby should never be allowed to lie on his back but always on his side so that the tongue tends to drop forward. The difficulty in respiration makes feeding difficult and it may be necessary to resort to nasal intragastric tube feeding for a while before the mother can be taught to manage the baby. A few severe cases may need a tracheostomy to save life. After some months the parts are big enough to allow normal respiration and feeding. The jaw also tends to grow relative to the baby as a whole so that these babies usually finish up as quite attractive small-featured children.

As they grow up a proportion of the children who have had clefts involving the alveolar arch develop a flat middle third of the face—dish face—due to undergrowth of the maxillæ and a protruding lower jaw and lip. This is in part the result of hypoplasia of the bones, but mainly due to the constricting effect of the scars resulting from repair of the hard palate.

Management

The objects of surgery as often stated are that the child shall look well, feed well and speak well. The infant should be seen during the first month of life by the surgeon who is to look after him. There is much individual variation in the timing of operations and the parents should have the opportunity of discussing the problem at an early age. If the baby has a complete cleft they must be told that two or three operations will be staged over the first 2 years but that further lesser procedures may be necessary in later years. The details need not be discussed at the first visit but the broad plan is outlined.

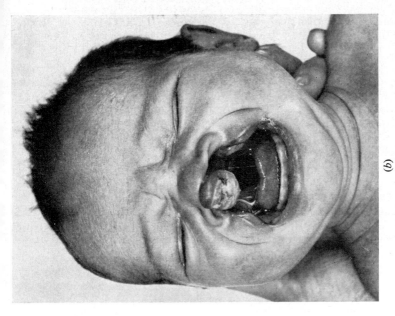

(a)

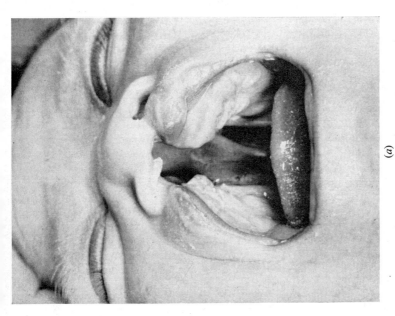

(b)

FIG. 28 *(a)* Unilateral cleft lip and palate. The nasal, labial, alveolar and palatal malformations are shown. *(b)* Bilateral cleft lip and palate. The protrusion of the premaxilla and consequent lack of columella can be seen.

The baby should be kept away from contact with respiratory infections. The mother may need encouragement to take him out in the fresh air for there is a natural tendency to hide the baby from the neighbours until the lip is repaired.

Feeding. The baby will not be able to feed from the breast if there is more than a mild cleft of the palate. A bottle with a big teat with a large hole in it so that the feed is poured into the baby rather than sucked out of the bottle is often quite satisfactory. Spoon feeding is advisable if this fails, and has the advantage that the baby is accustomed to the method he will need after the operations.

The special teats with a flange to block the cleft are unsatisfactory. They may cause ulcers by rubbing the borders of the cleft and nasal septum. They are also more difficult to keep really clean and thrush infestation may follow. Anæmia is not uncommon and many infants require an iron-containing supplement.

SURGERY. When the baby is gaining weight well and is 2 to 3 months old the lip should be repaired. The most important parts of this operation are the junction of the two halves of the orbicularis muscle and repair of the nostril floor. The nasal cartilages are mobilized so that they can re-set themselves as the septum is drawn towards the midline. A straight cut across the lip gives a reliably adequate appearance. Various flap procedures give an improved outward pout of the lip in severe cases. "Dental orthopædic" measures have been introduced to align the alveoli of severe clefts in early infancy before operation by the use of corrective sucking plates. They make surgery simpler and should improve long term facial development. Alveolar bone grafting at the time of lip closure is sometimes used to stabilize the improved position. These measures are by no means universal practice but do hold promise for the future.

The repair of the palate is usually performed at about 12 to 18 months of age. This time is a compromise between an earlier operation to achieve good soft palate development and a later procedure to minimize interference with maxillary growth. By repairing it before the child learns to speak he will usually be able to develop speech in the natural manner by learning from his parents. The operation is not done earlier because the smaller structures make the procedure more awkward. The important part of the operation is the repair of the levator sling in the soft palate. This enables the palate to be drawn up and back against the nasopharyngeal wall for the closure essential to speech. Various flaps are used to free the mucoperiosteum of the hard palate and close the gap. Length of the palate *per se* is less important than efficiency of the oronasal sphincter and this is achieved by free mobilization in the lateral spaces between the pharyngeal and cheek muscles and liberation of the tensores palati from their pulleys, the pterygoid hamuli.

Spoon feeding may begin a few hours after each operation and each feed should finish with a drink of clear water as a "mouth wash". Splinting of the elbows is almost the only restraint required.

Speech Therapy. If the child is still speaking poorly after a period at school, speech therapy may help him to acquire correct use of the mechanism. Speech therapy improves articulation in most cases even where the nasality persists. If there is persistent nasal escape a secondary pharyngoplasty operation may help. Persistent nasality may be due to nasal escape or a habit of speech as heard in some Americans. Three-quarters of children with cleft palate should learn to speak well with the primary operation and parental instruction alone.

Deafness. When the child persists in poor articulation, the possibility of deafness as an underlying cause must be borne in mind and audiometry may be required to reveal a high tone deafness preventing the child from recognizing what is required. Probably 10 per cent have severe impairment and 30 per cent have some disability. Middle ear infection is the usual cause, but quite a number have a congenital hearing defect.

Tonsillectomy and adenoidectomy. These operations should be advised with some caution in children with cleft palate. The scarring from a tonsillectomy can further reduce palatal movement, while the removal of large adenoids may cause the speech to deteriorate by removing the pad which the short palate touched to close off the oropharynx. The inevitable atrophy of the adenoids in adolescence does not produce the same deterioration.

Orthodontic treatment is required by many of the grosser cases. It is usually delayed until about 8 years of age, when many of the permanent teeth are through.

Soft tissue secondary corrections of the nose and lip may be needed at 4 years of age before going to school. Apart from the cosmetic aspect they may be required to improve the nasal airway. A few may need more elaborate rhinoplasty with division of the nasal bones at adolescence.

Gross failure of growth of the maxillæ may justify rapid expansion by cap splints with bone grafting to retain the gains, or maxillary osteotomies.

CONTINUING AFTERCARE. It will be clear that the surgeon must be prepared to keep in touch with a patient treated for hare lip and cleft palate throughout the patient's childhood. He must work in conjunction with the orthodontist, the dental surgeon, the speech therapist, pædiatrician and schoolteachers so that all aspects of the child's care can be dealt with at the correct time. In this way it is expected that the need to call on the Child Guidance Department will be rare.

The term "teamwork" is much abused today. It must be remembered that every team needs a captain and the parents must know that one person has a continuous interest in their child's progress. It is not enough to be bandied from expert to expert as problems arise to worry the parents. The general practitioner can help a lot, but inevitably lacks the experience necessary to know when to reassure and when to call further aid.

REFERENCES

Holdsworth, W. G. (1963) *Cleft Lip and Palate*, 3rd Edition, Wm. Heinemann, London.
"Treatment of the Cleft Palate: Scientific Symposium," (1959) *Ann. roy. Coll. Surg. Engl.*, **25**, 225.

CHAPTER 14

SURGICAL ASPECTS OF JAUNDICE

OBSTRUCTIVE JAUNDICE IN THE NEWBORN

ONLY a few of the conditions causing jaundice in the newborn require surgery. The majority have a "physiological" jaundice lasting only a few days. Hæmolytic jaundice (usually due to rhesus factor incompatibi)ulyitcan be readily confirmed or excluded on clinical or serological grounds.

In practice there are two uncommon causes of persistent obstructive jaundice which it is important to differentiate. These are *neonatal hepatitis* and *atresia of the bile ducts*.

The rarer causes of jaundice at this age include mucoviscidosis, pericholangitis, cytomegalic inclusion disease, syphilis, congenital spherocytosis, galactosæmia and toxoplasmosis.

Atresia of the Bile Ducts

This condition should be suspected in an infant who develops jaundice of the obstructive type *after* the first day of life and remains jaundiced for a month or more. The urine is dark with bile, the stools are clay coloured from its absence and the serum bilirubin is largely conjugated. However, *neonatal hepatitis* or *giant cell hepatitis,* although it causes hepatocellular jaundice, *cannot in its severe form be distinguished from extrahepatic obstruction either clinically, by all present liver function tests, or even with certainty by punch liver biopsy.* Presumably this is because the canaliculi are blocked by bile thrombi. The jaundice may fluctuate in either condition and some bile may enter the stools even in complete atresia. The frequency of the two conditions is ab ot the same.

Because of the diagnostic difficulties, wide surgical exploration to assess the condition of the bile ducts was used in the past. This approach carried a real mortality and morbidity. Though the majority of patients suffering from hepatitis have a poor prognosis, many might have recovered without treatment and, even when atresia was found, only a minority were amenable to surgical correction. Hence a resistance developed to any form of surgery and, by the time exploration was accepted as a last resort at 3 or 4 months of age, the liver was already cirrhotic and the outlook very poor even when repair was possible.

OPERATIVE CHOLANGIOGRAM. A safe limited type of surgery has now been evolved. By using it as early as the fourth week of life it is possible to save the repairable atresias without significant risk to the infants with hepatitis. Using one of the anæsthetics which do not damage the liver a small right subcostal incision is made. The gall-bladder is sought out. If it is present a small tube is inserted, the duct syringed with saline, diodone injected and a *cholangiogram* made during the injection. If the dye is seen to flow into the duodenum and back up the hepatic ducts the diagnosis is intrahepatic obstruction, usually due to hepatitis, though occasionally due to other causes such as pericholangitis. The injection has done no harm and indeed may hasten the clearance of jaundice if there was inspissation of bile in the ducts.

If it demonstrates a dilated duct system with an obstruction above the duodenum there is an atresia amenable to surgical correction by anastomosis to the alimentary tract. The best method is anastomosis to a Roux loop of jejunum. The lower end of the common bile duct may be grossly dilated. This so-called *choledochus cyst*, with its diagnostic triad of mass in the right hypochondrium, pain and obstructive jaundice is treated similarly. If the dye flows into the duodenum but not back into the liver, then atresia of the proximal extrahepatic ducts is suspected. No gall-bladder may be found—or it may be represented by a fibrous cord. This is suggestive of a widespread atresia. A gall-bladder filled with clear or pale yellow fluid means nothing, since all the secretions of the body may be stained yellow. Functional continuity is indicated by deep *green* bile.

In all cases a generous liver biopsy is performed. If no dilated obstructed duct or cyst has been demonstrated the abdomen is closed. The biopsy will make the diagnosis. If it confirms atresia then a full laparatomy can be carried out later. For the prognosis is hopeless without treatment, and it is then justifiable to explore the porta hepatis thoroughly in the knowledge that one is not endangering a baby who may only have a hepatitis with collapsed and tiny unrecognizable ducts. The dilated proximal duct may be found buried in the porta hepatis.

RESULTS. Biliary atresia is a rare condition occurring in perhaps 1 in 10,000 live births. Of these perhaps one in ten will have a gall-bladder or bile duct suitable for anastomosis. The surgical dividend is small and few people will have more than a handful of successes in a lifetime, but this method is the only one which can save this small proportion.

Untreated or untreatable cases of atresia usually live 9 or even 12 months and are deceptively well looking for a long time. In the rare intrahepatic atresia the child may live several years. This phenomenon is not explainable. Another mystery of the atresias is that the onset of jaundice may be delayed for some weeks. Recently there have been reports of biopsy showing intrahepatic ducts and later biopsy showing their disappearance. Perhaps there is such an entity as acquired atresia of the bile ducts. Much remains to be learned about these conditions.

The customary terminology is confusing. 'Extrahepatic' atresia involves the ducts outside the liver but usually also involves those within the liver back to the intralobular ducts, which are proliferated. 'Intrahepatic' atresia involves the intralobular ducts but the other ducts within and outside the liver are present.

HEREDITARY SPHEROCYTOSIS (ACHOLURIC JAUNDICE)

Jaundice is the usual presenting symptom of hereditary spherocytosis, although the hæmolytic anæmia may overshadow it. Being a hæmolytic jaundice the unconjugated bile does not enter the urine (hence "acholuric") and the stools remain coloured by bile; this is in clinical contradistinction to obstructive causes. The spleen is the important site of hæmolysis and splenectomy produces 100 per cent clinical cure although the abnormal biconvex shape of the red cells, and therefore their fragility, persists. It is now realized that splenectomy, particularly in infancy, may reduce the resistance to infection in some way and, since the operation is rarely urgent, it is best postponed until the age of two years. It is the one blood dyscrasia in which splenectomy is consistently effective.

Hereditary spherocytosis is the commonest cause of gall-stones in childhood. The stones are pigment stones resulting from the increased excretion of bilirubin. Two points follow from this. The gall-bladder should always be palpated during the splenectomy. If stones are present they are treated on their merits. Cholecystectomy is not always necessary and simple removal of the stones may suffice since the causative factor is being corrected. The second point is that children presenting with cholecystitis and gallstones should have a red cell fragility curve performed to investigate this possible underlying cause.

Acute cholecystitis is distinctly uncommon under the age of 16 and is usually misdiagnosed as high appendicitis. The pain in infective hepatitis can be severe and it would appear that many cases of alleged cholecystitis were really hepatitis.

REFERENCES

Clatworthy, H. W. and McDonald, V. G. (1956) The diagnostic laparotomy in obstructive jaundice in infants, *Surg. Clin. N. Amer.*, (December) 1545–1554.
Dacie, J. V. (1960) *The Hæmolytic Anæmias: Congenital and Acquired* (2nd. Edition), J. & G. Churchill, London.
Danks, D. M. (1965) Prolonged Neonatal Obstructive Jaundice: A Survey of Modern Concepts. *Clin. Pediatrics*, 4. 9. 499 (Sept.).

CHAPTER 15

THE SPLEEN

IN *thrombocytopenic purpura* splenectomy is a last resort. But it still has an important part in treatment. Spontaneous hæmorrhages usually begin when platelets go below 100,000 per c. ml. Most cases settle on blood transfusions with cortisone during crises. There may be further episodes which usually respond similarly. Those cases which follow an acute infection are probably particularly likely to settle. If the disease persists for over 6 months it may be labelled idiopathic rather than symptomatic, and splenectomy should be considered. The result of the operation is variable, but usually it is dramatic. The thrombocyte count rises within hours and the bruising and bleeding tendency ceases before the operation is over. The platelets should be counted 7 days after operation because there may be a marked overswing. If the level reaches over a million there is some danger of venous thrombosis and anticoagulant treatment may be needed until the count settles. Unfortunately there does not yet seem to be any clinical or hæmatological criterion which will surely pick out the cases which will respond to splenectomy. The spleen is not usually enlarged in idiopathic thrombocytopenic purpura.

The spleen is enlarged in a wide variety of conditions, but in only a few of these is splenectomy definitely beneficial to the patient.

Hereditary spherocytosis has already been dealt with in the chapter on the surgical aspects of jaundice. Its alternative names, including congenital hæmolytic anæmia, remind one that the condition may present clinically as an anæmia, overshadowing the jaundice. The condition responds consistently to splenectomy. If clinical cure is incomplete then the diagnosis is suspect, or the presence of a spleniculus must be considered.

Splenectomy is sometimes justified in *acquired hæmolytic anæmias.* But here the mechanism of the defect is different, and the results are variable. In acquired hæmolytic anæmia the red cells are normal. They are more readily hæmolysed due to the presence of a toxic substance or antibody on the cells which is demonstrable by the Coombs test. Splenectomy is successful in less than half the cases.

Splenectomy is sometimes helpful in reducing the rate of hæmolysis in various incurable diseases. These include thalassæmia, in which the defect is an abnormal hæmoglobin and aplastic anæmia if uptake of radio-chromium in the spleen from tagged red cells shows much destruction there, and in myelosclerosis.

In all these hæmolytic anæmias splenic enlargement is usually slight.

The operation may also be of value in *hypersplenism*. Varied causes of great enlargement of the spleen may result in overaction of the spleen and reduction of some or all of the cellular elements of the blood. It may also be used to relieve distress due to the sheer size of a very large spleen, e.g. in Gaucher's disease with its abnormal lipoid storage.

PORTAL HYPERTENSION

The spleen is enlarged in all forms of portal hypertension. The two main groups are those due to *extrahepatic* (prehepatic) obstruction of the portal venous system and those due to *intrahepatic* obstruction. The commonest type of extrahepatic obstruction is the so-called caverno-matous transformation of the portal vein, which is usually the end result of portal vein thrombosis rather than a real malformation. It occurs early in childhood and there is often a history suggestive of neonatal umbilical sepsis. The intrahepatic type is usually due to cirrhosis. Cirrhosis may occur at any age, but the development of portal hypertension with symptoms is more commonly seen in later child-hood or adult life.

The only clear indication for surgery in either type is severe hæmor-rhage from œsophageal varices. It can do little or nothing for the liver condition in cirrhosis. Porto-systemic venous anastomoses develop at several sites in an attempt at natural decompression of the portal system, e.g. the veins of Retzius between the colonic and the retro-peritoneal veins and between the superior and inferior rectal veins (piles). But the only dangerous site of the anastomoses is the lower œsophagus and upper stomach. Here the veins are unsupported and subject to the action of acid peptic juice, and hæmorrhage may be severe. It is a frequent cause of death in this condition. The hæmorrhage may be sudden and profuse, presenting as hæmatemesis or it may be more insidious presenting as anæmia, melæna being revealed by investigation.

Management. The initial treatment of the hæmorrhage is sedation and blood transfusion. If hæmorrhage persists a balloon catheter should be passed via the nose into the stomach. The balloon is inflated and then the tube is pulled upon so as to draw the balloon firmly up into the cardio-œsophageal junction and shut off the blood flow into the œsophageal varices. The blood can be aspirated from the stomach. This is probably as effective as the special double balloon "Sengs-taken" tube designed also to press on the varices themselves. But the veins sometimes occupy the upper end of the stomach as well and this treatment may be ineffective.

Vasopressin injections frequently stop the bleeding for an hour or more and this gives the veins time to clot. The dose is 1–3 ml. sub-cutaneously divided into three doses given at short intervals.

If these conservative measures fail to arrest the bleeding (which is not common) then urgent surgery may be required. The usual procedure is the transthoracic, trans-œsophageal ligation of the varices as advocated by Crile. This procedure only gives temporary relief but it may be lifesaving.

The definitive treatment of bleeding from œsophageal varices is still under discussion. The mortality from recurrent hæmorrhages is so high that something must be done.

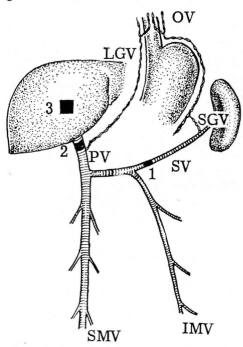

Fig. 29. The portal venous system.

SMV	= superior mesenteric vein.	SGV	= short gastric veins.
IMV	= inferior mesenteric vein.	LGV	= left gastric vein.
SV	= splenic vein.	OV	= œsophageal veins.
PV	= portal vein.		

Sites of obstruction.

Extrahepatic (1) Splenic vein thrombosis causing only splenomegaly and
(Prehepatic)   curable by splenectomy.

(2) Portal vein thrombosis causing hypertension throughout the portal system and hence development of dangerous portal-systemic anastomoses through the œsophageal veins.

Intrahepatic (3) Intrahepatic obstruction (e.g. cirrhosis) causing similar hypertension throughout the portal system.

The most popular operations are those to shunt portal blood into the systemic veins and hence reduce the hypertension. The two accepted procedures are splenectomy with anastomosis of the splenic vein to

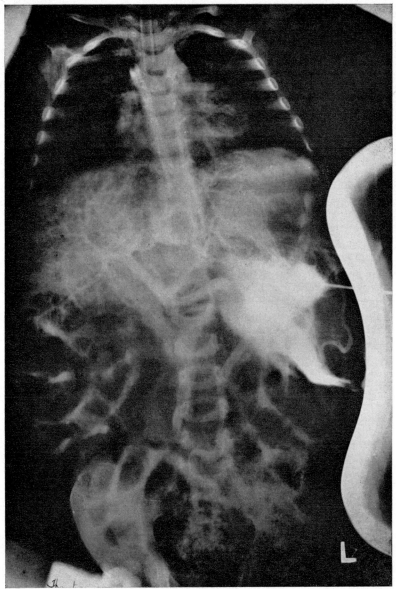

FIG. 30. Splenic portogram showing œsophageal varices and large azygos vein in a case of intrahepatic obstruction.

the side of the renal vein, and anastomosis of the divided portal vein to the side of the inferior vena cava. The risk of thrombosis in a shunt is dependent on the size of the opening (as well as the rate of flow through it). Thus the spleno-renal shunt is less valuable in young children and is unlikely to remain patent in patients under ten years of age. The portal vein is adequate in size in most cases caused by intra-hepatic obstruction. But these are mostly the cirrhotics in the more severe of which by-passing of the liver may lead to "ammonia intoxication" with confusion, flapping tremor and coma or even death from liver failure. When liver function is well preserved it is an effective operation.

The results of the various porto-systemic disconnection or transection operations have been disappointing in the long run, even where transection has been accompanied by extensive devascularization of the œsophago-gastric region. Simple transection of the œsophagus with reanastomosis is as satisfactory as more elaborate procedures as a temporizing procedure, although it can do nothing to prevent bleeding from gastric varices. It may allow the child to grow old enough for a splenorenal shunt to become practicable. Recent experience suggests that a central splenorenal shunt or inferior mesenteric-caval shunt may be applicable to younger children. Œsophagogastrectomy with inter-position of an isolated loop of colon is probably the best available procedure if a major shunt cannot be performed. Splenectomy alone is to be condemned because it destroys the splenic vein, which might be used in a subsequent shunt.

REFERENCES

Lynn, H. B. (1964) Surgical treatment of esophageal varices in children, *Surg. Clin. N. Amer.*, Vol. 44, No. 6 (December).

Shaldon, S. and Sherlock, S. (1962) Obstruction to the extrahepatic portal system in childhood, *Lancet, i*, 63.

Clatworthy, H. W., Jr. and Lorimier, A. A. (1964) Portal decompression procedures in children, *Amer. J. Surg.*, **107**, 447.

CHAPTER 16

SCROTAL SWELLINGS

SCROTAL swellings are common in infancy, and correct diagnosis is important to decide the relative urgency of the conditions. There are four key questions in the taking of the history.

1. How long has it been present?
2. Does it vary in size?
3. Does it sometimes go away?
4. Does it hurt him?

The answers to these questions will often give a diagnosis before the pants are removed. For example, a hernia is often present from early infancy, gets steadily larger as time goes on, but varies in size. It may temporarily disappear, this usually being noticed in the morning after a nights recumbency. If it seems tender or if the baby cries with it then one knows it has been incarcerated and that prompt treatment is needed to avert recurrence of this serious complication.

HERNIA

A complete hernia is the type which reaches the scrotum. The processus vaginalis has never closed, and the sac reaches right down to the testis, the body of which projects into it. The swelling is intermittent, disappears at night, and often on lying down. On examination it is a soft swelling which arises in the inguinal region and extends down into the scrotum. It gives an expansile impulse on coughing and is almost always completely and rapidly reducible. It is not tender or painful. Trusses are of little use and operation should be performed as early as is convenient after diagnosis—providing the baby is mature and otherwise well.

Hernia is discussed further in Chapter 17.

HYDROCELE

A hydrocele is an excess of fluid within the tunica vaginalis. Hydroceles are the commonest scrotal swellings of infants and children. The crucial finding is that *one can get above the swelling*. It is a scrotal swelling and above it the spermatic cord can be clearly identified. (The swelling of a congenital hernia, however, extends up the cord to the ring, i.e. it is inguino-scrotal. Even when the hernia is reduced a thickening of the cord can be felt with a characteristic "rustling of silk" feeling as the edges of the empty sac rub against each other.) Hydroceles transilluminate but herniæ in the young may also do so, and the only diagnostic value of the test is to differentiate from the uncommon hæmatocele, or from tumour of the testes (Fig. 29).

There are two types of hydrocele in children. Those which typically appear under the age of a year are different from those in the older patient. In early infancy the common hydrocele is slack and is often bilateral. There is no difficulty in palpating the testis through it. The scrotum is elongated but not tense or distended. The slack hydrocele needs no treatment. It can be expected to disappear within the first year of life. The parents should be confidently told that the condition is painless, that there are no possible complications and that there is nothing to be lost by observation.

Hydroceles which arise after the first year do not often disappear spontaneously. They are typically tense and may also be bilateral. In these a *narrowly patent processus vaginalis* allows peritoneal fluid to drip slowly into the hydrocele sac. The tunica fills up tensely and in doing so it usually seems to kink and obstruct the lumen of the processus in a valvular manner so that the hydrocele cannot be emptied by pressure. This in time may lead to its obliteration, but it usually persists. Tense hydroceles in children beyond infancy usually need surgical treatment because there is evidence that in the long run they are associated with diminished spermatogenesis and the swelling itself may be an embarrassment.

The operation is similar to that of hernia. The patent processus is freed from the cord in the inguinal region and ligatured and divided at the level of the extra-peritoneal fat. It is analogous to the sac of a hernia and is similarly treated. The hydrocele sac is merely opened to evacuate the fluid. There is no need to excise it. Direct operation on the hydrocele sac leaving the processus behind leaves the possibility of a recurrence.

Tapping of hydroceles is never curative. It is a waste of time as a method of treatment, but may on occasion be required to allow examination of the underlying testis.

ENCYSTED HYDROCELE OF THE CORD. Encysted hydrocele of the cord is quite a common swelling. It may be in the scrotum above the testis (when it has given rise to unfounded hopes that the baby has a third testis) or it may lie above the scrotum in the more proximal part of the cord. Again in these hydroceles it is possible to get above the swelling and palpate the upper reaches of the cord, unlike the findings in the presence of a hernia. The swelling transilluminates and is not tender. Treatment is similar to that of hydrocele of the tunica vaginalis.

Hydrocele of the canal of Nück is the analogous condition in the female. The only important differential diagnosis is from an ovary in a hernial sac. Of course the latter would not transilluminate, but this test may be difficult to apply to such a small swelling in a plump baby.

TORSION OF THE TESTIS
TORSION

Anatomically: INTRAVAGINAL
EXTRAVAGINAL (= T. of the CORD)

Clinically: ACUTE
SUBACUTE
RECURRENT
T. in Miniature (= T. of the *hydatid of Morgagni*)

Torsion of the testis is not rare. A number of cases with a less dramatic onset are missed and misdiagnosed as epididymo-orchitis, especially in infancy.

There are two types of torsion: the more common *intravaginal* type in which the testis twists on a long mesorchium suspending it from the epididymus, and the *extravaginal* type also called torsion of the spermatic cord, which is the type occurring in infancy.

Torsion occurs without warning, and may be discovered on the routine examination of a pyrexial, crying, vomiting infant. An older child will complain of severe pain and acute local tenderness. The pain is classically described as being so severe that the patient will always vomit. *But there are lesser degrees of torsion in which the onset is less dramatic.* It is in these that delay may seal the fate of a testis which had some hope of recovery.

On examination there is a red, brawny, tender swelling of half of the scrotum and œdema occurs rapidly. If the torsion is of the cord, the shortening draws the testis into the upper scrotum or to the inguinal region. It may thus be mistaken for a strangulated hernia. Intravaginal torsion presents with a swelling still occupying the lower scrotum but with the outline of the testis masked by the secondary hydrocele around it. It may be mistaken for an acute epididymo-orchitis.

Delay in treatment means subsequent atrophy of the testis—the fate of the vast majority of torsions. In the classical case with a dramatic onset the organ is probably destroyed before the child is seen. But in the less severe ones prompt operation gives some hope of survival of the organ. It is therefore imperative that every case in which the diagnosis is entertained should have a prompt exploration. No harm will come if the case turns out to have been inflammatory in origin— indeed by splitting the tunics the pain will be greatly relieved as tension is reduced.

An oft-described distinction between torsion of the testis and acute epididymo-orchitis is the relief of pain on elevation of the organ in the latter condition. We have not found this to be of much value in practice. Unless there is some clear predisposing cause, such as a chronic urinary obstruction or infection, epididymo-orchitis is very unlikely and it is unwise to delay exploration. In chronic epididymo-orchitis however, the outline of the craggy epididymus may be clearly palpable.

The operation consists of exploration of the cord and testis from an inguinal incision. The torsion is unwound and the tunica albuginea split to allow expansion of the congested contents and minimise pressure atrophy. The testis is then sutured to the scrotal lining to avoid recurrence. Exploration may reveal torsion of the pedunculated hydatid of Morgagni. The clinical signs and symptoms have been aptly described as those of "torsion in miniature".

It is important that the congenital variation which predisposes to torsion is often bilateral. The other testis should therefore be fixed as a prophylactic measure, either at the same time or later, depending on the circumstances. Torsion of the cord may occur in an incompletely descended testis. In this case fixation of the opposite testis may need to be done in association with some form of orchidopexy, and this is better left for another occasion.

EPIDIDYMO-ORCHITIS AND EPIDIDYMITIS

It may occur in boys of all ages. By far the commonest variety is that called *non-specific*. No organism can usually be isolated. The cause may be a virus. Reflux of urine through the seminal vesicles and vas deferens causing an irritative inflammation has also been suggested as a cause.

The findings on examination are a swelling which is tender and mainly involves the epididymis. The body of the testis is also somewhat enlarged and may be hidden by a secondary hydrocele. It seems likely that many cases diagnosed as non-specific epididymo-orchitis are really missed subacute torsions.

Tuberculosis of the epididymus is now rare. The swelling is craggy, hard and becomes attached to the overlying scrotum in the later stages. A sinus will develop if treatment is not instituted in time. Calcification may occur. The lesion is always secondary to a tuberculous focus elsewhere.

Mumps orchitis is usually easy to diagnose because the acute painful swelling of the bodies of the testes occurs during the course of the fever with its typical salivary gland swellings. Occasionally the mumps virus may produce testicular inflammation in the absence of parotid involvement, and the swelling may be unilateral. The diagnosis may then easily be missed. The presence of other cases of mumps in the family, or the presence of an epidemic may give a clue.

There is a great hazard of sterility following mumps orchitis. Cortisone has not been shown to be of value. The testes should be explored and the opportunity taken to split the tough tunica albuginea and allow the œdematous contents to expand. This will reduce the risk of atrophy from pressure necrosis though not from any direct effect of the mumps virus. It relieves the pain.

Acute suppurative epididymitis may occur in association with obstruction or infection of the lower urinary tract.

Acute suppurative orchitis. This hæmatogenous, usually staphylococcal infection of the testis may occur in early infancy and may progress to abscess formation requiring incision and drainage.

HÆMATOCELE

Hæmatocele is a collection of blood in the tunica vaginalis. It is usually due to direct trauma. It may occur in the course of a bleeding dyscrasia, such as leukæmia. It should be left alone and it will absorb.

IDIOPATHIC SCROTAL ŒDEMA

Idiopathic scrotal œdema is not rare. It is a puzzling lesion if one has not seen it before. One half of the scrotum swells up rapidly and has an alarming appearance. It develops within an hour or two and may subside almost as rapidly. It is not usually associated with any deeper lesion. There is no known cause but it often recurs. Support of the scrotum is all that is required.

Rapid development of scrotal œdema may also arise as a manifestation of *angioneurotic œdema*. There are likely to be urticarial lesions elsewhere and it should respond to the injection of adrenaline. An uncommon cause of scrotal œdema is *extravasation of urine*—which occasionally occurs in apparently healthy children for no obvious reason. These lesions are not acutely painful as are the typical torsions and acute infections.

TUMOURS OF THE TESTIS

Tumours of the testis are rare in childhood. *Teratomas, seminomas* or *interstitial cell tumours* may occur. The latter may secrete androgens causing the infant hercules type of premature development.

Teratomas may be simple or malignant; seminomas are always malignant, and interstitial cell tumours may be either.

Treatment is by orchidectomy with excision of the spermatic cord. Subsequent deep X-ray therapy is given if the histology confirms the malignant nature of the neoplasm.

REFERENCES

Angell, G. C. (1963) Torsion of the testicle: a plea for diagnosis, *Lancet, i,* 19.
Hanstead, B., John, H. T. (1964) "Idiopathic scrotal œdema of children". *Brit. J. Urol.,* **36,** 110.
Ross, J. G. (1964) Treatment of primary hydroceles in infancy and childhood, *Brit. J. Surg.,* **49,** 415.

CHAPTER 17

HERNIÆ

THERE are four types to be considered. The inguinal hernia is common and important. The umbilical is common but not important. Diaphragmatic herniæ are less common but important, and the femoral hernia is rare in childhood.

INGUINAL HERNIA

Inguinal hernia is the commonest cause of elective admission to the surgical wards of a children's hospital. About 1 in every 50 boys gets an inguinal hernia, and about 1 in every 500 girls is so affected.

The hernia is practically always an indirect one and is due to the presence of a congenital sac. The pathology is that the processus vaginalis testis fails to obliterate and the abdominal contents are allowed to enter the groin and may reach the scrotum. The failure may be complete in which case the sac extends to the base of the scrotum and in the male contains the testis. More commonly the sac is incomplete and the contents are allowed down for a limited distance which increases as the contents expand the sac.

The clinical onset may be at any time from the day of birth whenever some strain causes abdominal content to enter the sac. But first sight of the hernia is particularly frequent at two periods. They are often first seen at about the age of 2 months, and again there appears to be a peak incidence at about 1 year when the infant begins to walk. The first thing that is noticed is an intermittent painless, non-tender swelling in the groin. The lump is usually best seen at the end of the day, but is often gone in the morning. Though there is no pain there may be a sense of discomfort which even a small infant may manifest, while the older child will be "pulling at himself", or perhaps limping. The hernia tends to get bigger the longer it has been present.

The usual contents are small bowel. The omentum is not usually long enough to reach the sac and the large bowel rarely has the mobility. In girls an ovary and Fallopian tube may frequently be found there.

DIFFERENTIAL DIAGNOSIS. The condition is sometimes mistaken for a *hydrocele*, but can be distinguished because one can palpate the cord above a hydrocele, whilst one cannot get above the swelling of a hernia; it reaches to and through the external ring. A hernia can be reduced by pressure and the swelling usually goes with a typical gurgle due to the air in the contained bowel, which makes the diagnosis incontrovertible. Transillumination is not of value in differential diagnosis as both

114

herniæ and hydroceles transilluminate brilliantly in infancy. A few hydroceles may have persistent communication with the abdominal cavity which is wide enough to allow reduction of the swelling by pressure, but it will not gurgle, and the differentiation is a somewhat academic one, for such a communicating hydrocele will need similar treatment by removal of the sac. For this reason Denis Browne calls them fluid herniæ. The usual hydrocele, although it may have a small communication allowing it to get smaller or disappear during the night's rest, does not have a free enough communication to allow of prompt emptying on examination.

Other conditions which may be mistaken for a hernia, simple or incarcerated, are a *retractile* or an *undescended testis*; *torsion of the spermatic cord*, or *torsion of the testis*.

A retractile testis is one that is pulled up into the superficial inguinal pouch at times but can be manipulated into the scrotum. An inguinal

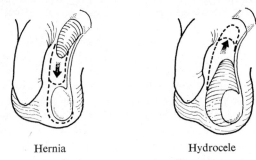

Hernia	Hydrocele

FIG. 31. The inguinal hernia is an inguinal swelling extending towards or into the scrotum. The hydrocele is a scrotal swelling which may extend up towards the groin but one can get above it on palpation.

swelling may be noticed whilst it is up in the pouch. The cord will be of normal thickness and texture. No treatment is required beyond categorical reassurance.

An undescended testis is one which cannot be manipulated into the scrotum. A concomitant hernial sac is usual and it may be difficult at times to know whether the lump described by the parents is merely the testis in the groin or whether there is also an intermittent hernial swelling. Repeated examination may be necessary. The point is of some importance, because if there is a hernia present it will be necessary to operate on it and then it will be necessary to bring down the testis at the same time or it will become adherent to the operation site. In the absence of a clinical hernia, operation for undescended testis is often delayed until about 9 years of age.

Torsion of the cord or of the testis may occur in a normally or incompletely descended testis. The diagnosis is an urgent one, because only prompt surgery to relieve the strangulation can give the testis any chance of survival. The swelling is usually of sudden onset; it is painful and tender and its size does not fluctuate. Later the overlying skin becomes œdematous.

COMPLICATIONS. The *dangerous complication* of inguinal hernia, which makes the condition so important, is *incarceration or strangulation*. The hernia becomes jammed and a vicious circle of vascular obstruction and œdema is set up in the contents. There is intestinal obstruction owing to the nipping at the neck. It will progress until the blood supply of the bowel is also impeded when the condition becomes a strangulation and even more urgent as gangrene will follow unless it is treated. The differentiation of incarceration and strangulation is an academic matter. The only safe rule of management is to treat every irreducible hernia of childhood as an emergency.

Strangulation is most common during the first year of life and its onset may be the first sign of the hernia's presence. Long term follow up has shown a 10 per cent incidence of partial or complete testicular atrophy due to nipping of the spermatic vessels at the external inguinal ring.

Strangulation can always (or almost always) *be reduced by continuous steady pressure* ("*taxis*") *with the baby well sedated*. The foot of the cot is raised and the patient sedated by morphine $\frac{1}{40}$ mg. per pound body weight, or an adequate dose of paraldehyde or chloral. After half an hour taxis is attempted. The fingers of the left hand are cupped around the neck of the sac, pushing it down towards the neck of the scrotum. The fingers of the right hand are then cupped around the fundus of the hernia and firm sustained pressure applied. Slowly the bowel content will begin to go back and then more easily the bowel itself will reduce with a gurgle. It is useless as well as dangerous to use great force in an attempt to overcome the baby's resistance. This will only make the baby continue to cry and strain and lock his inguinal shutter the harder. If constant pressure is maintained the baby will relax after a few minutes and it is then that reduction will begin. Denis Browne prefers repeated gentle pressures to a sustained one. But the fundamental of safe taxis is *persistence* in its *gentle* application, taking up to a quarter of an hour if necessary. If it is unsuccessful the sedated baby may be left to sleep with the foot of the cot raised for two hours when the hernia may slip back or a further attempt may be successful.

With this procedure it will rarely be necessary to operate on the hernia as an urgency. The baby can then be left for a few days before the hernia is operated. The œdema of the sac will settle and there will be less risk of the ligature cutting through the neck of the sac.

In girls an ovary may be strangulated or undergo torsion in the sac. This will be irreducible by the gentle taxis described and will be discovered at the operation which then becomes urgently necessary.

The rare syndrome of testicular feminization is sometimes discovered when operating for an 'ovary' in a 'girl's' hernial sac, so the gonad should be carefully scrutinized.

Treatment of Uncomplicated Inguinal Hernia. It may be said that an inguinal hernia never permanently regresses and that definitive surgery is eventually necessary. The dangers of infant surgery and particularly of anæsthesia have been reduced now to a point where early surgery is advocated. This avoids possible complications, for incarceration is commonest in the first year of life. In practice the patient's name is put on the list for operation at the time of diagnosis. Serious systemic disease is the only contra-indication.

All infant trusses are difficult to apply, troublesome to keep on, dangerous if mis-used and almost impossible to keep clean. The best of them is the rubber horseshoe truss with straps in the crotch. It remains in place better than a "single" truss and is used for unilateral as well as bilateral cases. They should be prescribed in pairs so that one may be constantly in position whilst the other is being washed and dried. The authors never prescribe them except for temporary control of a reduced incarceration, or until some other illness is treated, i.e. an acute bronchitis during which a hernia has incarcerated due to coughing and during which recurrent incarceration may otherwise occur. Clearly, they should never be applied until the hernia is first completely reduced.

THE OPERATION

Under general anæsthesia a transverse incision is made in a suprapubic skin crease over the region of the external ring and deepened to clear the ring. The spermatic cord is elevated and the sac eased out. It is dissected from the other structures of the cord. An opening is then made in the fundus and a probe passed up into the peritoneal cavity to confirm that the structure is in fact the sac and that there is nothing caught in its neck.

A hæmostat is then placed across the sac and this is withdrawn until the ring of properitoneal fat at the neck can be clearly seen. It is essential to see this landmark and be sure that the entire sac is removed or recurrence is likely. The sac is twisted to keep it empty. A transfixion ligature of linen thread is put in at the neck and the sac cut away. When the sac is cut away after ligature of its neck this then slides back through the external ring out of sight as though on a piece of elastic. The inguinal canal of a child is so short that there is no need to open it in order to do a complete herniotomy as would be done in an adult. A complete hernial sac is divided across the middle after dissecting it free. The lower part is left *in situ* after division across the sac and the proximal part treated in the usual way. The subcutaneous tissue is closed with catgut and the skin sutured with conventional sutures or by subcuticular catgut. The latter technique with a collodion seal dressing is a convenient method for the infant.

One or two technical points will make this simple but often delicate operation easier. The sac should always be dissected intact when possible. It is a stout structure as a whole, but if a hole is made in it, it will tear up to the internal ring and beyond with the utmost ease. If an opening is made, either accidentally, or deliberately to divide a complete sac and make a false fundus, forceps should never be applied to the cut edge. A fold of the sac should be picked up proximal to the hole and forceps applied across the fold. They will then hold without tearing.

If the sac is not found towards the front of the cord as soon as the external spermatic fascia is split open it will facilitate matters to draw the testis up and out of the wound. The assistant holds it down towards the scrotum so as to put the cord gently on the stretch, It is then much easier to dissect around the cord to isolate the sac, using two pairs of non-toothed forceps. This avoids waste of time in futile exploration in the wrong direction.

Blunt-pointed forceps and hæmostats should be used. The more delicate looking instruments with finer pointed ends are more likely to tear the sac than those which take a broad grip.

UMBILICAL HERNIA

This is a common enough condition in white children but it is so usual in Africans that it can be regarded as normal. There are two different types with different features and outlooks. The commoner of the two is the true umbilical hernia through the central cicatrix. It is a

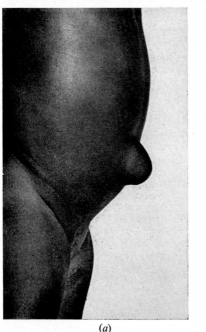 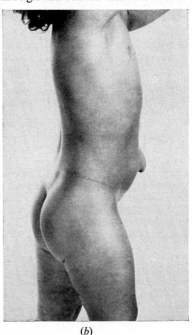

(a)   (b)

Fig. 32. (a) True umbilical hernia
(b) Supra-umbilical hernia

globular bulge and the skin over the umbilicus is pushed straight out. It is readily reducible; the tip of the little finger fits into an opening which is circular and has smooth edges. Some hernias are much bigger and may accommodate two or three fingers when reduced.

The outlook in *true umbilical hernia* is excellent. Strangulation is virtually unknown and spontaneous cure is certain even in the bigger ones. The hernia is painless and does not even cause discomfort, as an inguinal hernia sometimes does. It bulges and goes blue when the child cries, but this is an effect and not a cause of the crying. The mother may need reassurance of this.

The *semi-umbilical or supra-umbilical hernia* is really a defect in the linea alba adjacent to the umbilicus through which omentum or small bowel herniate. Its neck is elliptical and has sharp edges. The swelling points down as the structures push out the skin above the centre of the umbilical cicatrix. It will not heal spontaneously and should be closed at about 4 years of age. It will not cause any trouble during childhood so that operation can be left beyond the toddler period when the child would be more likely to be upset.

The subject is discussed further in the chapter on the umbilicus (Chapter 19).

DIAPHRAGMATIC HERNIA

Congenital herniæ through defects in the diaphragm have been discussed in Chapter 6 as the great majority give trouble in the neonatal period.

Œsophageal Hiatus Hernia

Hiatus hernia, which is herniation of part of the stomach through the œsophageal opening in the diaphragm, is not uncommon and may be a diagnostic problem in early life. Male infants are more often and more severely affected. The principal symptom of the condition is vomiting or regurgitation of feeds. This usually occurs from the first week of life and there is often some blood in the vomitus at first. The infant fails to thrive, weight gain slows down and there is often anæmia due to malnutrition and bleeding. The cause of the trouble is a lax cardia allowing regurgitation of acid pepsin into the œsophagus causing œsophagitis. The inflammation causes erosion which accounts for the hæmorrhage which may accompany the vomiting. If the erosion continues the lower portion of the œsophagus goes into spasm which may after a time become a fibrous stricture in about 5 per cent of cases.

The diagnosis may be made on the history which, it must be emphasized, is almost always from the first weeks or even days of life. The mother may have noticed that propping up the infant relieves the vomiting. However, a barium swallow and meal are needed to show the hiatus hernia itself. It may be difficult to demonstrate, but a small hernia may cause severe œsophagitis. Œsophagoscopy allows direct observation of the degree of œsophagitis.

The vomiting may be projectile and then differentiation from hypertrophic pyloric stenosis is needed. Other cases may need care to differentiate them from feeding problems.

TREATMENT

The treatment of hiatus hernia is primarily medical and the outlook is basically good. Symptoms subside in the first year or two of life in the majority of children, though they may recur in adult life. Perhaps 90 per cent of those discovered under one year of age do well.

POSTURAL TREATMENT. Adequate postural treatment is by far the most important point in the management of this condition. It must be maintained over a long period and adequate postural therapy means twenty-four hours a day in the upright position. Most damage to the

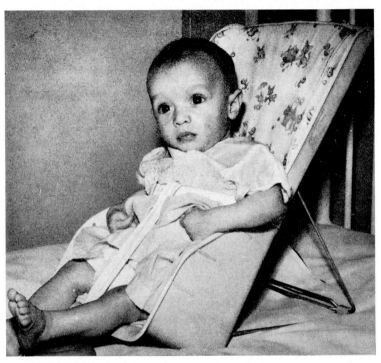

FIG. 33. Infant in "Hiatus Hernia Chair".

œsophagus may be done at night if the patient is lying flat and re-gurgitation is allowed to take place freely. Hence the need to sleep propped up. It is important to employ a chair, whether or not it is designed specially for the condition, and not to depend on pillow propping. A plastic 'Baby Sitter' (Ekco) with side pieces gives a 60° tilt. Babies too young to sit will only slump forward in a chair, squeezing the stomach, and making it useless. In the first weeks of life the baby may need to be fixed on a "cardiac slope".

Thickened Feeds. The feeds are thickened as much as possible and they are reduced in quantity but increased in frequency.

With treatment one-third will respond clinically within two weeks, while the remainder respond much more slowly.

The upright posture and thickened feeds should be continued until the infant has been free from vomiting for three months. There is usually a considerable improvement with the introduction of solids and again when the child spends more of his day standing and walking.

Progress may be assessed clinically by gain in weight, less vomiting and a rising hæmoglobin. The weight may remain stationary even in the absence of vomiting and the mechanism of this is obscure.

Repeated œsophagoscopy and examination of the stools for occult blood may be needed to check the healing of the œsophagitis. The hiatus hernia may disappear radiologically but the œsophagitis persist due to reflux through the incompetent cardia ("chalasia").

Exacerbations are common during intercurrent illnesses, even the common cold, and may necessitate further periods of postural treatment in cases which have been progressing well.

SURGERY. Surgery for hiatus hernia in infancy is not a panacea and should not be undertaken lightly. If surgery is confined to those who have failed to improve during a long course of medical treatment the results are only fairly good. The principal indication for surgery is severe persistent œsophagitis with failure to thrive. Probably all those with œsophagitis persisting to the age of two years should have the hernia repaired regardless of symptoms or lack of them.

The hernia has usually been reduced and repaired from within the chest with the assistance of a diaphragmatic incision, and the cardio-œsophageal angle reconstructed. Unfortunately a satisfactory anatomical repair is no guarantee of relief. Most of the children improve after a hernia repair but a minority still have a severe persistent œsophagitis which may or may not lead to stricture. Other approaches are on trial and it may be that fixation of a segment of the lower œsophagus below the diaphragm away from the swinging thoracic pressures is the important factor in success. With recognition of the pylorophrenic syndrome the addition of pyloroplasty in some cases has improved results.

Severe persistent œsophagitis, with or without stricture, is a grave problem. It may go on to produce a shortened œsophagus so that the œsophagogastric junction cannot be restored to its normal position below the diaphragm or a stricture which cannot be dilated. The outlook is then bad and the surgeon may be forced to replace the strictured area with an isolated loop of colon. This is a really major procedure but the results have been very good.

FEMORAL HERNIA

Femoral hernia is extremely rare in infancy and childhood. A simple repair from below the inguinal ligament is eminently satisfactory.

REFERENCES

Belsey, R. (1965) Reconstruction of the esophagus with left colon, *J. Thor. Cardiovasc. Surg.*, **49**, 133.

Burke, J. B. (1959) Partial thoracic stomach in childhood, *Brit. med. J.*, *ii*, 787.

Carre, I. J. (1959) The natural history of the partial thoracic stomach ('Hiatus hernia') in childhood, *Arch. Dis. Childh.*, **34**, 344.

Carre, I. J. and Astley, R. (1960) The fate of the partial thoracic stomach ('Hiatus hernia') in children, *Arch. Dis. Childh.*, **35**, 484.

Carre, I. J. (1960) Postural treatment of children with a partial thoracic stomach ('Hiatus hernia'), *Arch. Dis. Childh.*, **35**, 569.

Herzfeld, G. (1938) Hernia in infancy, *Amer. J. Surg.*, **39**, 422.

Swenson, O. (1964) Diagnosis and treatment of inguinal hernia, *Pediatrics*, **34**, 3, 412.

Waterston, D. J. (1964) Colonic Replacement of Esophagus (Intrathoracic), *Surg. Clin. N. Amer.*, **44**, 1441.

CHAPTER 18

RECTAL BLEEDING

THIS symptom is particularly alarming to the parents and perhaps to the child. But most of the conditions which cause bleeding are not at all serious, and the investigation of an isolated bleed does not have the same urgency as a similar occurrence in an adult. However, a few of these conditions have in certain circumstances proved serious or even fatal and the elucidation of the cause deserves careful consideration. Amongst children, rectal bleeding is particularly common in late infancy and the toddler, the pottie age.

The answers to a few questions will give a strong clue about the source of the hæmorrhage. Is the quantity lost a cupful of blood, a tablespoonful of blood, a teaspoonful of blood, or a saltspoonful of blood? How long has the bleeding been going on? Is the blood dark red, bright red or tarry? Is it mixed with the motion, streaked on it, or does bleeding occur before or after the motion? Is there any pain associated with the bleeding? Is there any constipation, diarrhœa, slime or discharge? A little blood staining the water in the pan or pottie may look a frightening amount to the mother.

SLIGHT RECTAL BLEEDING

In most cases the bleeding is slight and by far the greatest number of patients are either straining or have an anal fissure.

Straining and Congestion. Simple straining at stool is a frequent cause of slight bleeding. There is congestion of the venous plexus and a few drops of blood escape. Abrasion of the anal verge following on diarrhœa or hard constipated motions may itself be the cause of some small bleeds. The baby who is allowed or even encouraged to sit for a long time on his pottie in the hope of getting a motion is likely to congest his plexus through straining with the same result. The ill-advised habit of coaxing a baby to stay on the pot by provision of books to look at, and playing games whilst he is there, is a potent cause of a congested anal plexus with a tendency to moisture and maceration of the anal verge with easy abrasion and spotting of blood. It is therefore important to enquire into the toilet habits of such a young child, and advice on this matter may be all that is required.

Anal Fissure. An abraded mucosa may progress to produce a superficial anal fissure. This is not uncommon in early childhood and the patient then finds it painful to open the bowels and tries to hold back the motion through fear. The result of this is further constipated hard motions which cause further pain on defæcation and so a vicious circle may be set up. The quantity of blood passed is small. Many fissures will heal rapidly without any attention, but if the staining persists the child will be brought for examination and the diagnosis can be established on inspection. Proctoscopy is not necessary. The buttocks must be parted firmly to see the fissure which is usually anterior or posterior. Satisfactory lighting is important and a hand torch is usually inadequate. Digital examination of the rectum in the presence of a fissure is usually painful and unnecessary. However some fissures in children although they look typical, appear to be painless and the reason for this is not known. The treatment of anal fissure in childhood is conservative because the fissures are usually superficial and can be expected to heal with suitable encouragement. If the patient is constipated, then in bottle-fed infants an extra teaspoon of sugar may be added to the feeds to make the motion softer, and constipation if present in older patients is combated with suitable aperients. A mixture of milk of magnesia and liquid paraffin is a suitable laxative for short-term use, but liquid paraffin should not be given alone. It has a tendency to ooze out at the anus and, by causing further irritation, may exacerbate the trouble instead of relieving it. If the child can be persuaded to take it, a bulk laxative such as "Cologel" or "Blandlax" with adequate fluids produces a large bland and soft stool which is easy to pass. (Children do not take well to raw tacky granule preparations.) "Contact" laxatives (Dulcolax, Senokot) act differently but are often effective in practice by initiating prompt evacuation without straining. If constipation is severe and the masses are scybalous then amethocaine suppositories are useful. Enemas are painful and unnecessary.

It should be noted, however, that these remarks on the use of aperients apply only to the child who is constipated. Many of these children are *not* constipated and then the use of aperients can do no good. By producing unduly soft motions they may cause more irritation and trouble. In many cases advice to take a diet containing adequate fruit and vegetables and fluid with regular twice daily short visits to the toilet is all that is needed. In children who have become particularly frightened by painful defæcation it may be wise to avoid local interference as much as possible, even the use of local anæsthetic ointments.

If there is no improvement after two or three weeks of conservative treatment the infant should have an anæsthetic and have the sphincter slowly stretched by the gradual insertion of two to four fingers into the anus. This will get rid of spasm and allow the fissure to heal from the bottom upwards. An older child may require excision of the fissure and internal sphincterotomy for a fissure which has become chronic and, fibrosed but this is rarely necessary.

Rectal Polyp. Rectal polyp is probably the next commonest condition with a presenting symptom of rectal bleeding. The history is of increasing quantities of blood being passed from time to time over a period of weeks or months. There may be long dry spells in between. Most of the polyps are in the ampulla of the rectum and some may appear outside the anus from time to time when a stool is being passed. Polyps in children are all benign, *are not premalignant*, and do not have the dubious prognosis of those in adult life. The majority are single polyps, but there may be two or three present.

The diagnosis is confirmed in the great majority of cases on carrying out a rectal examination when the typical soft cherry-like tumour will be felt. In some cases where the lesion is higher up in the bowel it may be necessary to use a proctoscope or sigmoidoscope to discover the lesion. It is uncommon in the proximal colon and it may only be possible to demonstrate a lesion there by double-contrast barium enema. Many are never found as auto-amputation is common and it is the final more severe bleeding that causes anxiety.

The common *juvenile polyp* is not an adenoma. It is cherry red, smooth, round and not lobulated. It is often covered by mucus. Histologically it is a *congenital cystic hamartoma*. True solitary adenoma is exceedingly rare in childhood.

In many cases it will be possible to coax the polyp outside the anus with the examining finger and it may be possible simply to tie a stout silk ligature around the base there and then. The polyp will slough off painlessly and without hæmorrhage within a few days. In other cases it may be necessary to give an anæsthetic in order to get at the polyp through a proctoscope, but in almost all cases it is then possible to withdraw the polyp outside the anus. A convenient instrument is a pair of tonsil forceps which get a grip on the fold of mucosa from which the polyp is growing and draw this down outside the anus. An assistant holds the forceps whilst a transfixion ligature is placed across the base and the polyp is nipped off. It is surprising how mobile these polyps are and even those which arise quite high in the rectum can usually be brought down in this way, presumably because persistent attempts by the bowel to pass the polyp have stretched the mucosa at the base and loosened it. Polyps higher up may require a diathermy snare for their removal through proctoscope or sigmoidoscope. It is not easy to palpate or even see a small seedling lesion and occasionally there is more than one polyp present.

MULTIPLE POLYPS. Multiple polyps are much less common but occur in two rare but important conditions.

1. *Familial polyposis or adenomatosis coli.* This is an hereditary condition transmitted by either sex as a dominant gene, of multiple small polyps in the colon and rectum. In the typical case several polyps will be palpable and visible in the rectum, and barium enema will reveal the widespread nature of the lesion throughout the colon. The polyps are true adenomata and are plum coloured. Neoplastic malignant change in this condition seems to be inevitable. Radical treatment is therefore indicated. In childhood this will usually mean a total colectomy with ileo-rectal anastomosis. The rectal

stump is examined from time to time and remaining or developing polypi removed by diathermy. The rectum is at least as liable to cancer as the colon. But it is unlikely that the parents will accept complete coloproctectomy and ileostomy in a young child unless there has been prior familial experience of the disease. It may therefore be justified to proceed with ileo-rectal anastomosis and continue surveillance of the rectum during childhood though excision of the rectum will be required later.

2. *The Peutz-Jegher Syndrome.* In this condition there is typically a combination of gastro-intestinal polyposis with buccal and circumoral brown pigmentation. The polyps are larger and more numerous than in polyposis coli. They primarily affect the small intestine, but may also be present in stomach or large bowel. The treatment is the removal of any polyps within reach of the sigmoidoscope. It is not practical to attempt complete removal of the lesions throughout the small bowel. The condition may give rise to trouble from bleeding of the polyps in the small bowel or from intussusception occurring at the site of one of them. It may then be necessary to treat the polyps causing the trouble. Malignant change has been reported several times in the small intestinal polyps though histologically they are hamartomata. These have usually been in cases presenting with obstruction, and the infiltrating appearance has been recognized on examining the resected specimen of small bowel and tumour. However, the survival of these children shows the lesion to be clinically benign. Associated large bowel polyps may, however, undergo true malignant change.

Juvenile Polyposis Coli. This is a rare diffuse affection of the colon and rectum in which the polyps are of the juvenile type. There would appear to be no hazard of malignancy, so colectomy with ileo-rectal anastomosis and fulguration of the rectal polyps is the treatment of choice.

EXSANGUINATING HÆMORRHAGE

Major exsanguinating hæmorrhage causing clinical anæmia and pallor may be due to Meckel's diverticulum, blood dyscrasias, peptic ulceration, drugs such as aspirin and cortisone, duplication of the intestine, intussusception and angiomas in about that order of frequency. In any of these conditions there may be premonitory small bleeds before a major hæmorrhage. (Polyps do not cause single exsanguinating hæmorrhage, but persistent bleeding may lead to gross anæmia.)

Meckel's Diverticulum

This remnant of the omphalomesenteric duct is present in 1 to 2 per cent of the population. It varies in extent from a simple small diverticulum of the bowel to a complete fistula opening at the umbilicus. Most of these remnants never give any trouble, but a minority can cause serious symptoms. The whole problem of Meckel's diverticulum is conveniently dealt with here, as massive rectal hæmorrhage is by far the commonest presentation in the pædiatric age group. Complications of Meckel's diverticulum present in four main ways: (1) *Massive rectal hæmorrhage.* (2) *Intestinal obstruction.* (3) *Inflammation of the diverticulum.* (4) *Umbilical Sinus.*

Hæmorrhage. In a "bleeding Meckel's" the child typically has little

pain but rapidly goes off colour and has a poor appetite. Then follows
the passage of typical dark red but fluid blood in quite copious amounts.
The nature of the bleeding, intermediate between the tarry stool of
melæna and the bright red blood of rectal bleeding, may be quite
typical. There is usually nothing abnormal palpable in the abdomen or
there may be some indefinite local tenderness. It is not possible reliably
to demonstrate a Meckel's diverticulum by the use of a barium meal or
enema. If the clinical picture suggests a Meckel's diverticulum then
laparatomy is the only way of confirming or excluding the diagnosis.
Before this course is taken a full blood examination should be carried
out to exclude a blood dyscrasia as a cause of hæmorrhage and
sigmoidoscopy should be carried out to see if there are any polyps
present to cause the hæmorrhage. The bleeding from a Meckel's
diverticulum is frequently profuse and the patient may bleed down to

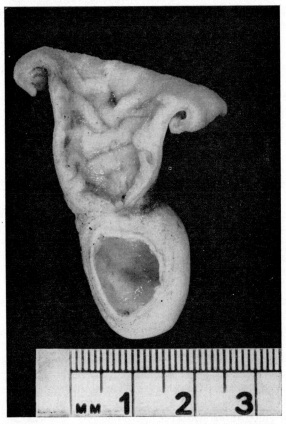

FIG. 34. Excised Meckel's diverticulum. The cavity is lined by gastric
mucosa. The gastric juice secreted has caused a bleeding ulcer in the
ileal mucosa.

30 or 40 per cent hæmoglobin quite quickly and require urgent transfusion to make him fit for operation. A laparotomy is carried out and the terminal ileum searched for a Meckel's diverticulum. This can easily be overlooked. The diverticulum always arises on the anti-mesenteric border, but it may be bound down to the mesentery by adhesions making it less obvious than one might think. There is frequently a tell-tale mesenteric adenitis at the site where the diverticulum is found bound down, apparently within the mesentery. It may be possible to clamp the base of the diverticulum, remove it and oversew the base without opening the bowel. But it will more often be preferable to carry out a wedge resection or a formal resection of the ileum bearing the diverticulum in order to remove it completely and avoid the risk of recurrent bleeding. The cause of the bleeding is the ectopic gastric mucosa in the diverticulum secreting acid pepsin which causes ulceration at its margin. It is the adjacent ileal mucosa which ulcerates under the influence of the acid secretion. It is therefore quite essential that the entire base of the diverticulum be removed or a residual islet of ectopic mucosa may produce recurrence of symptoms. If a Meckel's diverticulum is not found then it will be necessary to explore the entire alimentary tract for the other sources of bleeding listed above. If the operation is carried out promptly as soon as blood loss has been corrected then the site of blood in the intestine may give some clue as to the site of the causative lesion.

Meckel's diverticulum may also present as a cause of *intestinal obstruction*. The diverticulum may be forming the apex of an intussusception, or, if it is attached to the anterior abdominal wall, then volvulus of the small bowel may occur around it. Alternatively, the tip of the diverticulum may become attached to another loop of bowel causing a band obstruction.

Simple inflammation of the diverticulum occurs, but it is seldom suspected preoperatively. The abdomen is opened for acute appendicitis; the appendix is found to be normal, and the routine exploration further up the small intestine reveals the acutely inflamed Meckel's diverticulum. A resection back to normal bowel is the safest method of dealing with it.

The presence of an *umbilical sinus* discharging mucus may result from persistence of the distal end of the omphalomesenteric duct. It will require excision as an annoying lesion in itself; and is also a warning that there may be a Meckel's diverticulum inside the abdomen as the result of the persistence of the other end of the duct. A complete fistula may be present, when the patient presents at birth with the passage of flatus and perhaps fæces from the umbilicus. The treatment is again resection.

If a Meckel's diverticulum is found incidentally during a laparotomy then it should be excised. For although the majority of Meckel's diverticuli do not give rise to any symptoms the complications of the minority which cause symptoms can be serious and endanger life.

Blood Dyscrasia

It is important to remember these "medical" causes of rectal bleeding. Henoch-Schönlein purpura may cause hæmorrhage into the bowel or into the bowel wall. It may precipitate a real intussusception, but more often the hæmorrhage into the bowel wall produces a mass which mimics one. Thrombocytopenic purpura or leukæmia may also produce hæmorrhage from the bowel. It is therefore important to investigate the blood fully before proceeding to laparotomy.

Peptic Ulceration

This may occur at any age and a severe hæmatemesis or a severe melæna may be the first indication of its presence. Management is primarily conservative and the majority settle on blood transfusion, sedation and frequent small feeds.

Drug Induced Rectal Bleeding

Cortisone or aspirin can cause severe gastro-intestinal hæmorrhage. This is particularly liable to happen in the starving patient on nasogastric suction leaving a layer of unneutralized gastric juice to encourage ulceration.

Duplication of the Bowel

Duplication of the bowel frequently presents clinically as a severe rectal hæmorrhage, especially in the first two years of life. The cause of duplication is not definitely known, but it is assumed to be due to a vacuolation abnormality following a solid stage in the development of the intestine which allows a second piece of the bowel to develop parallel with the normal lumen. Duplication may occur anywhere from the mouth to the anus, but is commonest in the ileum, jejunum, stomach and colon, in that order.

Duplications may be either *globular* of which the majority have no connection with the lumen of the bowel to which they are attached or *tubular*. Tubular duplications cannot usually be felt and they are often only diagnosed at laparotomy for bleeding. A barium meal, however, may demonstrate the lesion. The globular duplication may be more easily felt and may give rise to much diagnostic argument because its position in the abdomen varies so much from time to time. This wandering characteristic of the duplication gives a diagnostic clue. (Most so-called mesenteric cysts turn out to be enteric cysts when the lining is examined.) Curiously enough, the lining mucosa is not always the same as the lining of the contiguous bowel but is quite frequently gastric in type in duplications of foregut or midgut, hence peptic ulceration can arise just as at the junction of a Meckel's diverticulum with the bowel. A duplication is occasionally associated with a malrotation.

The attachment of the duplication to the adjacent bowel and the relationship of their blood supply is such that resection of both portions of the bowel is necessary in treatment. A duplication is occasionally associated with malrotation.

Rectal hæmorrhage may also occur from *Volvulus Neonatorum* in a baby born with malfixation of the bowel and the condition of "mesenterium commune". The child will present signs of obstruction in that it will also be vomiting bile-stained fluid, but abdominal distension may be absent until late in the condition long after the volvulus has become tight enough to strangulate the loop and allow bleeding. There is therefore a real danger that the condition may be mistaken for dysentery.

Dysentery is another important cause of rectal bleeding, but in the usual case the clear signs and symptoms of the acute inflammation of the bowel make the diagnosis obvious. Sonne dysentery, however, may present with some abdominal pain and quite marked bleeding with no gross diarrhœa, and then it enters into the differential diagnosis of rectal hæmorrhage.

Mesenteric thrombosis in the neonatal period, associated with septicæmia, may cause severe rectal hæmorrhage in a collapsed baby.

Ulcerative colitis is a rare condition but seems to be becoming more common in pædiatric practice. It generally presents in a sickly child with frequent bloody and watery stools over a period. The diagnosis is made on the history, sigmoidoscopy and barium enema. The initial signs may be a little blood in the stools with perhaps an excess of mucus. At that point there may be no ulceration visible on sigmoidoscopy, but the mucosa is congested like red velvet, rather than the normal pink, and it bleeds easily. Diarrhœa may be slight in ulcerative colitis of atypical onset which seems not too rare in children. Medical treatment is certainly the first approach to this condition, but it is not always successful even at this early age and it may be necessary to resort to surgery. General measures are a bland, low residue diet, rest, sedatives and fluid and electrolyte control. Psychological factors may require attention. Local or systemic cortisone is of value in acute flares and the fear that it would render later surgery dangerous appears to be unfounded. Salazopyrine is of more value in chronically persistent cases. When surgery is required in childhood it seems that the outlook for successful restoration of rectal control by colectomy with ileo-rectal anastomosis is greater than one would gather from the reports of adult proctologists. This at least postpones a permanent ileostomy even though it may later become necessary if the disease persists in the rectum. Nevertheless the postponement of ileostomy until schooldays are past is obviously worth while when possible and the risk of carcinoma in childhood is negligible. The risk of carcinoma developing is now accepted as considerable in ulcerative colitis of ten years' duration even during clinical quiescence and this may be a further indication to resort to surgery. The usual indications are failure to respond to medical treatment or complications such as perforation, anal fistulæ or arthritis.

Hæmatemesis and melæna in the newborn may be due to swallowed blood or a coagulation defect.

Intussusception can cause severe rectal bleeding in its advanced stages when the diagnosis will be obvious from other signs and symptoms. But the passage of blood per rectum or on the examining finger may occasionally be the first obvious sign of this condition.

Perhaps a third of rectal hæmorrhages in childhood are never accurately diagnosed, even after full laboratory investigation, sigmoidoscopy, barium enema and laparotomy. The only thing that can be said about these cases is that happily the prognosis is good even if the bleeding goes on intermittently for some time.

Some time has been spent in this chapter discussing uncommon but nevertheless important causes of rectal bleeding. It may therefore restore a sense of proportion to state the following: By far the commonest cause of rectal bleeding is anal abrasion resulting from a transient abnormality of bowel habit. The three most important causes of the significant rectal bleeding are, Meckel's diverticulum, polyps, and blood dyscrasias.

MINOR CONDITIONS IN THE ANORECTAL REGION

"Something coming down" from the anus is a common complaint. True prolapse of the rectum—all layers of the wall or of the mucosa—is not uncommon and usually begins in the second year of life. But one must enquire carefully into the nature of the "prolapse" because other types of protrusion also occur. How far does it come down? Is it a complete ring or separate pieces ("blobs like cherries")? Does it only occur on defæcation? Does it go back itself or has it to be replaced? Is replacement easy or painful?

Prolapse of the whole rectal wall presents as a ring of bowel protruding about 2 inches from the anus. It usually occurs in the "bowel training" period in fit plump babies who are difficult about their potting—perhaps because of unnecessary fussing over their bowel habit. The achievement seems to be due to disordered use of the muscles controlling defæcation. Watching the baby in action one gets the impression that the prolapse is almost deliberate, even though the baby becomes upset after he has achieved it, and it has been suggested that it is a trick for gaining mother's attention or that the baby obtains some satisfaction in its performance. At all events it usually occurs in healthy, well fed though pernickety babies. Certainly wasting diseases with associated straining (e.g. cystic fibrosis) may be complicated by prolapse. Neurological disorders such as spina bifida may also cause prolapse. But these are not the usual type and most of the babies seen with this complaint will have no other physical defect. Pre-existing constipation is uncommon. Straining at stool is the underlying trouble and this seems usually to be habitual although occasionally it may follow an attack of constipation or diarrhœa.

Management is by avoiding straining. The baby is given a small seat on the adult lavatory, or a raised pottie if younger, to avoid the squatting position. The child is sat out say twice daily, after meals, for a few minutes and then taken off the seat whether a motion is passed or not. Further bowel training should be postponed and the mother impressed with the inadvisibility of prolonged sessions. Aperients are not used unless there is a definite evidence of constipation—indeed their unnecessary use probably perpetuates straining and prolapse in many cases. If they are needed the bulk forming laxatives are better than those which might produce semi-fluid irritant stools. An emulsion or tablet form is more likely to be acceptable than the commoner granular preparations. *Most important, the mother must be reassured that the condition is not as serious as it looks and is almost always outgrown with such handling within a few months or a year.* For the appearance is alarming to the layman.

Only about one in ten fail to respond to this regime. A perianal catgut suture tied tight enough to grip an assistant's little finger in the anus will break the habit in most of the others. It probably works by producing sufficient discomfort to discourage straining rather than producing fibrosis and should only be used when the regime has failed both at home and on a trial period in hospital. Perirectal injections of hypertonic saline to stimulate fibrosis are successful but may result in unpleasant abscesses if infection occurs. (Submucous injections are of less value in complete prolapse, but being painless and safe are worth trying.) The major abdominal interventions used for adult prolapse are virtually never needed in uncomplicated infant prolapse.

OTHER "PROLAPSES". *Prolapsed mucous membrane.* A ring of mucosa up to 1 cm. or so in length may come down. More often one or more localized bulges of mucosa appear over the *congested external hæmorrhoidal plexus* on defæcation. There may be a little bleeding from the congested plexus. The usual reason is prolonged squatting and straining —either because of constipation or just by habit. Regular but short visits to the lavatory and perhaps attention to the diet are all that is likely to be needed and submucous sclerosant injections help in the few persistent mucosal prolapses. Anything that comes out of the anus is apt to be called "piles" by the layman and it may be necessary to reassure the mother that these "external hæmorrhoids" are not the same as the internal piles so common in adults and not likely to progress to the same troublesome complications of which they may have had personal experience.

Polyps. A polyp low in the rectum may prolapse from the anus on defæcation. Management has been discussed in the previous chapter on rectal bleeding.

Intussusception. The head of an intussusception may protrude from the anus but can easily be distinguished from prolapse on anything more than the most cursory examination. The condition is discussed in a separate chapter.

Postanal Pits

A depression in the skin of the midline behind the anus adherent to the underlying coccyx is common. The name *postanal dimple* or *coccygeal dimple* is a good one for it conveys the trivial nature of the lesion. A few of the deeper ones are difficult to keep clean and may be worthy of excision to avoid recurrent infections. Although they are often called "pilonidal sinuses" there is no nest of hairs in the pre-pubertal patient and no conclusive evidence that they are the precursors ot this troublesome lesion of hairy adults. They must be differentiated from the rare but important *dermal sinus*. As a practical guide, if the edges of the pit can be pushed back to reveal the blind apex of the depression the condition is a postanal dimple which can be left alone.

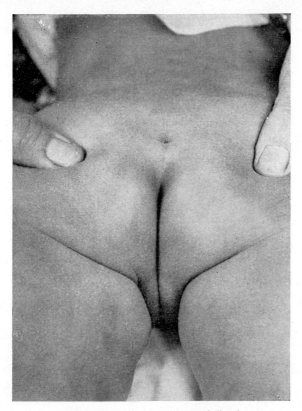

Fig. 35. Postanal pit or coccygeal dimple.

If the blind apex cannot be seen the lesion is either a dimple so deep as to be liable to get infected from retained fæcal debris or a dermal sinus. It should therefore be excised and a deep track looked for at this time. The postanal dimple sometimes overlies a back tilted coccyx and in this case the lower part of the coccyx should be excised to avoid a scar which may be uncomfortable to sit on.

DERMAL SINUS. This is a developmental tract which may lead down to a dermoid cyst within the spinal canal. It has a punctum through which infection can easily occur and it is a potential cause of recurrent spinal meningitis. The only external evidence may be a tiny dimple which can arise at any level over the spine. The caudally placed ones are more often over the lower sacrum than the coccyx. They should be excised on diagnosis.

REFERENCES

Todd, I. P. (1964) Juvenile polyps, *Arch. Dis. Childh.*, **39**, 166.

CHAPTER 19

THE UMBILICUS

THE umbilicus is the cicatrix left by the healing of the stump of the umbilical cord. It is thus liable to abnormalities resulting from defects of healing and also from failure to complete the embryological processes resulting in the formation of the umbilicus. These processes are narrowing of the ring itself, closure of the urachus, resorption of the allanto-enteric canal, and obliteration of the umbilical arteries and vein.

The most frequent lesion of the umbilicus of importance is *infection* of the stump after birth. The organism responsible is usually the staphylococcus. Infection may spread for some distance over the anterior abdominal wall as described in Chapter 7. It may also spread along the course of the obliterated umbilical vein causing an abscess in the region of the falciform ligament and the liver, or along from the tracks of the arteries causing cellulitis or abscess of the lower abdominal wall. It is treated by local application of a drying antiseptic lotion such as gentian violet 1 per cent, and the systemic administration of an antibiotic to avoid the risk of distant spread. Healing of the cord stump after infection may leave behind a little ball of granulation tissue, the so-called *granulomatous polyp*. This produces a slight persistent discharge. It can usually be treated by tying a silk ligature tightly around its base. The lesion is insensitive and no anæsthetic is required. The granuloma will drop off in a day or so. A flatter granuloma may be more easily removed by curettage and touching the base with a silver nitrate stick.

UMBILICAL HERNIA

The commonest anomaly is the presence of a *hernia*. The contradictory accounts given of the natural history and treatment of these herniæ at the umbilicus results from confusion of two lesions.

A true umbilical hernia is a protrusion through the weakened umbilical cicatrix. It presents as a skin-covered, almost spherical protrusion about the size of a cherry—though it may be smaller or much bigger. It reduces easily on pressure and the neck is felt as a thick-edged circular ring. There is often a gurgle on reduction indicating that the content is bowel. When the baby cries it bulges owing to the increase in abdominal tension. This often gives the mother the mistaken impression that the bulging hernia is causing pain and hence the crying. The thin skin may be stretched and bluish looking on straining. The mother may genuinely fear that it might burst. The first treatment of an umbilical hernia is therefore the assurance of the mother that they do not cause pain and cannot rupture. For practical purposes incarceration is also unknown so that there is no need to keep the hernia reduced. If left alone these true umbilical herniæ will heal spontaneously within the first year of life, as the delayed narrowing of the umbilical ring proceeds to completion. Virtually the only exceptions to this rule are those rare cases in which the umbilical hernia is an expression of an underlying condition. For example, the hernia may be an indication of the raised abdominal pressure in ascites. It may also occur in association with cretinism or with gargoylism.

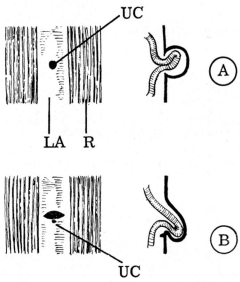

Fig. 36. (*a*) True umbilical hernia—through the umbilical cicatrix. (97 per cent).
(*b*) Para- or semi-umbilical hernia—through the linea alba adjacent to the cicatrix with the sac protruding under the skin of the umbilicus. (3 per cent.)
UC = umbilical cicatrix. LA = linea alba. R = rectus abdominis.

MANAGEMENT. No treatment is required in the great majority of umbilical herniæ. The parents are told of the high incidence of spontaneous closure and that, as there is nothing to go wrong, there is everything to be gained by patient expectancy. Most will close in the first year, but healing may occur at least up to ten years of age.

No truss or belt is advised. Strapping the hernia has been shown to hasten healing. It is often said to be worth while to keep the mothers happy but an explanation seems to be more sensible in most cases. If used, long strips of plain (not elastic) zinc oxide strapping should be employed, drawn tight enough to cause a fold of skin down the midline and relieve the muscle pull on the umbilicus with no attempt to "plug" the hole. If irritation of the skin does nevertheless ensue, treatment can be withheld without any anxiety regarding final healing.

A somewhat similar protrusion of the umbilicus may be seen in infancy. This is the *para-umbilical hernia*. It is usually supra-umbilical although occasionally it is infra-umbilical. The protrusion takes place through a split in the linea alba immediately adjacent to the umbilical cicatrix and the hernial sac itself protrudes into the skin of the umbilicus. Denis Browne therefore prefers to call these lesions semi-umbilical, a more accurate name. The result of this manner of protrusion is that the hernia tends to be conical and pointing downwards, and the neck is a transverse elliptical thin-edged slit, points which distinguish it from the true umbilical hernia. The importance of the distinction is that this para- or semi-umbilical hernia does not heal spontaneously *unless it is small to begin with*. Like the true umbilical hernia it gives rise to no symptoms in childhood. But it is thought to be akin to the para-umbilical hernia of adult life and may be its precursor. Operation is therefore advised for its cure. There is no urgency about this. As it is an elective operation it is better left until the toddler period is over. The psychological effects of hospitalization and separation at the toddler age are more likely to be persistent than at a greater age, when some explanation can be given to the child. Four years of age, before schooling starts in earnest, seems a reasonable compromise. But in any event hospitalization for this small procedure can be reduced to an overnight stay or "day case" status, and postoperative restriction of activity is pointless.

The operation is carried out through a curved incision following half the circumference of the umbilicus. The umbilicus is preserved and the scar becomes inconspicuous. This is a cosmetic point of some importance. Through the incision the aponeurosis is cleared and its tubelike prolongation around the hernial sac is freed all round. A blunt dissector is passed below the hernia. An incision is made through the upper half of the aponeurotic coat and then the neck of the peritoneal sac itself A blunt-pointed artery forceps is then attached to the edge of the two layers together. When a firm hold has been obtained in this way the forceps is held aloft so that the omentum and other contents of the sac fall back within the abdomen. The lower half of the sac and the aponeurosis can then be divided and clipped similarly. There is usually a bleeder to catch in the edge of the neck of the sac. The trick of managing this simple but potentially awkward procedure is to have a strong forceps hold on the aponeurosis so that it can be lifted upwards and allow the contents to fall back within the abdominal cavity. Otherwise the omentum can hinder a proper repair. The use of a probe and relaxation alone are inadequate to keep the omentum away from this focal point of the abdomen. If the surgeon should allow any tongue of omentum to protrude through the repair then recurrence is sure.

The closure is usually carried out by one or two mattress sutures of doubled 60 linen thread to overlap the borders of the defect reinforced by one or two simple sutures. Although small, the defect must be strongly closed, for it will be subject to considerable force from the pull of the abdominal muscles. There does not seem to be any need to suture the sac and aponeurosis in separate layers. When the skin is closed the redundant skin of the umbilicus is tucked in and the hollow maintained by inserting a little roll of gauze. If the skin is allowed to heal hanging outwards a most unsightly persistent tag may remain. The recurrence rate of this operation should be negligible.

EXOMPHALOS

A much more serious type of hernia is the truly congenital umbilical hernia or *exomphalos*, in which the contents are covered only by thin amnion-like membrane. Without prompt care this membrane ruptures allowing evisceration, and infection easily enters the abdominal cavity.

Obviously the replacement of contents within the abdomen will be much easier before the gut has distended with air, so that urgent management of this condition within the first few hours of life can facilitate treatment. There are two kinds of exomphalos.

(*a*) *Hernia into the Cord.* The mass may be as large as an orange and its contents may be the whole of the midgut loop, but the neck is narrow. It is basically a persistence of the physiological umbilical hernia. The cord will be ligated beyond this hernia before it is divided. If the cord is then slowly twisted the contents of the sac will gradually be forced back into the abdomen. Strapping is then wound round the base of the twisted cord and stuck to the abdominal wall to prevent unwinding. Normal healing of the umbilicus will follow and hospitalization and operation can usually be avoided. Theoretical objections have been raised to this simple procedure, but it has been proved to be safe and satisfactory.

(*b*) *Omphalocele.* Basically this is a failure of the umbilical ring to narrow down in the later stages of fœtal life. The swelling is broad-based. A relatively small defect, say 2 cm. across the base, can be closed by excision of the sac, replacement of the contained bowel in the abdomen, and primary closure. Primary closure of a large defect, which often contains liver as well as bowel, may be impossible owing to tension. It will then be wiser to retain the sac intact and to mobilize skin from the abdomen laterally to cover and protect it. As the baby grows the rectus muscles will tend to pull straight and narrow the defect. At 12 or 18 months of age it should be possible to replace the contents and to repair the abdominal wall soundly without undue tension. This two-stage procedure of Gross avoids many of the hazards of the actual lesion. Muscle relaxants may make a single stage repair easy in a large omphalocele, but once they have worn off there may be dangerous pressure on the diaphragm, limiting the abdominal respiration so important to neonates, or on the inferior vena cava hampering venous return.

It must be remembered that most cases of exomphalos have incomplete rotation of the gut associated with the incomplete closure of the umbilicus, but this rarely leads to intestinal obstruction. Other serious congenital defects may be present in as many as 30 per cent of omphaloceles large or small. An alternative method of treatment of the uncomplicated omphalocele which is too big for primary closure is to dress the sac with 2 per cent solution of mercurochrome in water for a day or two, to form a hardened membrane. The dressings are then continued as necessary to protect the membrane whilst cicatrization and epithelialization progress until the whole lesion is covered with modified skin. This has been found to be quite a practical alternative to operative skin closure, although it requires a longer period of careful nursing. In some cases where the hernia is smaller the lesion may shrink and become so flat as not to need any further repair, but in the larger cases a secondary repair at 12 or 18 months of age will be required as above. The contraction due to healing with fibrosis may make this easier.

In a large omphalocele where only the skin can be closed, sloughing of the skin flaps may occur. Two per cent mercurochrome dressings may help form a hardened membrane over the necrotic patches.

Umbilical Anomalies

Apart from true herniæ a protuberant umbilicus may simply consist of a skin-covered tube. This is the so-called *cutis navel* in which normal skin has grown along about half an inch of the cord so that separation takes place here instead of flush with the abdominal wall. It may require trimming for cosmetic reasons.

Occasionally the umbilicus may be displaced downwards as the so-called *pubic umbilicus*. This may be associated with urinary troubles such as bladder neck obstruction. Owing to the underdevelopment of the subumbilical abdominal wall the bladder apex is held down and this organ takes on a transverse sausage-like shape.

Umbilical Discharge

Far and away the commonest cause of umbilical discharge is *umbilical granuloma* following infection of the cord stump. If ligated at the base it will fall off and, if necessary, can then be touched with silver nitrate.

Fistulæ of congenital origin may present at the umbilicus but they are rare. If the *urachus* fails to close a discharge of urine may be observed. Such urinary discharge almost certainly indicates obstruction to the normal passage as well as patency of the urachus. If the *allanto-enteric canal* remains open flatus or bowel content may be passed from persistent connection with the terminal ileum and the umbilicus. Occasionally this bowel-like structure may be prolapsed through the umbilicus as a mucosa-covered, horn-like tube.

Cysts may arise beneath the umbilicus or adjacent to it. They result from partial persistence of developmental channels. A urachal cyst lies in the anterior abdominal wall just below the umbilicus. It may pass unnoticed for years until it becomes infected and presents as an abscess. After primary incision and drainage it will be necessary to dissect out the residual cyst wall to prevent recurrence.

A cystic remnant of the allanto-enteric canal may similarly underlie the umbilicus and require excision. A remnant of the distal end of this canal may open onto the umbilicus as a mucous polyp. A remnant of the proximal end of the channel (i.e. Meckel's diverticulum from the terminal ileum) may coexist. So the unimportant surface lesion may be a clue to the presence of the more serious internal one.

The umbilicus is one of the sites at which the veins of the portal and systemic systems meet. So any cause of portal hypertension such as cirrhosis of the liver or thrombosis of the portal vein may give rise to a *caput medusæ* of dilated anastomotic venous channels around the umbilicus as the portal vein drains into the lower pressure systemic veins.

Rarely the umbilicus may be the site of a *congenital arterio-venous fistula*. The enlarged veins are then associated with a machinery murmur.

REFERENCES

Grob, M. (1963) Conservative treatment of exomphalos, *Arch. Dis. Childh.*, **38,** 148.

CHAPTER 20

RECURRENT ABDOMINAL PAIN

THE differential diagnosis of acute abdominal pain is discussed in the chapter on appendicitis. Appendicitis is not the commonest cause of such pain but it is the most important because of the serious or fatal consequences of delay in its diagnosis.

Recurrent abdominal pain may be even more difficult to diagnose or to manage. The problem is mainly one of school age children.

Detailed History

The most important factor in the diagnosis is the careful elucidation of an accurate, detailed history from mother and child. Physical signs are usually absent. Much useful information will be volunteered and the mother should be encouraged to give a full account of the story and her opinions. The child should be similarly encouraged. A family history may uncover anxieties that the child's symptoms may be the precursor of some serious condition. Specific questioning is necessary to supplement the story. Where is the pain? Is it sharp, aching or sickly? How long do the pains last? How long do the bouts of trouble last? What brings it on? Is it when she is tired, excited, worried about school? Are there associated symptoms, e.g. vomiting or headache? Does she suffer much from sore throats, coughs, catarrh? How much school has she missed? Does it come on when she runs? How does it affect her appetite? It may help to ask the mother if she considers the child placid or nervous. Apart from their intrinsic value, these questions often stimulate the mother to further comments revealing her attitude to the problem.

Classification

It is convenient to classify recurrent abdominal pains as *functional* or *organic* but to realize that both factors may operate. People vary greatly in their reactions and there seems to be a constitutional type that reacts to stress with abdominal symptoms. The stresses may vary and be psychological or physical at different times. The child's reaction to those symptoms will be dependent largely on the parents' attitude.

FUNCTIONAL

EMOTIONAL STRESS. This is probably the commonest problem, though one sees a selected group in surgical outpatients. Two factors are common. The *mother* may be unduly anxious about the child and this may become apparent only as she is encouraged to talk. She may believe the child delicate because he is not as well covered as a sibling or a neighbour's child and may feel guilty about this.

The second factor is the attitude of child and parents to *school*.

PERIODIC SYNDROME. The *periodic syndrome* is a label attached to a group of disorders in which there is usually a more persistent pain associated with feeling off colour for several days. There may be fever, and vomiting may be more impressive than the pain. There are no specific physical signs. Many of these children may give a history of allergic conditions such as hay fever, asthma or eczema. The patient is more frequently a pale, thin girl who gets circles under her eyes and may develop travel sickness. Dizziness, headache and changes of colour may also be complained of. The family history may suggest abdominal migraine in some cases and epileptic equivalents have been suggested in a few with positive E.E.G. findings. The former labels of acidosis and cyclical vomiting are démodé.

ORGANIC

NON-SPECIFIC MESENTERIC ADENITIS. The pains are central or right-sided. They may be alarming in their apparent severity yet the mother will agree that they last only a few minutes. The child typically goes white with this kind of short, sharp pain, which may occur several times a day in bouts lasting a few days. There may be vomiting and there is usually loss of appetite. There is probably no fœtor oris but there may be a smell of acetone on the breath. The bowel habit may be unchanged. On examination there may be diffuse and variable tenderness in the right iliac fossa, with no guarding, but sometimes with an indistinct mass. Such a clinical picture is often associated with chronic catarrh or other upper respiratory infections, including frank tonsillitis. It is remarkable that appendicectomy sometimes relieves the pains even though the organ removed is normal and it is difficult to ascribe the lasting effects entirely to the psychological effects of operation. Perhaps the colic results from blockage of the narrow appendicular lumen as a result of its participation in the generalized lymphoid reaction to infection. The condition usually recurs over a year or two and is then outgrown.

Periodic syndrome and mesenteric adenitis are convenient labels to attach to clinical entities. They have little support from the morbid anatomist but are of use in discussing the matter with parents. For example when a patient has mesenteric adenitis it may be said that the pains are due to glands in the abdomen; that these glands are not serious, are not tuberculous and do not require surgery or medicines, diets or tonics. Parents are best told that the pains will probably come back again from time to time but that they will eventually go away. If the pain lasts more than 3 hours the child should have an aspirin and if it lasts more than 6 hours the doctor should be called.

In the case of the periodic syndrome it may be said that this is a common condition in girls (or boys) at this age, that it will be often relieved by an aspirin and a glucose drink and that the attacks usually disappear at the age of 12 to 14 years.

It may be stated that chronic or recurrent appendicitis (attacks going back more than say a year) is rare in childhood. Unfortunately, it cannot be said that the condition is unknown nor can a child with periodic syndrome be guaranteed against the future development of appendicitis. The need to introduce reasonable caution into one's assurances and advice may reduce its effectiveness. But there is little doubt that the easy and largely unsupported suggestion that "it might be a grumbling appendix" leads many a mother to such a state of anxiety and doubt that in the end the child loses a normal appendix.

RECURRENT APPENDICITIS. The genuine attacks are usually longer than those of "adenitis", the pains more persistent and the signs more consistent under observation.

Certainly it is better to take out one too many than one too few appendices and one should not be influenced by a desire to avoid looking foolish before one's medical colleagues by removing a "lily white" appendix. But a careful history-taking and discussion will avoid many unnecessary operations. Often the mother only wants reassurance from a surgeon that the story is *not like* appendicitis. However, the spectre of recurrent inexplicable attacks of pain during holidays, at Christmas, away at boarding school, at examination times or when abroad may lead intelligent parents to an understandable desire to "have it finished with". Removal of the appendix in these circumstances may fail to relieve the pain in some but simplifies management in many.

RENAL PAIN. If the pain is localized to one side, a renal cause should be considered. Urinalysis may show infection. But an obstructive uropathy in the upper urinary tract will often produce no abnormality of the urine, nor will the micturition be abnormal if the bladder and its outlet are normal. This often leads to delay in the diagnosis of, for instance, hydronephrosis. The kidney is not usually large enough to be palpable in the early stages and an intravenous pyelogram is necessary to make the diagnosis. It is an important one because in the early stages the kidney can be saved by a plastic operation on the pelvis and its outlet.

UNCOMMON ORGANIC LESIONS. Though the physical causes of recurrent abdominal pain have been played down in this chapter because of the innumerable examples without them, there are several of uncommon but important organic lesions which may cause trouble.

Usually physical examination is negative. But a *mass* may be felt, e.g. a chronic intussusception or a mobile mesenteric cyst or enteric duplication and it should be remembered that malignant abdominal tumours occur even from birth. Recurrent pains may result from hæmorrhage into the substance of a Wilms tumour or a neuroblastoma.

Visible peristalsis may be a clue to intermittent or incomplete intestinal obstruction as a cause of recurrent pain, here usually associated with vomiting. Every children's surgeon of experience must have had the satisfaction of operating on a child labelled periodic syndrome through the years and curing the condition by correcting a *Malrotation* or removing a *Meckel's diverticulum*. It is not always easy to keep these occasional triumphs in perspective with the frequent and more mundane troubles of the little belly-acher (Apley's telling phrase).

The *specific mesenteric adenitis of Tuberculosis* must still be borne in mind. Recurrent abdominal pains with vague, ill-localized tenderness and malaise may occur during the course of an abdominal primary infection and later breakdown of glands or intestinal ulceration may occur. The Mantoux test, the persistently raised E.S.R. and perhaps the social history may lead to the diagnosis or to a laparotomy which confirms it.

Ulcerative colitis in childhood may have an atypical onset with recurrent pains and nothing impressive in the way of diarrhœa. The parents will usually comment that the child seems ill and tired out during the bouts.

The pain from *Infective hepatitis* may continue for as long as a year or more.

Girls at the *Menarche* will often get recurrent pains not necessarily at fixed intervals.

If the child has an irregular bowel habit with his pains then stool examination may reveal a chronic infection such as *Salmonella typhimurium* or Sonne dysentery.

Constipation is rather an overworked diagnosis in accounting for recurrent abdominal pains. Chronic constipation is surprisingly painless even when it reaches the state of rectal inertia and overflow incontinence. Acute constipation in a child who usually has regular motions is quite a different matter and can cause a severe acute lower abdominal pain.

Finally, one must remember that pain felt in the abdomen may only be referred there. The primary lesion may be elsewhere, e.g. a *Spinal* lesion giving root pain as in the now rare Pott's disease (tuberculous spondylitis) or a basal *Chest* lesion irritating the diaphragm from the upper side.

Scheme of Approach

A careful history is the most valuable single tool. The details of the *type* and *timing* of the pains; possible onset factors, and attention to the background of the family and their attitude to the condition are all important. Apley has said that the farther the pain is from the umbilicus the more likely it is to have an organic cause.

INVESTIGATION

In most cases a full *blood count* will be justified to exclude such conditions as glandular fever (infective mononucleosis), to note the eosinophilia of some allergic conditions, and to rule out a polymorph leucocytosis from some hidden infective lesion (even appendicitis). A *Heaf test* is also more or less routine as is a *urinalysis.*

Plain radiography is unlikely to be rewarding—an occasional renal calculus may be seen, but in these cases lateral pain and other signs and symptoms will probably be specific pointers to proceed further to intravenous pyelography. Abdominal distension, visible peristalsis or copious vomiting will suggest an obstructive cause and be a specific indication for plain X-ray. The demonstration of calcified glands on plain X-ray is not uncommon, but it is really of no help, for it tells one nothing of their possible activity or quiescence.

A barium meal and follow-through is in general an unrewarding investigation. Obviously, pain or tenderness in the epigastrium or a relationship to feeding may be specific indications and may reveal a peptic ulcer even in this age group. However, the rare peptic ulcer of childhood often presents without specific features in the pains, though a positive family history is usual. Crohn's disease is a rarity which might also be demonstrated in this way.

Intravenous pyelography is the contrast examination most likely to help in childhood. It should be performed in all cases where the pain is lateralized. But many young children fail to localize renal pains to the side. Clearly it would be impracticable as well as unwise to perform a pyelogram on all children with recurrent abdominal pains. But in those in which continued observation suggests the likelihood of an organic cause the investigation should be done. Campbell has stressed that uropathies in children may be missed because of the alimentary symptoms of urinary disease, i.e. presentation with anorexia, malaise, vague abdominal pains, perhaps vomiting and fever.

Throat swabs may reveal pathogens in children with little complaint referable to the throat and response to treatment suggests that this recurrent tonsillitis or pharyngitis may be the underlying cause of some recurrent pains.

Similarly a stool culture may reveal pathogens such as *Shigella sonnei* in occasional cases without frank diarrhœa.

SURGERY. Sometimes one has to open the abdomen as a final investigation. Often this ends in the removal of an apparently normal appendix. Sometimes a Meckel's diverticulum, tuberculous adenitis or other cause of symptoms is revealed. It may become the last resort to relieve anxiety of all concerned. If the child has been fully investigated a McBurney incision is quite adequate for the necessary exploration.

Conclusion

It is particularly important to avoid becoming over-enthusiastic in investigating these pains as one just possible rarity after another is considered and every bodily avenue explored. Particularly should one be chary of raising the bogey of the grumbling appendix. The story of the functional pains described earlier in the chapter is usually a typical one. When the diagnosis is made commonsense advice on coping with the attacks must be given as well as explanation and reassurance that the trouble is usually self-limiting. Very few will need formal child guidance.

If doubt persists as to the nature of the attacks, it is often helpful to arrange for *admission to hospital during an attack*. Observation, exclusion of physical signs and simple investigations will then usually enable one to pin-point a physical cause or be more confident in excluding one. This is preferable to repeated outpatient attendances between attacks at which little further information may be gleaned and confidence is bound to be undermined.

REFERENCES

Apley, G. and Mackeith, R. (1962) *The Child and his Symptoms*, Blackwell Scientific Publications.
Kempton, J. J. (1956) The periodic syndrome, *Brit. med. J.*, i, 83–86.

CHAPTER 21

ACUTE APPENDICITIS

APPENDICITIS is the commonest cause of urgent admission to the surgical wards of a children's hospital. Though it may occur at any time from birth to old age the incidence in children rises as they get older and reaches its peak in the mid-teens. Deaths from appendicitis in childhood are now rare, but tragedies still occur, especially in children under the age of 3 years where the diagnosis may not be entertained until the condition is advanced. It must be emphasized that appendicitis is not rare in children of 2 and 3 years of age, and that it occurs even in infancy.

Pathology

Acute appendicitis is an infection of the vermiform appendix. In some cases there is definite evidence that the infection reaches the appendix by the blood stream, for example, from a focus in acute tonsillitis, but in the majority of cases it seems likely that the infection is the result of coliform organisms in the bowel content entering the bowel wall through some breach in the mucosa.

There are two factors involved in acute appendicitis, one is the *bacterial infection* and the other is *obstruction*. The lumen of the appendix is a narrow one. It may be blocked by a fæcolith, by a fibrous stricture the result of previous inflammation, or by the acute swelling of lymphoid tissue in the wall. When the lumen is blocked the pressure rises in the blind end distal to the obstruction and interferes with the venous return from the organ. The result is to add tissue necrosis to the infective element. The condition may thus pass through the stages of acute catarrhal, suppurative and then gangrenous and perforated appendicitis. A fæcolith may cause a localized area of necrosis and perforation at the actual site of obstruction.

In the young infant the omentum is thin and filmy and it has been said that it thus provides little protection against the spread of infection. However, the localization of infection from a perforated appendix is usually largely performed in this age group by adhesion of surrounding coils of bowel, rather than by the omentum alone, and these will frequently be seen to be carrying out their localizing function efficiently. It has been said also that generalized peritonitis more readily occurs in these young children and that it may be the first indication of intra-abdominal upset. However, careful studies have suggested that the increased danger to life which used to exist at this age and the increased proportion of cases complicated by the presence of a mass or peritonitis can largely be ascribed *to delay in diagnosis.* This results from the unfortunate traditional teaching that the disease is rare under the age of 3 years. *It is not rare under the age of 3, it is merely less common than in older patients.*

When the infection reaches beyond the wall of the appendix it may result in spreading peritonitis and eventually generalized peritonitis, or it may be walled off, producing an appendix mass. The term appendix mass is preferable to that of appendix abscess because exploration of these cases reveals that most of the mass consists of a wall of adherent bowel, omentum and thick fibrinous deposits, whilst the central core of pus around the appendix is usually surprisingly small.

DIAGNOSIS

J. B. Murphy's triad remains a sound basis for the diagnosis of acute appendicitis:

PAIN
VOMITING
FEVER

Pain is almost always the first symptom. In the very young it may not always be specifically complained of, and then the first sign may be a spell of irritability followed by continuous crying. The pain is typically a continuous one, although there may be waves of increased severity. It starts in the centre of the abdomen and moves to the right iliac fossa. This is first of all a tension pain in the inflamed, distended organ felt centrally through the splanchnic nerves, and then, as the infection spreads through the wall, the parietal peritoneum is irritated producing a local pain at the site of the appendix.

Vomiting usually follows within a few hours of the onset of pain. It is typically of stomach contents and only repeated once or twice. Vomiting may be more persistent in the obstructive form of appendicitis. There may be no vomiting, but if not there is almost always anorexia. *The child who is hungry virtually never has appendicitis.*

The *fever* associated with appendicitis is typically moderate, perhaps 37·7° or 38·3°C (100° or 101°F). It may be absent early in the disease. It becomes higher when the stage of peritonitis is reached, but unfortunately at this stage diagnosis is much less likely to be in doubt.

On examination of the typical case the child will be lying quietly in the bed, looking ill. He will have a brown furred tongue and a fœtor oris. Examination of the abdomen will reveal localized tenderness and involuntary rigidity over the appendix area.

Such a typical case is clearly easy to diagnose. Unfortunately, in appendicitis a typical case is uncommon. This account has been given to form a basis on which to form a picture of appendicitis in childhood, and this common and important disease will now be discussed more fully.

The diagnosis is based on the sum of the symptoms and signs. There may be no clear symptoms in the young patient, for the child may not specifically complain and the mother will describe an irritable spell followed by persistent crying. The history is crucial and time should be spent on piecing it together from the parents and from the child. If little history can be obtained there must be some definite signs if the diagnosis is to be upheld. The aphorism that either the history is a good one or the signs are definite is a reliable saying. One is fortunate, indeed, to have both typical. The chronology of the illness is important and it is often wise to begin by asking when the child was last perfectly well. Then specific enquiries should be made regarding any previous simlar episodes and it is always wise to enquire about possible dietary iniiscretions and the presence of infections in other members of the family, before going on to the remainder of the history.

Two small practical points may help. The first is that the history should be taken sitting down. The full story may often take 20 minutes or so to collect and is less likely to be rushed when every one is comfortable. The second is to make notes of the story as it is obtained. This makes for greater accuracy, allows easier recall and gives everyone time to collect their thoughts.

The Symptoms

Pain. Pain is the first and most important symptom in appendicitis. It may be difficult to analyse a child's pain in detail, but it is usually possible to get some idea of its duration. In the older child it is useful to have a series of questions to obtain such particulars. A normally talkative child will usually be less communicative when ill and the doctor may also be an inhibiting influence. Indeed, the loquacious young patient more often than not does not require surgery because he does not have appendicitis. It is important to phrase the questions in a language the child will understand and to give him alternatives as far as possible. For example, Have you got a pain in your tummy? When did it start? Did it come on suddenly or gradually? When was it at its worst? How is it now? Has it been in the same place or has it moved about? Has it kept you awake or do you think it will keep you awake? It it coming and going or is it there all the time? Have you ever had a pain like it before? Does it hurt to sit up?

Pain may even be absent if the condition has been slow to develop; if the infection has been masked by antibiotics given earlier, or if an abscess is already forming. The old aphorism of Rutherford Morison that if it lasts more than six hours it is not green apples is a good one. The typical pain of appendicitis is a continuous central pain moving to the right iliac fossa. There may be waves of increased severity. On direct questioning the child will, however, usually admit to persistent pain. In obstructive appendicitis the pain may indeed be intermittent, but intermittent pain is more commonly due to some transient infection than to appendicitis.

The pain may also arise in the right iliac fossa from the beginning. This is more likely to occur in a child who has had previous attacks of appendicitis which have already sealed off the organ. But the story of pain beginning in the right iliac fossa should always make one more suspicious of a urinary cause than appendicitis.

Vomiting. Vomiting is rarely present before the pain in appendicitis. Vomiting as a first symptom is more suggestive of an acute gastritis than appendicitis. *In young children, however, the pain may not be complained of and vomiting may then be the presenting symptom.* It is usually only repeated once or twice and the vomitus is not bile-stained. The patient may only have nausea (feel like being sick). Loss of appetite in a healthy child is a danger signal. The child with appendicitis is not hungry but may complain considerably of thirst.

BOWEL MOVEMENTS. Constipation is frequently present but a history of diarrhœa is not uncommon. So many parents give laxatives routinely that it is worthwhile to ask when the last laxative was given. A history of chronic constipation which is so often obtained in children of all ages is of no real significance in making a diagnosis.

MICTURITION. The urinary system must be investigated by question and answer because disturbances of micturition are less likely to be noticed by the mother than disturbances of defæcation. Does it hurt to pass urine (do a wee-wee)? Have the parents noticed any increased frequency of micturition or any change in the character of the urine?

MENSTRUATION. In any girl over 11 years of age details of the menarche and recent menstrual periods should be sought out.

PREVIOUS ATTACKS. Previous attacks similar to the present complaint should be gone into in detail.

Headache is rarely present in appendicitis before the stage of peritonitis. Its presence should lead one to suspect some other diagnosis. Sore throats often occur in cases of acute mesenteric adenitis and the presence of recent respiratory infection may provide a clue to this condition. Children prone to travel sickness often have a tendency to recurrent abdominal pain and vomiting, and this feature should be borne in mind.

The time taken in obtaining this history will also serve to accustom the child to the presence of the doctor. He sees that the doctor is on good terms with his parents and this helps to establish rapport. This in turn makes the physical examination easier and more valuable.

Examination

The pulse is taken for a full minute to serve as an introduction between the child and the doctor It is usually raised and rates of over 120 per minute mean peritonitis if the condition is in fact an abdominal one. However, in the older child the pulse rate may be normal in the presence of early acute appendicitis. A rectal temperature is the most reliable in infants. In toddlers the axilla is usually used and in older children an oral temperature is preferred. *It is important to take the temperature for a minimum of two minutes.* The fever is usually a moderate one of 37·7°C (100°F) or perhaps 38·3°C (101°F). In older children there may on occasion be no pyrexia. This usually means an obstructive appendicitis, but it may only mean the hurried taking of the temperature before the child has settled in after his journey to hospital.

The colour of the facies can be misleading. There seems to be a tendency for the constitutional colour of the child to be deepened—the ruddy child is a brighter red while the pale child appears even paler. The sclera should always be examined. Many cases of infective hepatitis presenting with abdominal pain and vomiting have been missed by neglecting this part of the examination. The alæ nasi may be working in young children with peritonitis. This is because their respiration is largely diaphragmatic. Fixation of the diaphragm by peritonitis hence causes respiratory distress and brings the accessory muscles into play. So this "sign of pneumonia" may be misleading.

An examination of the mouth is useful. The lips are often dry and cracked from voluntary fluid limitation and dehydration. Examination of the tongue will usually show a dry brown coated tongue, which may, however, be present in many digestive upsets. There is a coliform fœtor oris which is often considered to be a characteristic sign of appendicitis. The presence of acute inflammation of the tonsils or pharyngitis is significant, being more common in acute mesenteric adenitis than in true appendicitis. Quite mild tonsillar inflammation may cause considerable cervical adenitis, and in children the presence of some shotty non-tender lymph nodes in the neck must be regarded as normal.

For examination of the chest and abdomen the pyjama jacket or nightgown must be removed, not just opened. The heart and lungs are always examined. There is usually tachypnœa in a young child with peritonitis. The abdominal wall and diaphragm are immobilized by the inflammation. As has already been said, children of this age breathe abdominally, so that this results in a raised respiratory rate. The lungs must be carefully examined. Basal pneumonia may cause abdominal pain. Pneumonia may also be associated with septicæmia causing a paralytic ileus and simulating appendicitis with peritonitis.

In the examination of the abdomen it is often helpful to begin by observing the movements of the abdominal wall. This takes time and is less frightening to the child than the immediate descent of a large hand on the abdomen. After observation for the presence of free movement of the abdominal wall the abdomen should be auscultated. The silent abdomen is classically considered a sign of peritonitis, but in young children at least bowel sounds may persist even in the presence of gross peritonitis.

Next, one should ask the patient to point to the most tender place on the abdomen. In the case of appendicitis the child will usually point with one finger to a small definite area. Other conditions, such as acute mesenteric adenitis, have a more diffuse tenderness and this can be recognized by the child's vague demonstration of the site of the pain.

Palpation begins in the quadrant farthest away from the pain, usually the left hypochondrium, and moves around the abdomen recognizing the presence of tenderness and involuntary rigidity. Care and patience are needed to distinguish voluntary guarding in a nervous child from true involuntary rigidity, the only sign of underlying inflammation.

The willingness or otherwise to move or sit up in bed may be helpful. Gurgling of the cæcum is often said to make appendicitis unlikely but it is not a reliable sign.

Point tenderness is important in an older child. But most of the very young children will not present as acute appendicitis, but as peritonitis or an appendix mass resulting from a perforated appendix. Localized tenderness is uncommonly seen under the age of 3 years because they are rarely recognized at the earlier stage of development of the disease. Tenderness is not so marked in generalized peritonitis, but muscle guarding is still a feature. Board-like rigidity rarely occurs in young children. The abdomen distends rapidly. With the onset of peritonitis vomiting may recur and may become green, bile-stained and copious as a result of paralytic ileus. The temperature becomes higher and the toxæmia and illness of the patient become more marked. The pulse rate rises.

If the child suspected of an abdominal lesion should be asleep it may be worth palpating the abdomen as the first step in examination.

Rectal examination may not be necessary if the diagnosis is already established beyond doubt, but where the cause is not obvious it should always be done. Pelvic abscesses are quite common in children. Localization may be excellent and there may be a gangrenous appendix in a pelvic mass with no abdominal tenderness at all.

Special Patterns of Appendicitis

1. **Between the Ages of One and Four Years.** It has already been said that it is uncommon to see an uncomplicated appendicitis at this age. Almost all present as a peritonitis, usually generalized, or as an appendix mass.

More often than not vomiting is the first sign or symptom to be noticed and the presence of pain is not recognized until later. *There is always a pyrexia and tachycardia.* The child is often sitting up with a flushed face and active alæ nasi when first seen. Even a normally good-natured child is irritable at this stage. The abdomen is warm and tumid. Even with gentle examination there is resistance to palpation in all quadrants. There are often active bowel sounds. Indeed they may be more active than normal. Distension soon occurs. Diarrhœa is rather more frequent than constipation as an early sign of peritonitis. The urine frequently contains a considerable number of pus cells and even organisms. The presence of pyuria leads one to suspect a urinary infection as the cause of the illness; but a degree of pyuria may occur in appendicitis, presumably because the inflamed organ irritates an adjacent ureter or bladder.

2. **Variations with the Position of the Appendix.** The appendix, particularly in the young infant, may be *high on the right side* due to an undescended cæcum. The subhepatic appendix when inflamed will produce tenderness under the liver instead of in the usual position at McBurney's point which is one-third of the way along a line from the anterior superior iliac spine to the umbilicus. In its early stages such tenderness may be mistaken for hepatic tenderness and give rise to suspicions of hepatitis. The appendix lying behind the cæcum produces tenderness well out in the flank which may be mistaken for renal tenderness. The presence of the overlying bowel prevents the inflammation from irritating the parietal peritoneum in the earlier stages and the typical localized point tenderness is frequently absent.

The pelvic appendix again is out of contact with the anterior abdominal wall and hence there may be no physical signs in the abdomen. However, a rectal examination will demonstrate a localized tender swelling in the rectal wall. Tenderness is difficult to evaluate in the young child, but the presence of a hot boggy swelling is usually unmistakable.

It should be remembered, however, that there is a no-man's land *behind the bladder* where the appendix may be adherent, too high to palpate from the rectum and too low to produce tenderness in the abdomen. In such a case one may be presented with an infant or child who is irritable and off colour, and who if young enough may not be complaining of pain. Yet there are no physical signs to account for the malaise and fever. A white cell count may show a high leucocytosis. Otherwise careful observation and repeated examination over a few hours are necessary, when signs per rectum or per abdomen will begin to show themselves and confirm the diagnosis.

The retro-ileal appendix may also produce an unusual picture. Protection from the anterior abdominal parietes leads to the absence of any localized or acutely tender point. Instead there is a vague discomfort in the centre of the abdomen associated with some distension of the bowel and a picture not unlike that of an early enteritis. In this type, vomiting may precede the presence of pain and may be persistent.

3. **Previous Attacks may Modify the Picture.** If the appendix has already been sealed off in the retrocæcal area then the next attack may present as a pain beginning out in the flank with anorexia, with or without vomiting.

4. **Appendicitis may Follow Respiratory or Enteral Infection.** Two of

the commonest imitators of acute appendicitis in their early stages are upper respiratory infections and gastro-enteritis. It is extremely important to remember that both these conditions can not only imitate appendicitis but may precipitate a true attack. If appendicitis occurs along with an upper respiratory infection it is usual for it to begin not at the onset of infection but after a day or two has elapsed. The story may be of a child who has an acute tonsillitis and after a day or two in bed complains of persistent abdominal pain and appears to be more ill and nauseated. Abdominal signs of appendicitis appear. The presence of the tonsillitis must be no deterrent to proceed to appendicectomy if the signs are such as would otherwise lead one to the diagnosis. It should also be remembered that measles is an acute respiratory infection which happens to have a rash on the fourth day. Like the other respiratory infections it produces frequent abdominal colics during its course, but also more rarely may precipitate an attack of appendicitis during the fever.

It is also possible for an attack of gastro-enteritis to be complicated by the presence of true appendicitis and one has on several occasions grown a pure culture of *Shigella sonnei* from the acutely inflamed or perforated appendix of such patients. Again, if the abdominal signs are typical of appendicitis the knowledge that there has been a gastro-enteritis in the family should not deter one from operation.

5. **Appendix Mass.** An appendix mass may be present insidiously at any age. There has usually been a spell at the onset when the child is off colour with anorexia, perhaps an isolated vomit and mild abdominal pain. A moderate pyrexia is usual but not invariable. The diagnosis is clinched by the finding of a mass in the right iliac fossa. It is usually acutely tender but may not be in some cases, particularly if it has been slow to develop or is a recurrent mass. A mass in the right iliac fossa even though not typically acutely tender should be considered as an appendix mass until proven otherwise. An appendix mass may be entirely within the pelvis. There may be no abdominal findings whatever, and it may only be palpable per rectum.

6. **Painless Appendicitis.** Though rare, this does occur for a variety of reasons.

Subacute onset. The patient's symptoms may date back a week in all and, in that time, the appendix has slowly become inflamed.

The inflammatory process is aborted by antibiotics. A misdiagnosis of urinary infection or pharyngitis may be followed by a short course of sulphonamide or oral penicillin which may mask the symptoms.

Pelvic position. It may lie out of contact with the sensitive parietal peritoneum. It is tender but this can be detected only on rectal examination.

Constitutional insensitivity. The stoic small boy who has been brought up to appreciate that "girls cry but boys don't" and the mentally retarded child present pitfalls.

Differential Diagnosis

It may be said at once that the diseased appendix presents some of the most difficult diagnostic problems in surgery. This does not mean that the majority cannot be readily diagnosed. In the past the dangers of the condition were so many and so serious that over-diagnosis was stressed and the "if in doubt have it out" school of thought had everything on its side. With the modern management of peritonitis and paralytic ileus in particular the mortality has dropped to 1 or 2 per cent in children. Furthermore the remaining mortality is principally in the really young children with peritonitis or an appendix abscess formed before they are first seen. In these the diagnosis is quite clear (and immediate surgery may not be indicated). There is therefore now much less justification for the practice of appendicectomy on suspicion.

It is important to have definite diagnoses—perhaps they are better called labels—to apply to conditions which simulate acute appendicitis. There are two reasons for this. The first is that it helps to clarify one's own thoughts in considering alternative possibilities, and secondly in the management of the parents. A diagnostic title must be produced if confidence is to be maintained in the majority of cases. Most parents prefer a positive diagnosis rather than a statement that "this is not appendicitis but I don't know what it is".

ACUTE NON-SPECIFIC MESENTERIC ADENITIS

This is perhaps the commonest condition to simulate appendicitis. It is also the one which may most closely resemble it. The differential diagnosis is usually easy, although sometimes difficult and occasionally impossible. It is more difficult to differentiate it in patients under 5 years of age. Mesenteric adenitis tends to be more sudden in onset and to reach its peak more quickly. The temperature rises rapidly and usually goes up beyond 38·3°C (101°F) within a matter of hours. The pain is severe within a short time. It is spasmodic and not persistent. There may be vomiting, but this is much less frequent than in appendicitis. Indeed the appetite is often unaffected by the trouble and this gives a strong suggestion that appendicitis is not present. Constipation is not a feature. There is frequently a history of a recent respiratory infection. Almost always there have been previous attacks of short duration. Usually all is well again within a day or two.

The pyrexia may be out of all proportion to the other physical signs and the child does not look ill. The pulse rate is often normal. There may be a mild conjunctivitis and a running nose or snuffles. A herpetic sore on the upper lip is common in mesenteric adenitis but rare in appendicitis. On examining the mouth, fœtor is not so commonly present nor is the tongue coated. The tonsils are often enlarged and inflamed, or they may have been recently removed. Cervical lymphadenitis is usually noticed.

When the child is asked to point to the most tender spot the fore-finger usually goes near the umbilicus, but the localization may be vague in contradistinction to the precise localization of the tender spot in the majority of cases of appendicitis. The abdomen is not distended and is usually scaphoid. Tenderness is more often medial to the outer border of the rectus abdominis than lateral to it. It is less accurately localized and may move from place to place on repeated examination. The reverse is true in acute appendicitis. True involuntary rigidity is uncommon. The enlarged mesenteric lymph nodes may sometimes be palpated and if they are low in the ileocæcal region they may be mistaken for an inflamed appendix. Rectal examination is inconclusive. One of the diagnostic features is the prompt way the illness abates. Often the patient is completely better in 24 hours. Its course is characteristically a fluctuating one. Observation over a period of a few hours distinguishes it from appendicitis by revealing a varying picture from time to time instead of the progressive picture of appendicitis which is usually accompanied by a rising pulse rate. During observation of a doubtful case a half-hourly pulse chart is invaluable. First, it ensures that a nurse sees the child regularly and, secondly, it will ensure that a serious progress to peritonitis following appendicitis is not missed. If one is still in genuine doubt between acute mesenteric adenitis and acute appendicitis after a period of 8 hours' observation then it is justifiable to perform an appendicectomy to settle the matter. Under present-day conditions it is perfectly safe to observe such patients in this way and there can be little justification for immediate appendicectomy in such doubtful cases.

PERIODIC SYNDROME

This is discussed in the chapter on Recurrent Abdominal Pain. However, even a periodic syndrome must have a first atack, and it is not uncommon for the patient during a more severe episode to be referred for consideration of acute appendicitis. The patient is more often a girl, usually intelligent, and aged between 9 and 13 years. The syndrome includes abdominal pain, nausea, perhaps vomiting, headache, pallor usually with dark circles under the eyes, and commonly a history of travel sickness. Not all the features of the condition are present together, but the pattern described is that of a type frequently seen. There is often a family history of abdominal pains, of asthma, or of migraine. The attacks of pain or vomiting usually last about 15 to 60 minutes, but may recur over a period of 2 or 3 days during which time the child is off colour. The stress of life is a factor and the school background is often a worry to the child. The differential diagnosis is made on the history of the person more than on the physical examination. There is almost never a pyrexia and constipation is not a feature. Any abdominal guarding is of the voluntary nervous variety and convincing localized tenderness is absent. This condition is less commonly seen, however, in the acute stage but is usually referred by the practitioner for an opinion on the attacks after they have passed off.

ENTERITIS

The early stages of this condition are frequently puzzling. There is crampy abdominal pain and vomiting. The diarrhœa may be much *delayed* but a sharp pyrexia frequently develops. The abdomen is soft, rumbling and yielding to palpation, although there may be a slight diffuse tenderness and the routine rectal examination may produce the first abnormal stool. Some recent unusual features in the diet or involvement of other members of the family may give a clue to the condition.

URINARY CONDITIONS

Urinary infection frequently presents as an acute abdominal condition and may readily be mistaken for appendicitis. Specifically urinary symptoms may not appear until quite late. The pyrexia is usually of rapid onset and it is often high. Vomiting is common and headache frequent. Sweating is a feature commonly seen. Abdominal tenderness is usually bilateral and most marked in the loins. But there is no true rigidity. Urinalysis reveals pyuria, organisms and in about half the cases, albuminurias.

Acute nephritis may also present with abdominal pain as the most marked symptom. Puffiness of the face might lead to the suspicion of this condition, and examination of the urine will reveal albuminuria, red cells and casts. The naked-eye appearance of scanty, smoky urine may be quite typical, and the blood pressure may be raised above the normal for the child's age.

Renal colic may also be a pitfall, but here the pain is all on one side and comes in severe waves which may be so marked as to cause vomiting. The patient is rendered restless by the pain. Sweating almost always occurs and terminal dysuria is common. The urine will contain red blood cells and frequently crystals of oxalate. An X-ray may show no stones, but a crystal the size of a pin-head can cause severe renal colic. Renal colic may also be the presenting symptom of hydronephrosis or other renal tract anomalies (see Chapter 24).

INFECTIVE HEPATITIS

Infective hepatitis often causes abdominal pain before jaundice has become apparent. Indeed, in abortive cases clinical jaundice may never arise. Vomiting is common and anorexia marked. The pain is usually vaguely localized and the site of tenderness is over the hepatic edge and higher than usual for appendicitis. Later on the presence of bile in the urine and a raised serum bilirubin, or frank jaundice first seen in the sclera may be diagnostic. There may be a local epidemic of hepatitis to draw attention to the possibility of this condition.

PNEUMONIA

Pneumonia is usually only a difficult problem in the young child under 5 years old. The septicæmia of a perforated appendicitis and the immobilization of the abdominal wall and diaphragm from the peritonitis renders respiration rapid in this condition as well as in pneumonia. Basal pneumonia may be present with abdominal pain. Physical signs in the early stages may be difficult to evaluate. The abdominal guarding will be greater in the upper abdomen than the lower. In the older child who will co-operate it will be found that the abdominal guarding becomes less when the breath is held in the case of pneumonia whereas it is persistent in the case of intra-abdominal infection such as peritonitis. An X-ray of the chest may be diagnostic before the physical signs are definite.

UNCOMMON DIFFERENTIAL DIAGNOSES

Anaphylactoid Purpura (Henoch-Schönlein). This condition may cause acute colicky pain and reflex vomiting. The purpuric spots can be overlooked, particularly in artificial light.

Iliac Adenitis. Acute pyogenic iliac adenitis may cause tenderness and a mass in the right iliac fossa. But it is much less acute in onset than appendicitis and the systemic upset is minimal.

Acute Constipation. Acute constipation may cause colicky abdominal pain and vomiting, but the tenderness is much more likely to be absent or left-sided. The child is fit and the condition is relieved by a suppository.

TREATMENT

The treatment of appendicitis is appendicectomy. In most cases the operation should be performed at once, but there are occasions when it should be delayed, sometimes for a matter of hours, sometimes for weeks.

An older child with acute appendicitis, even with the presence of some localized peritonitis, will need little special preparation prior to surgery. Only if the child is markedly dehydrated need an intravenous infusion be set up. It is rarely necessary to give more than half or 1 litre of half-strength plasma before the patient is fit for surgery.

Preoperative Management

When the appendicitis has become complicated by spreading or generalized peritonitis the preparation becomes much more important. It is more particularly in the very young child that the disease is likely to be seen at this late stage and it is in this age group that most of the childhood mortality occurs. There is usually a rising pyrexia with an increasing tachycardia associated with the septicæmia, and dehydration. If surgery takes place in this phase there is a danger of hyperpyrexia and peripheral vascular failure on the operating table as the induction of anæsthesia raises the temperature and accelerates the pulse rate. The important point is to begin treatment quickly but to *delay surgery until the temperature and pulse are under control*. It is a valuable rule not to operate immediately on a patient with a pulse rate over 120 beats per minute, or a temperature of more than 38·3°C (101°F). If either of these limits are exceeded preparation should take place prior to surgery.

The two essential points in preparation are the control of the septicæmia by antibiotics and the correction of dehydration by intravenous fluids.

Gastric Suction. A polyvinylchloride gastric tube should also be passed to empty the stomach. In addition to repeated aspirations, continuous suction drainage should be applied. This prevents the onward passage of more swallowed air. Such swallowed air is the main cause of the abdominal distension which develops when peritonitis has reached the stage of causing adynamic ileus.

Antibiotics. Ampicillin and streptomycin, two bactericidal drugs convenient for injection, are usually used; 250 mg. ampicillin every six hours with streptomycin 40 mg. per kilogram body weight daily in four divided doses are given.

Intravenous Fluids. A readily accelerable intravenous infusion is started. The needle or stab technique should be used if possible, but in chubby children of the younger age group it may be difficult to introduce a needle with an adequate bore. If it cannot be done there should be no hesitation in cutting down on a vein and putting in a wider bore piece of polythene or nylon tubing. The left antecubital fossa is a preferred site for infusion as it is near to the anæsthetist, away from instruments and surgeon. The initial intravenous fluid infusion can be given quite rapidly as the deficit is usually of 500 to 1,000 ml. Our practice is to give 250 to 500 ml. half-strength plasma within the first hour and the same amount over the next 4 hours. It may be felt that these are large quantities of intravenous fluid for say a two-year-old but a patient with peritonitis will have a large deficit. An indwelling catheter is invaluable to collect the urinary output and judge the effect of treatment by observation of quantity and specific gravity. These measures, antibiotics and fluid infusion, are the principal weapons in combating the ill effects of peritonitis, but other measures are of value.

Sedation. Sedation is important even if the child is not complaining of pain, and morphine may be given in doses of $\frac{1}{20}$ mg. per kilogram body weight. The atmosphere should be kept cool. When the temperature has broken and is below 38·3°C (101°F) and the pulse is dropping *pro rata*, the patient is premedicated for the operating theatre.

The Operation

Anæsthesia is most commonly achieved by the use of nitrous oxide and oxygen given by endotracheal tube with small divided doses of short-acting muscle relaxants, or fluothane may be used.

The abdomen is palpated once more under the anæsthesia. It is frequently a help in siting the incision, for a small mass may be felt when the muscles are relaxed.

A McBurney incision is most widely used. We have not had occasion to regret it. Even if a diagnostic error is made then it is possible to excise an inflamed Meckel's diverticulum or to reduce an intussusception through this incision. Other lesions mistaken for appendicitis are unlikely to require any further operative procedures. If there is doubt about the site for the McBurney incision then it should be made high up in the flank rather than in the pelvis to allow the exposure of an incompletely descended cæcum. The pelvic appendix usually presents no difficulties in removal unless there is an abscess present and the real problems are the high retrocæcal organs. Furthermore, the high incision can be readily converted to a wider exposure should this be required. The split may be continued laterally, or medially by dividing the rectus sheath and retracting that muscle to the midline.

The appendix is removed and the stump invaginated with a purse-string suture. Retrograde appendicectomy, i.e. removal from base to tip rather than the reverse, is frowned upon as it frequently means that the exposure is inadequate. If the appendix is found to appear normal then it should not be removed until other pathological conditions have been sought. The right uterine tube and ovary should be felt in girls and the small bowel is routinely searched for a Meckel's diverticulum. In a fit patient a symptomless Meckel's diverticulum observed *en passant* during operation should be removed at appendicectomy. When inspection of the right uterine tube and ovary is required during such an operation they may be found to be somewhat elusive. A pack is put into the medial end of the wound to keep away the coils of small intestine. A dry swab is pushed into the pelvis and then withdrawn. The uterine tube comes up with the gauze and can be held in a pair of intestinal forceps and delivered into the field of vision along with the ovary.

If there is a localized or generalized peritonitis as much pus as possible is sucked out of the abdomen, using a properly guarded abdominal suction tube so as to avoid unnecessary trauma to the bowel which may result from the unprotected orifices of a simple suction tube. A swab is taken for culture. Some surgeons use a solution of penicillin and streptomycin in the peritoneal cavity and also use antibiotics in the wound layers, but others are unconvinced of their value. If any intraperitoneal solution is used care must be taken that it is a suitable one which cannot produce adhesions.

No drainage of the peritoneal cavity or the wound is employed.

Ampicillin and streptomycin are given for 5 days after the operation if the appendix has been gangrenous, or peritonitis present. Even in the presence of generalized peritonitis severe postoperative paralytic ileus is infrequent in children and it is rare that intravenous fluids and gastric suction need to be continued for more than 60 hours. We never use long intestinal tubes for bowel decompression. The patient is usually up and about after the second day or as soon after that as he is taking fluids by mouth.

COMPLICATIONS

Serious complications are uncommon. Superficial *wound infection* is not so uncommon. It occurs in about 1 in 10 cases of appendicectomy and this is probably because in pædiatric practice about 40 per cent of cases of acute appendicitis are already perforated by the time they reach the hospital, so that contamination of the field becomes inevitable in a proportion of cases. The wound infection is almost always in the sub-cutaneous layers. The usual story is that the wound heals and that towards the end of the first week it then begins to look red and pus collects beneath the healed wound. Probing at the tender spot will usually break open the wound and release it.

A pelvic abscess is particularly likely to follow a gangrenous pelvic appendix or a fæcolith liberated in the pouch of Douglas. Spontaneous resolution or discharge into the rectum is the usual solution in children. If there are signs (abdominal tenderness or guarding) suggesting the presence of spreading infection around the abscess then antibiotics should be used to control this.

Subphrenic abscess is rare. It should be suspected when fever, leuco-cytosis and malaise persist for more than two weeks in the absence of evidence of infection elsewhere. X-ray screening of the patient will give help in diagnosis. It will show fixation of the diaphragm by infection and later may demonstrate a frank abscess cavity with a fluid level in it. If a posterior abscess is found it should be drained through the bed of the twelfth rib. An anterior one may be drained through a subcostal incision at the most tender point.

The use of antibiotics has removed almost completely the danger of death by spreading peritonitis in the postoperative management of these cases. It is important to realize, however, that their use can vary the clinical picture of infection by pyogenic organisms. If pus is already sealed off by an abscess cavity wall then the antibiotics cannot reach the centre and they may thus mask an infection instead of curing it. The result is that pyogenic organisms can produce a slowly developing lesion with much less general upset. The lesion is a cold abscess similar to that seen as the result of tuberculous infection. It is important to recognize this altered clinical picture. Any patient who has been on antibiotic therapy must be observed for at least 48 hours after every-thing appears to have settled, and a thorough examination made for residual masses. These may be clinically quiescent when the patient is discharged yet flare up within the next week or month after the anti-biotic control is removed. In an extreme case one of us has seen a girl who had a persistent non-tender thickening in the pouch of Douglas for 2 years after the removal of an acutely inflamed pelvic appendix. Only then did the enlarging mass become a typical acute abscess with central softening and spontaneous discharge into the rectum.

Intestinal obstruction as the result of adhesions following surgery occurs in about 1 in 200 cases. The patient develops colic, vomiting and abdominal distension with increased bowel sounds. An X-ray of the abdomen in the upright position shows fluid levels in dilated bowel. These cases should be operated on to relieve the obstruction. Such a case is easily recognized, but occasionally the earlier onset of mechanical obstruction by bands is masked by the presence of postoperative ileus of the adynamic type in a patient with peritonitis. The established adynamic obstruction is gradually overcome, but mechanical obstruction persists. If this possibility is not recognized then persistence in conservative measures (intravenous infusion and gastric suction) may lead to deterioration of the patient's condition to a stage where the necessary surgery will not be withstood. If the possibility is borne in mind and X-rays are taken these should distinguish the diffuse even distension of all the coils of bowel in adynamic ileus from the progressive distension of the loops down to the level of a mechanical obstruction.

Appendix Mass (Appendix Abscess)

If a mass is clearly palpated at the first examination of the child then the treatment is primarily conservative. Antibiotics are given in full dosage, strict bed rest is enforced and the diet is restricted to fluids and light, easily digested foods. If there has been much vomiting then aspiration of the stomach and continuous gastric suction with intravenous fluid replacement is also used. This régime continues as long as the gastric aspirate remains copious and bile-stained (green). In the vast majority of cases the gastric tube can be taken up within 2 days and fluids started by mouth. The abscess starts to regress and is often gone within a week. The child is kept in hospital until the temperature, pulse rate and tenderness have also settled. A definite date not more than 8 weeks ahead is fixed for interval appendicectomy.

There is almost always a *response* to conservative treatment in 48 hours, the pulse and temperature falling and abdominal guarding over the mass diminishing.

If the mass has not settled satisfactorily within a week on this antibiotic and conservative régime then it is unwise to continue antibiotics indiscriminately. Streptomycin is a quick-acting drug and if it is able to reach the organisms it will destroy them within 48 hours, so that a week's course gives an ample margin. If resolution has not taken place the abscess is so walled off that the drugs are unable to reach the organisms, or the organisms are insensitive to them. Under these circumstances it is better to withold further antibiotics and await natural resolution. If this fails the abscess may be drained by a short muscle-cutting incision overlying it. The important but rare indication for the further use of antibiotics is the development of tenderness and rigidity around the abscess. This is evidence of spread of infection beyond its walls. In the unlikely event of this condition arising antibiotics should be given again and under their control the abscess should be drained, and the appendix removed if this is not too difficult.

Prolonged courses of antibiotics may indeed be successful on occasion in allowing resolution of the abscess, but sometimes they can give rise to a condition which is difficult to manage. A chronic mass with a thick wall may be formed; the patient's general health degenerates with the onset of anæmia, and attempts to withdraw the antibiotics are followed by further extensions and flares of the intra-peritoneal infection. Furthermore, streptomycin is itself a drug with toxic risks, although these are so slight as to be considered negligible in comparison with the risks of the disease itself when it is given with discrimination and by weight as has been described here. It was the introduction of streptomycin in particular that made this conservative régime safe. Other newer antibiotics may be used in combination, but we have no reason yet to prefer them to streptomycin though ampicillin has proven a most useful adjunct.

CHAPTER 22

CONSTIPATION

CONSTIPATION literally means a packing together. In general, the term is used to mean an infrequent bowel habit, although it is sometimes used to describe hard stools. There has been a tendency to blame constipation, without much foundation, for many and varied ailments. Now the pendulum has swung, as it so often does in medicine, to a widespread inclination to consider constipation as never of importance. This is equally untrue.

The passage of hard stools is usually of *dietary* origin. The child may have come to the doctor merely because of maternal anxiety, or because he has painful defæcation or anal fissure (see Chapter 18). It is unlikely to require more than reassurance of the mother and advice to include a variety of fruit, vegetables and *adequate fluid* in the diet. Children are often encouraged to drink so much milk—the excellent food value of which is so widely advertised—that they have little appetite for other foods which would give a more bulky residue. It is a particularly common cause of constipation in the toddler who still insists on a bottle perhaps last thing at night. Milk should be considered as a solid food rather than a mere fluid-supplying beverage.

Transient constipation is common and may be due to dietary changes, dehydration, unaccustomed recumbency or deliberate failure to respond to the call to stool. It is of no importance. Uncomfortable lower abdominal colic may arise and indeed this usually stimulates further attempts at defæcation and solves the matter. It is unlikely that the many cases of recurrent abdominal pain attributed to *chronic* constipation have any connection with the bowel habit. Rather is it surprising how symptomless chronic constipation can be when the bowel has learned to adapt itself to large volumes by adjustment of its plastic tone and eventually by real enlargement of the bowel.

The danger of constipation which has become chronic is the development of incomplete evacuation. Once it begins it is progressive by a vicious circle.

It is therefore sensible to train children to a regular daily habit so as to avoid the tendency for a proportion to develop these troubles. A regular habit of going to the lavatory daily after a meal for a short time should be encouraged. Attempts to coax a child to produce results by leaving him sitting there with toys, books or blandishments are not helpful. The visit should be short, regular and habitual and not become part of a game with emotions involved.

RECTAL INERTIA (ACQUIRED MEGACOLON)

Many people have gone through a long and healthy life habitually opening their bowels every 4 or 5 days. But it is unjustified to take this as meaning that bowel habit training is of no importance. Providing that the bowel is completely emptied no harm ensues. But there is a tendency for the bowel to become overstretched so that some of these children will develop the *rectal inertia syndrome*. The enlarged rectal ampulla does not empty completely and the residuum collects to form a hard impacted mass of fæces which may eventually reach up above the umbilicus. At this stage liquid fæces is likely to leak around the mass in an uncontrollable fashion.

The typical clinical story of rectal inertia is of progressive constipation without serious interference with general health (though irritability and loss of appetite are quite common). Then overflow incontinence of fæces occurs. It is at this stage that anxiety arises and medical advice is sought. Unfortunately the condition at this stage may be mistaken paradoxically for diarrhœa and treated by chalk and opium and antibiotics, making matters worse. On examination, the mass in the lower abdomen is usually palpable and sometimes visible. Rectal examination will reveal a capacious rectal ampulla with a mass of fæces reaching down to the pelvic floor. There may be perianal soiling. At this stage barium examination will show a dilated rectum and distaꞌ colon. The labels megarectum, megacolon, dolichocolon have been applied to the pictures seen and were erroneously thought to be evidence of a primary colonic abnormality, whereas they are merely the results of chronic overloading.

CAUSES OF RECTAL INERTIA. Habitual constipation or rectal inertia arises from various causes.

Some arise from an organic cause; for example, anal stenosis, or spina bifida with a neurological defect resulting in the absence of the sensory stimulation to the defæcation reflex. Many seem to follow a transient cause such as a painful anal fissure. This encourages holding on to the fæces and hence produces an even more painful defæcation next time, and so the circle may go on, ending in rectal inertia with overflow incontinence long after the original fissure has been healed.

Others follow functional causes. For example, prolonged recumbency such as may be needed in the treatment of osteitis. Defæcation in the supine position is difficult and leads to failure to respond to the urge, and then with stretching of the bowel the urge fails to arise.

The majority date from the toddler training period, even though the complication of overflow incontinence may not bring them to the doctor until some years later. Holding back is a common reaction to overstrict or overpermissive training, or it may result from fear of defæcation due to anal fissure or prolapse. It usually settles down after a period but may persist and result in gross constipation with mega-colon and overflow incontinence.

A few cases are associated with really important psychological upsets requiring specialized treatment. But in the majority the functional upset is in itself merely a training problem due to a negative phase which may have settled long before the child is seen. If the condition is explained to the mother as psychological in these days she (and even the doctor) is likely to feel very worried and to lose even more of her confidence in her ability to handle her child. It is usually better to call the matter one of habit training.

Management of Rectal Inertia

Management consists of emptying the bowel; keeping it empty for long enough for it to recover its tone, and then training in regular attempts at defæcation whether the call is felt or not.

Hard, impacted masses may need manual evacuation under general anæsthetic. (The mass may be so hard that the authors have had cases referred as malignant tumours of the pelvis.) Then daily rectal washouts are given until the bowel is *empty* (*not* only until the child starts to have actions). Enemas are useless because the dilated bowel cannot return them efficiently and may be dangerous because water intoxication by absorption from the enlarged bowel may be so rapid as to be fatal. A few ounces of saline are run in by funnel and then syphoned out and the process repeated according to the child's tolerance; 10 to 20 pints a day are usually used. The use of retention enemas of olive oil or detergents beforehand may help the washouts. This procedure can only be carried out without undue upset to the child by practised nurses with plenty of time. It is unfair to expect a district nurse to cope at home unaided, and the upset of hospitalization under modern children's hospital conditions is less than attempts to carry out adequate treatment at home.

When the hard masses have been removed a regular aperient is administered to help evacuation (Senokot, Mixture of Neostigmine, Dulcolax) and these children require and tolerate remarkably high dosage. A tumbler of *warm* water first thing in the morning before breakfast is a most satisfactory, safe and inexpensive laxative. A follow-up has shown that the fear of developing lifelong dependence on aperients by regular dosage is unfounded.

The bowel is kept empty for two more weeks by alternate day and then twice weekly washouts. A weekly washout is continued for a further 2 weeks at least, to prevent re-loading and at this stage *habit training* in regular defæcation (after a meal, twice daily) is begun. This last is the most important part of the management.

Hypertonic phosphate enemas may often be substituted when the hard masses have been removed. They are more convenient—and in milder cases may allow a modified regime to be carried out at home avoiding hospitalization.

The parents of many of these children are poor copers—and this is often the basic reason for the development of the syndrome—so that a tediously prolonged and sympathetic follow-up is essential. Even then, relapse may occur in more severe cases but responds to a further course of similar management.

When the barium enema shows a large megarectum it is tempting to suggest surgical removal. Very rarely this may be necessary. But even then it is utterly useless unless carried out as a relatively small part of a training programme. It should never even be considered until one believes the child will co-operate in such aftercare. Otherwise things seem to go wonderfully well for 6 to 12 months and relapse then occurs.

It has been reasonably said that in a condition where psychological factors are common such physical treatment will have the bad effect of fixing the child's interest on his bowels. But his interests are already fixed on his bowels. These are the children who get the nickname "stinky" at school. Their sense of smell and their schoolfellows will soon make them bowel-conscious, and psychological factors soon follow even in those cases with an organic origin. The quickest way to get their interest away from the bowel is to cure the condition.

ENCOPRESIS

This name, analogous to enuresis, is intended to refer to a condition of loss of control of defæcation (soiling) without any organic local or neurological cause; it is *always* of psychological origin and usually needs expert psychiatric care. Before the convenient label is applied to a child it is essential to know that the condition is not really the commoner overflow incontinence resulting from habitual constipation as described above. The position is analogous to the child with organic urinary retention and overflow incontinence (due to, say, congenital urethral valves) being mistaken for an enuretic.

HIRSCHSPRUNG'S DISEASE (CONGENITAL MEGACOLON)

Hirschsprung's disease is a form of chronic intestinal obstruction now known to be due to absence of intramural ganglia in the distal bowel—usually the rectum and lower sigmoid.

The common presentation used to be as a gross chronic constipation in a puny, pot-bellied child; with crises of tense abdominal distension, increased peristalsis and vomiting. There is an impressive megacolon. Since the work of Swenson, first published in 1948, attention has been focused on the distal undilated bowel as the cause—here again the megacolon is secondary; the normal colon becomes enlarged and hypertrophied in an attempt to overcome the obstruction caused by the

inability of the distal aganglionic bowel to produce a co-ordinated wave
of contraction.

Hirschsprung himself had noticed the undilated distal bowel as long
ago as 1888, and in 1920 Dalle Valle of Naples recognized the aganglionic lesion and familial nature of the disease. Here is an example of
the necessity to make the right discovery at the right time. It fell to
Swenson to make his brilliant observations at a time when infant
surgery was developing and they could be put to practical use.

Bodian studied the specimens of over 200 cases comprising the
Great Ormond Street series. In every case the same lesion was found
—extending from the anus upwards for a varying distance—the
place of the absent ganglia being taken by abnormal clumps of non-
medullated nerve fibres, apparently the searching ends of post-

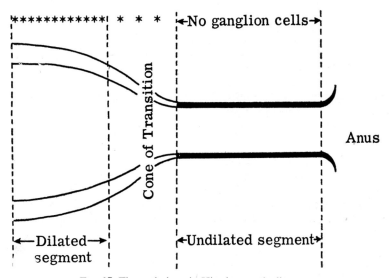

FIG. 37. The pathology in Hirschsprung's disease.

ganglionic fibres. About 70 per cent involve the rectum and lower sigmoid, 15 per cent the rectum only, and 15 per cent extend further up
the colon and may even involve the ileum.

Carter's investigations of the families has confirmed its familial
nature with a preponderance of 5 to 1 of boys to girls in the ordinary
length segments. Long segments arise equally in male and female.
The ordinary and long segment types usually breed true in families.

It is not a common disease, but increased understanding by pædiatricians has brought to light many cases who may in the past have died
in early crises before the underlying condition was recognized. It occurs
in at least 1 in 5,000 births.

PRESENTATIONS

The disease presents a varying clinical picture at its onset. Some symptoms almost always arise *within the first days of life*, though they may be mild.

1. A neonatal low intestinal obstruction may present with repeated bouts of gaseous distention and vomiting; this may be relieved spontaneously or by medical measures (i.e. digital examination of the rectum or rectal washout).

2. Mild remittant obstructive symptoms through infancy following a neonatal obstruction as above, or rarely following a normal neonatal period.

3. Recurrent obstruction may be severe and need continued medical care by daily rectal washouts (which can only be safely carried out in hospital) or colostomy.

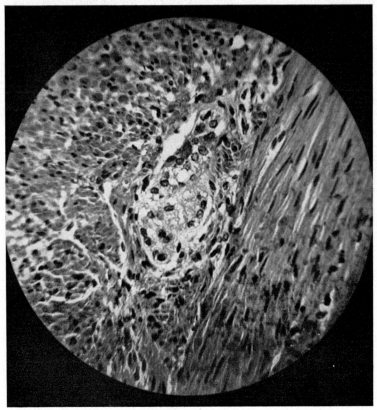

FIG. 38. Photomicrograph of normal bowel to show a ganglion in Auerbach's plexus. (× 300.)

4. Neonatal intestinal obstruction may persist requiring operation forthwith, at which the cause is recognized and a colostomy performed above the aganglionic segment. Frozen section control may be needed to identify the extent of the segment and in a few with long segments ileostomy will be required.

5. Diarrhœa. Paradoxically the disease may present in infancy with frequent loose stools. The baby becomes rapidly ill and dehydrated

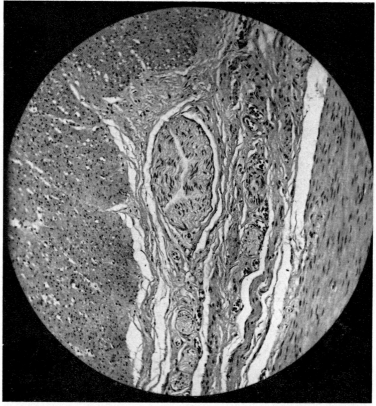

Fig. 39. Photomicrograph of aganglionic segment to show abnormal nerve trunks in place of a ganglion between muscle coats. (× 112.)

and the abdomen is tensely distended. In the past these babies often died under the diagnosis of gastro-enteritis with toxic distension of the bowel. If the possibility of Hirschsprung's disease is borne in mind the passage of a rectal tube will usually produce prompt passage of fluid fæces and amelioration of the baby's condition though colostomy may be urgently required. Without relief of the distension mucosal gangrene and death may rapidly ensue. These crises have been called "putrefactive diarrhœa", or "enterocolitis" but the exact cause of the bouts of production of copious fluid stool is not yet known.

DIAGNOSIS

The survivors of this infant period will usually present the classical picture of Hirschsprung's disease as it used to be seen, though early consideration of the diagnosis has resulted in the majority of the children now being seen in a relatively early phase before gross malnutrition is established. The classical picture is of a stunted, pot-bellied child with flat buttocks and wasted limbs, flared ribs and visible peristalsis in his grossly enlarged colon. Interference with diaphragmatic movements makes chest complications common. The abdomen is grossly distended with wind and *difficulty in passing flatus as well as fœces is distinctive of Hirschsprung's disease* because it is a true though incomplete intestinal obstruction. Rectal examination reveals a clean anus and usually an empty rectum—the fæcal masses may be palpable

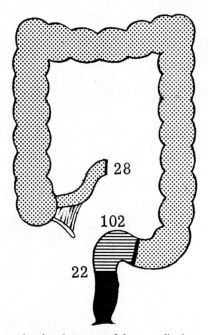

FIG. 40. Diagram showing the extent of the aganglionic segment in a series of 152 cases of Hirschsprung's disease (after G. G. Wyllie). In 22 cases the segment was confined to the lower rectum below the pelvic floor where it cannot be seen from within the abdomen. In 102 cases it reached the usual level up to the lower half of the sigmoid colon. In 28 it reached higher up the colon and occasionally involved the ileum; in these cases an extension of the standard pullthrough resection is required. In every case the aganglionosis extended from the anal margin.

through the bowel wall since they are impacted at the upper end of the segment. Soiling is virtually unknown in Hirschsprung's disease and certainly excludes any but an extremely short affected segment, although diarrhœa may occur during crises of "enterocolitis".

The mortality in untreated cases is about 40 per cent in the first year of life and few will reach adult life. They succumb to obstructive crises with enterocolitis or to intercurrent chest or other infections.

The picture contrasts strongly with that of chronic constipation due

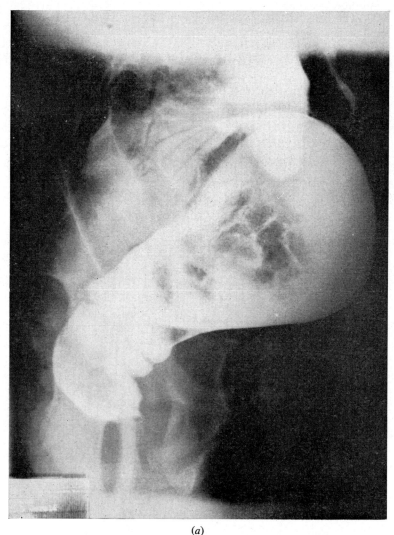

(a)

FIG. 41. (a) Barium enema of Hirschsprung's disease.

to rectal inertia. In the latter the child is not seriously ill; the abdomen is generally flat so that fæcal masses are easily felt or seen. Peristalsis and gaseous retention are not prominent. Rectal examination reveals a capacious ampulla loaded with fæces and the anus may often be soiled by overflow incontinence.

The most useful confirmatory investigation is the *barium enema*. But this must be done by a special technique to demonstrate filling of the unexpanded terminal gut and then the expansion through the cone to the enlarged bowel above. Routine filling of the colon may miss the

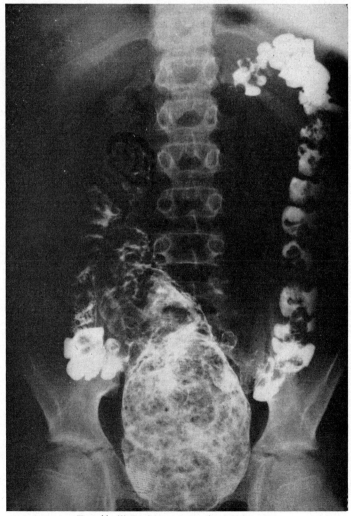

FIG. 41. (*b*) Barium enema of rectal inertia.

lesion as the dilated sigmoid falls into the pelvis and hides the un-expanded rectum. It may also be dangerous as fatal water intoxication has followed absorption from the enormous colon. *Preparation by the usual methods to empty the bowels should be omitted* because the deflation may temporarily relieve the contrast between dilated normal bowel above and undilated rectum below and lead to misdiagnosis.

Some of the milder cases may present similarities to severe rectal inertia. *Rectal biopsy* is a convenient means of settling the matter. Microscopy shows the neurological lesion.

Treatment

Swenson's operation remains established as a sound procedure with good results recorded in follow-ups reaching over 10 years. It is a testing operation and simpler alternatives are being evaluated, e.g. Duhamel's retrorectal, transanal pullthrough; Soave's endorectal pullthrough; and Rehbein's anterior resection with sphincter bou-ginage.

The operation consists of resection of the aganglionic segment right down to the anal canal. This involves a tedious and difficult dissection in the pelvis to preserve the pelvic splanchnics (unlike the adult resections for cancer). The bowel is then intussuscepted through the anus and divided there, so that an accurately placed anastomosis can be made outside the perineum and then pushed back through the anus into place. This is essential, for as little as an inch of retained agang-lionic bowel can cause complete relapse.

Most operators like to carry out a colostomy at diagnosis if the child is seen in infancy, proceeding to the resection at about 6 to 12 months of age. If the child is seen later it is usually possible to prepare him by wash-outs and proceed direct to the resection.

RESULTS. The mortality has been about 5 per cent. About 75 per cent become normal in general health and local condition. About 20 per cent have some residual symptoms. Many of these are so slight as only to be elicited on direct questioning, but some have residual symptoms of Hirschsprung's disease or constipation which may need medical management, and a few have difficulties in control.

REFERENCES

Benson, C. D. and Lloyd, J. R. (1964) An evaluation of the surgical treatment of Hirschsprung's disease, *Surg. Clin. N. Amer.*, **44**, 6, 1495.

Bodian, M., Carter, C. O. and Ward, B. C. H. (1951) Hirschsprung's disease, *Lancet*, i, 302.

Nixon, H. H. (1964) Review article: Hirschsprung's disease, *Arch. Dis. Childh.*, **39**, 204, 109.

Swenson, O. (1950) A new surgical treatment for Hirschsprung's disease, *Surgery*, **28**, 371.

Wyllie, G. G. (1957) The course and management of Hirschsprung's disease, *Lancet*, i, 847.

CHAPTER 23

URINARY INFECTION, HÆMATURIA AND CALCULI

URINARY INFECTION

URINARY infection is a common problem in pædiatric practice. It has become more important in recent years because long term analyses have shown a worse picture than had been anticipated with many patients proceeding to renal failure in childhood or adult life. These reviews have stimulated a more aggressive attitude to early and precise diagnosis and more thorough treatment.

Not every case requires a complete urological investigation. This would be an unpractical approach but *complete investigation should always be undertaken in persistent or recurrent infection.*

There will frequently be some underlying abnormality of the urinary tract. Urinary infection is much commoner in girls but the incidence of important anatomic abnormality causing persistent or recurrent infection is about equal in the sexes. In practice, girls should be investigated if they have more than one attack of infection and boys if they have one. Some abnormality can be expected in about half the children fully investigated.

Terminology. The term "urinary infection" is preferred to pyelitis, pyelonephritis, trigonitis and particularly to cystitis. The urinary tract is in continuity and few infections are as localized as these latter terms suggest.

Presenting Features of Urinary Infection at Different Ages

Infancy. Urinary infection is more likely to present in the first two years of life than at any other time in childhood. It is important to realize this because urinary symptoms are uncommon at this age compared with constitutional symptoms and the majority of severe infections have a remediable anatomical abnormality. Indeed, at this age, the cardinal features are usually anorexia, vomiting and unexplained fevers with inevitable failure to thrive, irritability and constipation or diarrhœa. (What Meredith Campbell has called the "alimentary symptoms of urinary disease in childhood".) The infection may closely mimic gastro-enteritis. These symptoms are common to many disorders of infancy but it is important to keep urinary infection in mind as a possibility in any infant with "failure to thrive". It may well happen that, when the infection becomes established, the symptoms become less prominent and the infant languishes in poor health.

During the neonatal period pyelonephritis may be part of a septi-cæmia with vomiting, refusal of feeds and sometimes a partially obstructive type of jaundice.

Girls from Two to Fourteen Years. Urinary infection is a common bacterial infection in this age group and, since organisms readily ascend the short female urethra, it is four times more common in girls. Because of this, most symptoms are *local* rather than general. Frequency, urgency and dysuria are commoner than an acute febrile illness with rigor, swinging pyrexia, loin pains and tenderness. The pain may not be localized to the renal area. In the younger group there is often wetting by day and perhaps reversion to bed wetting. (Bed wetting without any other symptoms is not caused by organic disease.) Again, the symptoms may become less prominent as the infection becomes established.

Boys from Two to Fourteen Years. Infection in this group is least common but important because it is so often due to a remediable anomaly. There may be loin pain and tenderness with pyrexia and dysuria or there may be a poor urinary stream. This is an important but neglected physical sign in boys with suspected urinary abnormalities. It is helpful in the diagnosis of the important obstruction below the bladder neck. Again the pain may be central rather than localized to the renal area.

Special Investigations

The Urine
Radiology
Endoscopy

The Urine. Bedside urine analysis is crude and the absence of protein in chemical tests is of little significance. In two thirds of proven infec-tions there is no clinically detectable protein in the urine. A fresh warm specimen of urine must be examined under the microscope and cultured within two hours of being passed unless it has been refrigerated to stop overgrowth of contaminants. Adhesive bags are used to collect infants' urine, and a clean midstream catch specimen is adequate in older children. Infection can be present without significant pyuria though this is unusual. It can, even less commonly, be present without bacilluria. Usually, both are present and must be looked for. An unspun drop of urine is examined and normally there should be less than 10 white cells per high power field, or per c.mm. if a counting chamber is used. Over 100 cells c.mm. indicates infection. Quantitative bacteriology is in-valuable if adequate facilities are available. For this the vulva or penis must be carefully cleansed before taking the specimen and the urine must be plated promptly. More than 100,000 organisms per ml., and particularly more than a million organisms per ml., is indicative of infection, while less than 10,000 per ml. probably indicates growth of contaminants. Fortunately, few colony counts fall between 10,000 and 100,000 and so confusion is rare. If the same organism is isolated from three consecutive daily urines, it is wise to assume that infection is present. Suprapubic needle puncture of the full bladder is a simple, safe and invaluable means of obtaining uncontaminated urine in cases of persistent doubt. Organism sensitivity tests to the drugs available are invaluable though *in vivo* results do not always correspond to the *in vitro* tests.

They should precede any but the most urgent and short term treatment and a specimen should *always* be taken before treatment begins. If this has not been done, treatment should be stopped for three days prior to taking such a specimen.

Radiology. The most useful investigations are the intravenous pyelogram and the micturating cystogram. An intravenous pyelogram must be performed in all girls who have had more than one urinary infection and in all boys who have had a single attack. This can be done when the temperature is normal before the infection is fully settled. It is unwise to await complete resolution of the infection before going ahead with the pyelogram because such resolution may not be achieved unless the underlying cause is found. Even high dosages of dye given intravenously are without increased risk in infants and children. Restriction of fluids is an important part of the preparation. The intravenous pyelogram is more informative about the structure and function of the kidneys, and perhaps the ureters, than of the lower part of the tract but useful bladder views and even voiding views can sometimes be obtained.

The Micturating Cystourethrogram. The investigation is of the greatest value in demonstrating structural and functional abnormalities of the lower urinary tract. The bladder is filled with dye by a urethal catheter and radiographs are taken with the catheter *in situ* (cystogram) and, with the catheter removed, during micturition (micturating cysto-urethrogram). Children over four years of age can usually co-operate, but under four years a general anæsthetic is kinder. It is then necessary to exert suprapubic pressure to get a voiding film and this is not so reliable in demonstrating reflux into the ureters. The structural abnormalities shown by this method have been known for a long time, e.g. trabeculation of the bladder, diverticula, ureterocele and posterior urethral valves. These can also be seen by the practised endoscopist. The most important contribution has been to demonstrate functional abnormalities, particularly incompetence at the vesico-ureteric junction, allowing vesico-ureteric reflux, and the less common functional rigidity of the bladder neck, causing a bladder neck obstruction. It also shows the true size of diverticulæ which may seem much smaller on a static film. Cineradiography is not essential though observation on the image intensifier gives more information than spot films. The two radiographs described are generally adequate for clinical purposes. Micturating cysto-urethrography is complementary to the intravenous pyelogram and in hospital practice it is used increasingly. *It is invaluable in patients with persistent infection in whom the intravenous pyelogram is normal*; to show vesico-ureteric reflux in patients with radiologically scarred kidneys; in patients where reflux is suspected for any reason, and in urethral and bladder neck obstructions. Some authorities would say that it is even more useful than an intravenous pyelogram when investigating children under five years of age, particularly girls. It can give information in cases with a high blood urea precluding intravenous urography. In these cases in particular the introduction of infection into an obstructed urinary tract may lead to a fulminating infection and the investigation should be carried out as an immediate preliminary to treatment of the lesion revealed.

Cystourethroscopy will show bladder trabeculation, diverticula or tumours, ectopic or dilated ureteric orifices, ureteroceles and posterior urethral valves or polyps. A ureteric catheter can be passed through the instrument and radio-opaque dye injected into the kidney pelvis or retrograde pyelography. In practice, with radiological improvements, cystoscopy is often used to confirm radiological appearances and it is now uncommon to see something which cannot be shown on an X-ray. Retrograde pyelography is becoming an uncommon investigation in pædiatric urology.

Primary Pyelonephritis and Vesico-Ureteric Reflux

There remains a group of bacterial infections of the kidney in which no anatomical abnormality of the tract is revealed and these may also

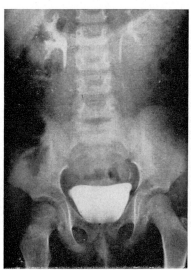

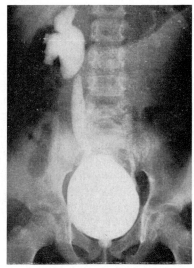

FIG. 42. Normal intravenous pyelogram of four-year-old girl with recurrent urinary infection.

FIG. 43. Micturating cystogram of same girl showing bilateral vesicoureteric reflux.

proceed to fibrosis and destruction of the parenchyma resulting in renal failure. Serial intravenous pyelography is invaluable in assessing their progress. Pyelonephritis may produce an irregular contracted picture of the pelvis or dilatation of the minor calyces due to parenchymal shrinking. More important is the thinning of the cortex recognizable in the early (two minute) film, the nephrogram, typically shown as irregular narrowing opposite certain calyces due to scarring. Serial films may reveal absence of normal growth in a kidney in which the disease is apparently quiescent and this is a bad prognostic sign.

Areas of *dysplasia* in the parenchyma account for at least some of these infections in apparently normal tracts—histologically one may for example see clusters of dilated tubules apparently unrelated to the glomeruli.

In some, the micturating cystogram shows *vesico ureteric reflux.* This may be the result of the infection and stop when the infection is treated. In others, usually with some dilatation of the lower end of the ureter, it persists and seems to be the result of antecedent weakness of the ureterovesical valve mechanism. Various antireflux operations to restore a flap valve such as reimplantation through an oblique tunnel have been devised. They may cut short the infections. But long term chemotherapy is the treatment of choice in the majority of patients.

Management of Infections

The treatment of the first acute attack of urinary infection is by a three-week course of an appropriate drug. There is a wide variety of drugs to choose from, many with overlapping effects.

Four types of drug have established themselves in treatment; *sulphonamides, nitrofurantoin, nalidixic acid* and *ampicillin.*

The sulphonamides (and sulphafurozole and sulphadimidine are the most widely used) are quite effective in milder infections but are unreliable where there is much pus or numerous organisms. Many infections are self-limiting and perhaps the drug gets some of the credit. Much of any sulphonamide is excreted in the urine but if one is used a full dose for the age and weight of the patient should be given (150 mg./kg./24 hours) because of the need to eradicate the infection in the kidney parenchyma and not merely to sterilize the urine. Sulphonamides are active against *Escherichia coli* and *Bacillus proteus* and are particularly useful in prophylaxis against relapsing infections. A small dose twice a day is adequate for this purpose.

Nitrofurantoin is effective against a wide range of urinary tract organisms which do not tend to develop resistance during treatment. It is rapidly absorbed and is present in high concentration in the urinary tract. It is a most satisfactory drug for long term prophylaxis. Nausea is occasionally a problem with full dosage and the drug should be given *with* food or milk if necessary. The dosage is 5 to 8 mg./kg./24 hours but it should be given every six hours in acute infections.

Nalidixic acid is a bactericidal drug effective against *E. coli* and *B. proteus*. Eighty per cent is excreted by the kidneys. It is most effective in acute infections, though resistance sometimes develops during treatment. It is well tolerated and has no serious side effects. The dose is 50 mg./kg./24 hours.

Ampicillin is derived from the penicillin nucleus but is bactericidal to most Gram-negative organisms. It is almost all excreted in the urine and side effects are minimal. Infants up to two years require 62·5 mg. 6-hourly and older children twice the dosage. It is not a suitable drug for long term prophylaxis since some organisms develop resistance during prolonged courses.

Streptomycin is effective but it has to be given intramuscularly not less than three times a day in acute infections. The dose is 40 mg./kg./day. It is most important to alkalinize the urine before and during treatment. Prolonged treatment is inadvisable.

The tetracyclines are little used in urinary infections and chloramphenicol should not be used at all. The latter is excreted in an inactive form as well as being dangerous to bone marrow.

The treatment of a persistent or recurrent parenchymal infection of the kidney must be *thorough and prolonged*. After a full three-week course of the appropriate drug, low dosage maintenance therapy should continue for at least three months and should be controlled by repeated urine examinations even in the absence of clinical symptoms.

Urinalysis monthly for three months and three monthly for a year should be the minimum follow up. Persistence of pyuria or bacteriuria merits treatment even without clinical signs of the infection if the tragedies of uræmic death from chronic pyelonephritis are to be averted. A sulphonamide or nitrofurantoin twice daily is the sort of maintenance dose used but culture and sensitivity tests guide treatment. *It is the duration of the infection rather than the severity of the symptoms that determines the degree of renal damage.*

CONCLUSION. Urinary infections in children should be regarded as potentially serious and prolonged supervision is advocated. Pyuria in infancy and childhood is *not* a simple and easily controlled condition. At least twenty per cent will go on having severe attacks and it will be a lethal condition in many.

Perinephric Abscess

Perinephric abscess usually arises from a blood spread infection, often by a staphylococcus. A focus in the cortex of the kidney may progress to form a carbuncle of the kidney or may discharge into the perinephric space. The patient is febrile with tenderness and eventually swelling in the loin. The lesion may be a closed one, so that the urine is sterile in about half of the cases. Treatment is by drainage and antibiotics.

HÆMATURIA

Hæmaturia is an alarming presenting symptom. The causes are discussed in the appropriate sections but the following comments should help in planning investigation.

1. The nature of the hæmaturia. Is it bright or dark? Is it copious or a trace? Are there clots? Is it evenly mixed with the urine or does it come at the beginning or end of the act? Are there associated urinary casts, albuminuria or pyuria?

For example copious bleeding usually comes from the kidneys. Dark (old) blood suggests glomerulonephritis as do albuminuria and casts. A meatal ulcer causes a typical story of passing a spot of bright blood at the beginning of micturition, with pain.

2. Is it really blood? Hæmoglobinuria also causes red urine. Examination of a fresh specimen for cells will distinguish true hæmaturia. Hæmoglobinuria may be seen after mismatched transfusion, after injuries causing muscle damage and in ischæmic lesions of the renal tubules. Urates may cause a brick red urine, especially in newborns. Beetroot and iced lollies contain dyes which may colour the urine bright pink.

3. Associated signs and symptoms. For example, in typical glomerulonephritis, there will be headache, raised blood pressure, a puffy face, and perhaps a history of a streptococcal sore throat a fortnight before. Loin pain and tenderness suggest obstruction or infection on the involved side. Agonizing loin pain suggests a calculus passing down the ureter. Pain and a constant desire to micturate suggest acute cystitis or bladder calculus. A palpable mass in the loin suggests a tumour (e.g. nephroblastoma) or a large hydronephrosis.

IMPORTANT OR COMMON CAUSES.

1. Medical.

Glomerulonephritis. (N.B. Focal nephritis may present as hæmaturia with little or no associated signs or symptoms. Renal biopsy may be necessary to confirm the diagnosis.)

Blood dyscrasias, e.g. leukæmia and thrombocytopenic purpura.

2. Trauma.

3. Infection. Usually infection of a congenitally abnormal tract, e.g. in hydronephrosis or megaureter.

Hæmorrhagic cystitis

Renal tuberculosis

(Schistosomiasis in endemic areas)

4. Tumour. Nephroblastoma
   Angioma ⎱ Rare manifestations
   Rhabdomyosarcoma ⎰ of rare conditions.
   (Urogenital sinus sarcoma)

5. Calculus. Nowadays usually secondary calculi in a tract which is obstructed or infected, or both.   Calculi also occur in metabolic disorders.

Investigation of Hæmaturia. Unless there is an obvious cause for the passage of blood it is wise to investigate the complaint although the basis will not be discovered in many patients.

It is convenient to do a physical examination, not neglecting blood pressure, full urine and blood analysis and an intravenous pyelogram in the first instance. If these investigations show nothing, it is safe to await events. If the hæmaturia recurs, a micturating cystogram and cysto-urethroscopy should be carried out. In the majority of cases they will show nothing abnormal. Bladder tumours, innocent or malignant, are really rare in the over-all incidence of hæmaturia. Retrograde pyelography is almost never indicated. Cystoscopic interpretations of small "papilloma" and "hypertrophied verumontanum" vary greatly but to pinpoint a convincing lesion is frequently impossible. One thorough investigation is enough and if nothing is found then the parents and child are reassured on the basis that a cause is not found for every case of hæmaturia but that, if there is any serious basis for the symptom, the cause is *always* found. They should be warned to expect further episodes and advised not to be alarmed by them. Minor episodes involving at most a few cubic centimetres of blood do not cause anæmia and this should also be made clear. Repeated complete investigations are rarely warranted and even more rarely productive.

Renal biopsy studies show that many are due to "local" nephritis which is not revealed by other investigations. However biopsy confirmation is not necessarily justified in clinical practice.

CALCULI

A calculus or stone in the urinary tract consists of salts deposited in a protein matrix. It may be symptomless or cause acute pain and hæmaturia and pyuria. A large stone in the kidney, such as the staghorn calculus which fills the pelvocalyceal systems, may be quite painless but a small calculus passing or attempting to pass down the urinary tract causes colic felt in the side. In the bladder it may cause a constant desire to micturate (strangury) and severe pain. In the urethra it causes severe pain in the penis and a tiny grain may initiate a reflex retention of urine.

IDIOPATHIC CALCULI. Uric acid stones in the bladder used to be common and have become very rare in these islands. The reason is unknown, though dietary factors are invoked. Primary renal stones may result from breaking off a plaques formed at the tips of the renal papillæ and vitamin A deficiency may be a factor in the causative epithelial degeneration.

METABOLIC CALCULI. In cystinosis and cystinuria soft olive green calculi form in the kidneys. Secondary infection may cause further renal damage. Although the inherited disorder is incurable copious fluids may prevent or even dissolve the calculi. Oxaluria may result in precipitation of small but rough surfaced calculi which are hence more likely to cause pain and hæmaturia. All cases of primary renal calculi should have the blood calcium, phosphate and phosphatase estimated. However, hyperparathyroidism causing calculi is exceedingly rare in childhood.

STASIS CALCULI. Recumbency calculi—soft collection of calcium phosphate—used to be a common complication of prolonged bed rest for orthopædic conditions, such as tuberculosis, until the importance of changing posture and copious fluids were recognized.

Stasis due to obstructions may also cause stones, for example in hydronephrosis or megaureter.

INFECTIVE CALCULI. Infection of stagnant urine in obstructive uropathies increases the likelihood of calculus formation. This is probably because the inflammatory exudate forms a protein matrix.

REFERENCES

Burke, J. B. (1961) Pyelonephritis in Infancy and Childhood. *Lancet*, *ii*, 1116.

Myers, N. A. A. (1957) Urolithiasis in Childhood, *Arch. dis. Childh.*, **32**, 161, 48.

Panel on Ureteral Reflux in Children (1961) Spence, H. A., Stewart, C. M., Marshall, V. F., Leadbetter, W. F., Hutch, J. A., *J. Urol.* **85**, 2, 119.

Smellie, G. M., Hodson, C. G., Edwards, D., Normand, I. C. S. (1964) Clinical and Radiological Features of Urinary Infection in Childhood. *Brit. med. J.*, *ii*, 1222.

Steele, R. E., Leadbetter, G. W., Crawford, J. D. (1963) Prognosis of Childhood Urinary Tract Infection: The Current Status of Patients Hospitalized between 1940 and 1950. *New. Eng. J. med.*, **269**, 17, 883.

Williams, D. I., Eckstein, H. B. (1964) Surgical Treatment of Reflux in Children. *Brit. J. Urol.*, **37**, 1, 13.

Wyllie, G. G. (1955) Hæmaturia in Children. *Proc. roy. Soc. med.*, **48**, 12, 1113.

CHAPTER 24

CONGENITAL MALFORMATIONS OF THE URINARY TRACT

MALFORMATIONS OF THE KIDNEY

THE commoner malformations of the kidney are:

APLASIA
HYPOPLASIA
HORSESHOE KIDNEY
ECTOPIA
CYSTIC KIDNEY
DUPLICATION
HYDRONEPHROSIS

The first four of these are particularly likely to be associated with the presence of *dysplastic* areas in the parenchyma. This is of considerable importance because of the role this lesion may play in causing resistant pyelonephritis.

Unilateral *aplasia* occurs about once in five hundred children.

Agenesis of kidney and ureter may be part of the syndrome of the absent umbilical artery when observation of the cord may lead to the diagnosis.

The pyelogram of a *hypoplastic* kidney shows the typically short stunted calyces and the renal outline is small because of the narrow parenchyma. This narrowing of the parenchyma on the pyelogram is similar to the picture seen in advanced pyelonephritis as the r esult of prolonged uncontrolled infection.

The *horsehoe kidney* is one in which the lower poles of the right and left kidney are joined across the midline. The pyelogram is typical in that the lower poles come closer together than the upper, and the lower calyces are directed medically. They are more prone to infection than normal kidneys, and also liable to obstruction at the outlet of the pelvis causing hydronephrosis which may require pyeloplasty but not division of the isthmus.

Ectopic kidneys are frequently found in a lower position than normal, usually in the pelvis, and in the condition of crossed ectopia both kidneys lie on the same side of the body.

Congenital polycystic kidneys show a typical pyelogram with elongated calyces bearing indentations where the cysts press on them. The condition is bilateral and it is inherited. The lesion will probably already have been recognized by palpation of the enlarged lobulated kidneys before pyelography confirms it. Clinically, polycystic kidneys usually produce renal failure with uræmia in the first years of life. Some remain symptomless until adult life and present a similar picture then. In addition to this familial type of bilateral polycystic lesion a similar lesion (called multicystic kidney) may occur affecting only one kidney, and this may be associated with atresia of the upper ureter. The apparently normal opposite kidney may later show signs of dysplasia.

Duplication. This is an important and common variation, present in 1 in 170 children. It is really a duplication of the pyelon (the collecting system, calyces, pelvis and ureter), and the parenchyma is in one piece, though often there is a waist between the two halves. The ureters may join anywhere below the kidney. They may join above the bladder or they may open separately into the trigone, or one ureter may open lower down into the posterior urethra or into the vagina in a girl. It will be realized that such an *ectopic ureter* may be a cause of incontinence. The ureteric orifice may be stenosed in which case a ureterocele (a cystic swelling) is likely to develop on it, and as a result of back pressure and stagnation infection in the affected half of the kidney is particularly likely to occur. The two ureters cross on their way to their outlets so that the ectopic ureter is almost always that draining the upper pole of the kidney, which is usually the inefficient part. It may be so inefficient that it does not secrete adequately to show on a pyelogram and its presence may only be suspected by the gap in the X-ray picture suggesting that some further part of the kidney must be present, although not demonstrable. In such a case cysto-urethroscopy will demonstrate the ectopic orifice and retrograde pyelography will demonstrate the extent of the abnormal portion. It may be possible to treat the condition by removing only the damaged half of the kidney. Often the infection will have spread to involve the parenchyma of both parts and a nephro-ureterectomy is required. The lesion may be bilateral.

It should be stressed, however, that although duplicated kidneys are particularly prone to infection, the majority of them are probably perfectly efficient in function throughout life. This is clearly seen from the fact that duplication is not uncommonly found by chance during routine post-mortem examination.

Hydronephrosis. Hydronephrosis is usually the result of an abnormality of the pelvi-ureteric junction. The junction may be stenosed or it may be kinked by congenital folds of adventitia, or it may have deficiencies in its muscular wall. The ureter may be found to be kinked over a renal vessel (usually the lower division of the renal artery) but these vessels probably play only a secondary role in the causation of hydronephrosis when one of the lesions mentioned causes the pelvis to distend and bulge over them. Hydronephrosis may also result from scarring and hence stenosis following urinary infection, or it may be secondary to some obstruction lower down producing back pressure. Hydronephrosis may be found during the investigation of a urinary infection, but the typical story is that of recurrent attacks of abdominal pain which may be so severe as to cause vomiting, or may be of a more persistent dull aching character. If the pain is localized to the renal area the diagnosis will not be difficult, although it should be recognized that in only a minority of cases is the distension sufficient to produce a clinically palpable kidney unless one is fortunate enough to examine the patient during an acute exacerbation. However, the abdominal pain

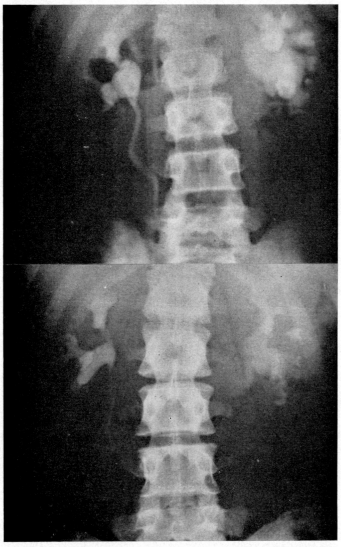

Fig. 44. Left-sided hydronephrosis before and after operation.

is sometimes vague and unlocalized, and often it is not until urinary infection supervenes that the renal cause of trouble is suspected.

Hydronephrosis is an upper urinary obstruction. There is no alteration of the bladder function and therefore micturition is normal. Unless infection has supervened there will be no demonstrable abnormality in the urine and therefore the lateralization of the abdominal pain may be the only clue to its urinary cause. This is an important point because *it means that in investigating cases of recurrent abdominal pain one cannot claim to have excluded a urinary cause by urinalysis alone.* It is necessary to carry out a pyelogram in addition. It is important that the diagnosis of hydronephrosis should not be delayed because in the early stages it is possible by a plastic operation on the pelvis and its outlet to conserve the kidney. If treatment is delayed then back pressure will have destroyed the renal substance and infection may have added its quota of destruction; the only treatment possible may then be nephrectomy. When it is realized that the congenital abnormality underlying the hydronephrosis is bilateral in a considerable proportion of cases, even though the symptoms arise much earlier on one side than the other, then it will be understood how important it is to conserve the kidney whenever possible.

Parenchymal atrophy behind the obstruction is irreversible and established infection may also become incurable. There are various types of plastic reconstruction at the pelvi-ureteric junction but that of Hynes and Anderson is almost always applicable. Chemotherapy should be kept up for three months after surgery in infected cases.

As many as 25 per cent of mild hydronephroses are non-progressive, so, in the absence of persistent symptoms or infection, reassessment after a year's observation may be justified.

ABNORMALITIES OF THE URETER

The common abnormalities of the ureter are:

> HYDROURETER
> MEGAURETER
> DUPLICATION OF THE URETER

HYDROURETER

The term *hydroureter* is usually used to denote a ureter distended secondarily as a result of obstruction lower down the urinary tract. If the outlet of the bladder is obstructed in early infancy or even fœtal life then the dilatation of the upper urinary tract begins in the lower third of the ureter and the ureter may become grossly distended before the renal pelvis and kidney suffers any damage. If left long enough, however, the back pressure will affect the kidney and produce a hydronephrosis. When the obstruction occurs later in life the ureter seems to have become less distensible so that back pressure affects the kidney earlier. Hence in the older man with prostatic obstruction one may see only a mild dilatation of a ureter with an enormous hydronephrosis above it. This altered reaction in the different age groups is interesting in itself and may be also of some value in enabling an expert urologist to decide when a particular lesion began.

MEGAURETER WITH AND WITHOUT VESICO-URETERIC REFLEX

Megaureter denotes a ureter distended as a result of some obstruction at its lower end, or some other malformation of the ureter itself. The urine stagnates in the megaureter and hence infection and stones are common complications. If the condition remains long enough the kidney becomes hydronephrotic. It may be possible to treat such a lesion by dividing the ureter above its narrow segment and re-implanting it into the bladder. The long-term results of this treatment have not been good and if the other kidney is normal it is often best to perform a nephro-ureterectomy. The cause of many megaureters is still not understood, for there is no obvious organic or neurogenic obstruction to account for them. In some the voiding cystogram shows reflux from the bladder. Reimplantation of the ureter through an oblique tunnel in the bladder wall—after narrowing the ureter by excision of a strip if necessary—may prevent this and hence the infection. A similar procedure may be required in secondary hydroureter after treating the primary cause, such as bladder-neck obstruction.

DUPLICATION OF THE URETER

Duplication of the ureter goes along with duplication of the renal pelvis and has already been discussed. It is important to remember that many duplications are functionally efficient, so that the mere presence of duplication must not be taken as meaning that it is therefore the cause of symptoms. If one half of the kidney or one ureter is dilated, then, of course, it is much more likely to be causing trouble.

ABNORMALITIES OF THE BLADDER

The bladder may present *congenital diverticulæ*, or it may be divided by a *septum*, but these are rare and the bladder abnormalities we see are usually the result of *obstruction to its outlet*.

Lower Urinary Obstruction

MARION'S DISEASE

The obstruction may be by the so-called *Marion's disease*, or *bladder neck obstruction* in which there is hypertrophy of the muscle around the bladder neck and some degree of fibrous infiltration. The bladder in this condition becomes hypertrophied, trabeculated and easily palpable. Back-pressure effects later spread to involve the upper urinary tract.

The treatment is by excision of a wedge of the bladder neck or a plastic Y–V operation to broaden it. The underlying cause is not known and the condition has been over diagnosed.

Chronic cystotrigonitis with œdema and thickening of the internal sphincter may cause a functional rigidity of the bladder neck which usually disappears with satisfactory antibacterial therapy.

POSTERIOR URETHRAL VALVES

In boys the obstruction may be the result of *congenital valves in the posterior urethra.* The usual valve is either a diaphragm with a small hole in it or two semilunar folds like an extension of the normal folds

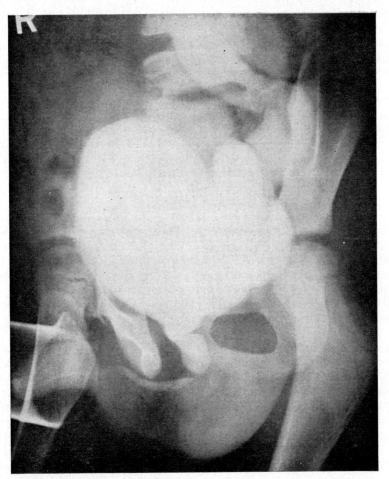

FIG. 45. Posterior urethral valves demonstrated by micturating cystogram. There is free ureteric reflux.

at the crista terminalis. It is important to realise that like the semilunar valves elsewhere in the body they are unidirectional in their effect. There is no obstruction to passage of a sound up into the bladder even though there is obstruction to the outlet of urine. The hypertrophied and trabeculated bladder will be palpable. If a voiding cystogram is carried out one will see the greatly distended posterior urethra down to the level of the valves. It may be possible to palpate the enlarged urethra by doing a rectal examination while pressure is exerted on the bladder fundus. The child with a severe obstruction may present with dribbling micturition and failure to thrive from birth, and with a high blood urea from that time. In milder cases the condition may be recognized only years later, either as a result of superadded infection or the effects of renal failure or micturition difficulties. The valves can usually be removed by a diathermy resectoscope. It may be necessary also to resect part of the secondarily hypertrophied bladder neck. The overstretching of the sphincter which has occurred may result in incontinence following treatment of the valve. Furthermore, owing to the insidious nature of the condition, irreversible back-pressure damage to the kidneys may have arisen before the child comes under surgical care. The outlook is therefore not good, even though it is one of the conditions of lower urinary obstruction which are pathologically fully understood. Indeed, in many of the cases presenting in the early infant period the kidneys have already been irreversibly damaged before birth, though in older patients the outlook is better.

Megaureter Megacystis

Another type of chronic enlargement of the bladder is that called the *megaureter megacystis* syndrome. These children have a greatly dilated bladder and greatly dilated ureters with easy reflux back from the bladder up the ureters. The pathology is not understood and there is no obvious obstruction causing it, even though a plastic widening of the bladder neck often does seem to help these children to evacuate. The history may reveal that the child has had infrequent micturition throughout life and may pass urine only once or twice in the 24 hours.

The mainstay of treatment is teaching the child to micturate frequently by the clock and not to wait for filling of the enormous bladder. The child is trained to pass urine 3-hourly and to micturate again a few minutes afterwards each time. The object of this *double micturition* programme is that when the child empties the bladder the first time he also empties a lot of urine back up the dilated ureters. This trickles back into the bladder and at the second micturition it is evacuated. Thus the retention of a stagnant pool of urine is avoided and the risk of infection reduced. With a regular system of micturition such as this, and perhaps a bladder neck plastic operation the condition, serious as it looks, may not in fact be greatly progressive. However, a proportion of cases will not be seen until secondary infection has occurred and greatly increased the renal parenchymal damage.

In a few of these cases in boys it has recently been discovered that the posterior urethra shows an extensive layer of fibro-elastosis in its wall. This is apparently an abnormal development of prostatic tissue and may produce an inelasticity which causes difficulty in evacuating the bladder. However, this alone would not explain the fact that these children have such a capacious yet not particularly hypertrophied bladder and large ureters with early reflux; so that the effect is different to that seen in other forms of obstruction, for example by urethral valves or Marion's disease.

Neurogenic Defects

It is important to mention here the group in which the urinary tract may be normally developed but incompletely innervated. The commonest cause is *spina bifida.* Neurological lesions are also seen in association with *sacral agenesis.* The matter is discussed in the chapter on spina bifida. These lesions affect the urinary tract mainly by their interference with control of the bladder outlet. There may be laxity of the outlet causing constant dribbling or there may be a tightness of the outlet resulting in distension of the bladder with vesico-ureteral reflux and back pressure effects on the upper urinary tract with overflow dribbling of urine. In either case there is an increased tendency to infection, but in the latter case the effects of back pressure make the outlook much more serious. A bladder neck resection or plastic operation will improve emptying and an operation at the ureterovesical junctions will prevent reflux, but the improvement will often be incomplete because there is frequently an interference with the function of the bladder wall itself. The situation is not as simple as the localized obstruction of Marion's disease or urethral valves. Local operations to produce continence are not of much value except in those cases where the neurogenic effect is so slight that the complaint is rather one of stress incontinence than complete lack of control. However, there is a tendency for spontaneous improvement up to the age of 7 or 8 and one should not be too hasty about advising radical surgical measures. Nevertheless many of the boys will require a penile clamp or a penile urinal. In the girls it may be necessary to resort to transplantation of the ureters into an isolated loop of ileum which is brought to the surface of the abdomen where plastic bags can be fitted to collect the urine and enable the child to remain dry and non-odorous. An ileal loop diversion may be required in either sex if infection cannot be controlled, quite apart from the problem of continence. Somewhat similar neurogenic defects of bladder emptying may result from neurological diseases such as transverse myelitis, and from injuries, or from the effects of intraspinal tumours.

Conclusion

It may be felt that much space has been given to rare conditions. But these conditions, although individually uncommon, make up a considerable body of urinary pathology, much of which is remediable, or at least in which destruction can be halted. In primary pyelonephritis much less can be done, particularly in the later stages. The importance of full investigation and vigorous treatment of pyelonephritis in its early curable stages must be reiterated. Recent studies confirm that the outlook in established urinary infection in childhood is serious, and the eventual mortality considerable.

REFERENCES

Williams, D. Innes (1958) *Encyclopedia of Urology*, Vol. 15, *Urology in Childhood*, Springer-Verlag, Berlin.

Johnston, J. H. (1961) "Urinary Tract Duplication in Childhood". *Arch. Dis. Childh.*, **36**, 180.

Hydronephrosis and Hydroureter in Infancy and Childhood: A Panel Discussion (1962) Culp, O. S., Rusche, C. F., Johnson, S. H. and Smith, D. R. *J. Urol.*, **88**, 4, 443.

CHAPTER 25

NOCTURNAL ENURESIS

NOCTURNAL ENURESIS is perhaps a label rather than a diagnosis. Bedwetting is the complaint. It is meant to convey the idea of involuntary micturition in the absence of an organic disorder. In most cases there is a tendency to spontaneous improvement with increasing age, but the sufferer and family may be caused much distress before this occurs.

The natural history differs from organic incontinence and a full history, clinical examination and urinalysis are sufficient to reach a presumptive diagnosis in most cases. A therapeutic test is then usually advised before further investigation is considered, and this avoids many unnecessary urological procedures.

Bedwetting before the age of 4 should not be regarded as enuresis. A fastidious mother may worry earlier through lack of appreciation of the natural variation in the age of development of control. The child may be wet most nights, but if there has never been a *single* dry night then an organic lesion should be considered. Severe enuretics often also have increased frequency or urgency of micturition by day and may have accidents. But severe diurnal symptoms are also suspicious of an organic cause. Most true enuretics become dry by day but do not achieve the same reliability by night. It is rare, if not unknown, for a patient to have an organic basis for nocturnal enuresis without some other symptom or sign.

Vertical incontinence is a name given to the condition in which the child is frequently wet by day but dryer in bed and at night. It is typical of the leakage from an ectopic ureter opening somewhere below the bladder sphincter.

Stress incontinence is also likely to cause more trouble by day. It may be due to sphincter weakness or a similar condition may arise from emotional causes. ("Giggle incontinence" is a specific condition and may originate from a cerebral lesion.)

Periodic recurrences and improvements are suspicious of an underlying urinary infection causing irritation.

The child (or baby) who is literally always wet also merits careful investigation. The constant dribbling may be the result of overflow incontinence secondary to bladder neck or posterior urethral obstruction. Observation of the stream for force and calibre may be helpful. Delay in treatment may allow irreversible renal damage to occur.

The usual enuretic has never achieved nocturnal control, but there is a group, the onset enuretics, who become wet again having previously achieved control. The trouble starts after some stress such as an acute illness or a period in a strange home. Enuresis sometimes follows an attack of pertussis and in such cases an electro-encephalogram may show abnormalities. This latter illustrates that the frequency of an organic cause may depend on the care with which the search is made.

But most enuretics show no organic signs and there may be strong pointers to a functional basis in the family history. Overstrict attention to cleanliness in early life may start some anxieties, but the commoner impression is of a feckless family with a mother unable to cope consistently with training problems.

Cystometrograms do usually show abnormalities such as a high tension bladder and perhaps uninhibited contractions. But these are indicative of immaturity rather than disease.

Management

As a first line of treatment day time training will often produce at least enough improvement to make one confident of the diagnosis and avoid the need for full urological examination.

It is explained to the mother that there is no actual disease, but that the child is maturing slowly in this respect—just as at first some children may be more clumsy with a spoon than others. The child is to be sent to the lavatory by the clock at regular times during the day and not left to go only when he feels the urge. His nights are not disturbed except by wakening to pass urine when the parents go to bed. Nor is his fluid intake restricted except to a reasonable supper drink. On this régime most frequent wetters become occasional wetters. Micturition may be hourly at first, beginning at a weekend, increasing to 2-hourly but never more. This can be maintained at school with the co-operation of the teachers.

A book with red and white stars to record wet and dry nights helps to keep up morale and give an opportunity for much needed encouragement.

The basis of this treatment (Ellison Nash) is that many children by postponing micturition habituate themselves to a full bladder and may only pass enough urine to be comfortable when they do go. For there are many more interesting things for a young child to do. Thus they come to respond to the urgent pain of an overdistended bladder rather than the sense of filling which becomes dulled. By keeping the bladder frequently emptied their sensation of filling should become more acute and improve their reflex control. It is thus quite the reverse of the kind of time training in which the enuretic was encouraged to hold out for increasing intervals. Yet this method may also produce results! Undoubtedly suggestion plays a considerable part.

It is useful to know at what part of the night the bed is wet. Some children are deep sleepers and wet themselves in the prolonged act of wakening in the morning. They may be helped by dextro-amphetamine sulphate 5 to 10 mg. in the evening.

Drugs are on the whole of little value. Probanthine may help, but must be given in doses starting with 15 mg. and then increased to maximum tolerance—and this may be surprisingly high. Methylephedrine sometimes helps. It is more convenient than ephedrine because it is longer acting; $\frac{2}{3}$ or $1\frac{1}{3}$ gr. may be required. Meprobamate 200 mg. at night for a month will break the cycle in many hardened wetters.

Posterior pituitary extract given in the form of a snuff (e.g. Disipidin 100 mg at night) will sometimes be extremely effective. Here again the element of suggestion is considerable.

In persistent cases admission to hospital for observation and urological investigation will sometimes be justified. The strange surroundings may produce a temporary cure. It will probably not persist on discharge, but at least obviates the need to proceed to investigations and encourages the parents about the possibility of dryness.

Much success has recently been achieved by the use of alarms by older children. These consist of a metal plate in the bed which when moistened by urine rings an electric bell. The child then has to get up, change the sheet and re-set the alarm. Although it seems crudely mechanical the device does seem to work and to produce no unfortunate psychological sequelæ.

In a few cases deeper psychological causes of the habit may be revealed and their treatment may be more important than that of the symptom itself.

Traditional measures such as frequent awakening through the night or severe restriction of fluid intake are ineffective in teaching the child to go dry throughout the night. A single awakening to pass urine at about 10 p.m. is often effective. This lifting must be complete awakening and the child should put on his slippers and dressing gown and go to the lavatory rather than half empty his bladder while half awake into a pottie in the room. One must take care that the management advised is not itself a source of misery.

Conclusion

The enuretic with no other symptoms than intermittent bedwetting does not have organic disease. It is important to look out for other leading symptoms such as dysuria, a poor stream, wetting by day or an infected urine, any of which may indicate an abnormality in the tract.

REFERENCES

Nash, D. F. E. (1949) Development of micturition with special reference to enuresis, *Ann. roy. Coll. Surg. Engl.*, **5**, 318.
Enuresis: Leader, *Brit. med. J.*, (1960) **1**, 1416.
Barber, R. F., Borland, E. M., Boyd, M. M., Miller, A. and Oppe, T. E. (1963) Enuresis as a Disorder of Development. *Brit. med. J.*, **2**, 787.

CHAPTER 26

GENITAL ANOMALIES

Hypospadias

HYPOSPADIAS is a condition resulting from failure to form a complete anterior urethra in the male. The external urinary meatus lies at some ventral position on the penis or scrotum. There are four degrees of hypospadias, *glandular, penile, peno-scrotal* and *perineal.* The glandular type is the commonest and the perineal opening the rarest.

GLANDULAR HYPOSPADIAS. This minor degree accounts for almost 80 per cent. In this the urinary meatus lies at the base of the glans ("glandular hypospadias"). The balanic urethra has failed to develop and is represented by a groove on the ventral surface of the glans. It is no disability. It may cause anxiety in regard to the newborn when it is noticed that the infant has not passed urine during the first day of life and the penis is examined. The infant will pass a stream whether or not a meatotomy is performed. Though there are operations to advance the meatus to the tip of the glans the condition is best left alone, except in those few whose glans is tilted ventrally causing annoying splashing on micturition. Like any ectopic orifice the displaced meatus may be stenosed and may then require a minor operation to enlarge it.

Browne has drawn attention to the almost constant presence of a tiny opening just distal to the functioning meatus. The blunt end of a needle passed into it reveals a sinus dorsal to the urethra. It may be short or extend as far as the scrotum. No embryological explanation has been brought forward—indeed this structure is neglected in standard texts. It has a practical use. If the blades of a pair of small scissors are passed into the functioning meatus and this dorsal sinus and the scissors closed, then the openings are converted into one larger opening. Thus meatal stenosis can be relieved without extending the opening proximally as in an orthodox meatotomy. The technique is particularly valuable in managing a stenotic meatus at the corona—for proximal extension of the opening may cause splashing and necessitate a formal repair of a minor degree of hypospadias which would otherwise require no treatment.

PENILE AND PENOSCROTAL HYPOSPADIAS. In these intermediate forms, in which the proximal part of the anterior urethra is formed, the distal part has failed to develop. "Chordee" (ventral flexion) is also present in these forms and meatal stenosis may be present.

PERINEAL HYPOSPADIAS. This is the most severe and rarest form. The urethral folds on the under surface of the phallus fail completely to

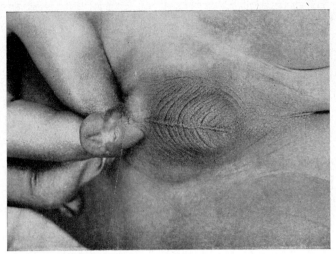

FIG. 47. Penile hypospadias.

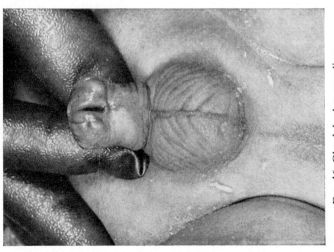

FIG. 46. Glandular hypospadias.

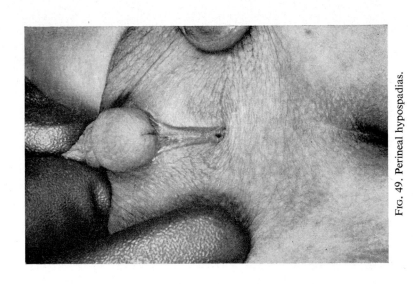

FIG. 49. Perineal hypospadias.

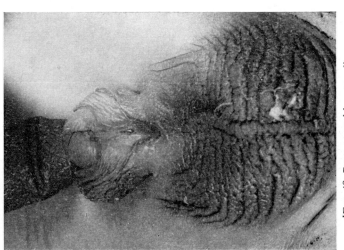

[FIG. 48. Peno-scrotal hypospadias.

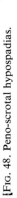

form a tube. The urethral orifice is behind the (cleft) scrotum. The phallus is flexed ventrally (chordee) with a tight fibrous cord in place of the corpus spongiosium. The perineum thus takes on a somewhat female appearance. If testes are palpable in the scrotum the diagnosis is clear. If they cannot be felt then prompt investigation is required to be sure that the condition is only a local defect and not a manifestation of an intersex condition (Chapter 26).

REPAIR OF HYPOSPADIAS

The treatment of penile and more severe degrees of hypospadias is required to allow controlled direction of the urinary stream in the

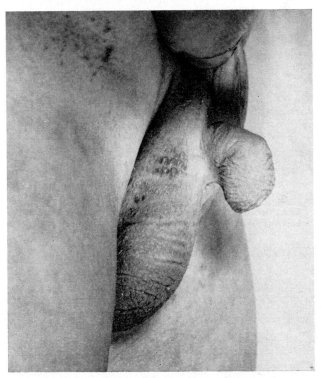

FIG. 50. Lateral view of hypospadias to show chordee.

standing position in childhood and also later ability to achieve satisfactory coitus and insemination. Two objects need to be achieved. First the phallus must be straightened and, secondly, a urethra must be constructed to reach the glans. There are several operations, none perfect.

The Denis Browne operation is widely used. It produces an untidy but effective meatus and has the great merits of reliability and of completion before schooling begins.

A first-stage operation is performed in which a transverse incision is made on the ventral surface of the penis in front of the meatus. By undercutting, the fibrous vestige of corpus spongiosium is excised allowing the penis to

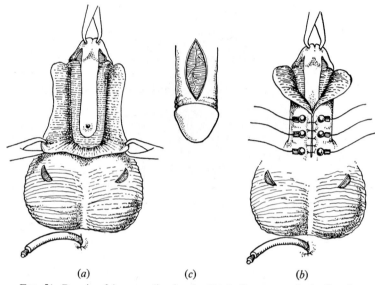

(a)   (c)   (b)

FIG. 51. Repair of hypospadias by the Denis Browne method. Chordee has already been corrected at a preliminary operation.

(a) Shows the flaps of skin mobilized laterally leaving a median strip about 1 cm. wide. Triangular raw areas on the glans help to bring the meatus forward. Crawford makes this advancement at the first stage and one of the authors finds this makes a better meatus.

(b) Shows the flaps drawn over to bury the median strip by means of non-strangulating double stop sutures (beads with *aluminium* cylinders to grip the suture on to which they are crushed with forceps). Epithelium grows around from the buried strip to form a urethral tube in about 10 days. The important principle is the burying of a *strip* without attempting to fashion a tube.

(c) Shows the dorsal relaxing incision along the shaft of the penis—essential to avoid tension and consequent breakdown. The perineal urethrostomy shown diverts the urine for 10 days and closes spontaneously in 3 days on removal of the catheter.

straighten, and the incision is then sutured longitudinally including a bite of the corporal fascia with each stitch to avoid the formation of loose folds of skin in the ventral midline which make the second stage awkward. This corrects the chordee. Meatotomy is often required at this stage. Although simple in plan, the procedure requires careful attention to details of technique for successful application. It is usually done at about 18 months of age and the penis then left to grow until about 4 years of age when the second stage is performed to construct the urethra to the tip of the penis. The boy is enabled to pass urine standing up before he goes to school.

An interesting principle is involved in this second stage. Most previous procedures have aimed at forming a tube, complete or incomplete, of rolled skin. Fistulæ were common owing to the extensive œdema and tension resulting from operative trauma to the penis. The buried split skin graft techniques did not have this disadvantage, but were prone to contraction and stricture formation, and involved unpleasant bouginage. Browne observed that once a fistula had epithelialized throughout its length there was no longer any tendency for it to close. Furthermore, he noticed that penile skin behind the coronal sulcus (unlike ordinary skin) healed without any permanent fibrosis. He therefore devised a simple technique of burying a strip of skin on the ventral surface of the penis from the functional meatus up to the glans. Epithelium extends around from its edges; it also curls up, and within ten days a tube has formed. Tension is avoided by a dorsal slit over the penile shaft and the urine is diverted for ten days by perineal urethrostomy, the wounds heal in a leathery fashion, but within six months or so this thickening settles down and fine scars are left which can stretch with growth. (Ordinary skin will not do this. Permanent fibrosis occurs so that growth of the resulting tube cannot be expected in other situations.)

EPISPADIAS

In epispadias the penile urethra is not formed and in its place a mucosal strip runs along the *dorsum* of the penis. It is much less common than hypospadias and again various degrees exist. A mere cleft of the glans may need no treatment. A defect extending down the shaft will require repair on similar principles to the hypospadias operation— the mucosal strip is buried by rolling the separated corpora cavernosa together dorsally over it, along with the skin.

The condition may extend further and be associated with a wide bladder neck and urinary incontinence. (Hypospadias does not interfere with the urinary continence as the posterior urethra is always normally formed.)

It is usual to delay repair to the third or fourth year when the question of continence will have been resolved. In the incontinent minority repair of the sphincter may be possible, but in most cases urinary diversion (implanting the ureters into the colon or an isolated ileal loop) will have to be performed later.

ECTOPIA VESICÆ

Ectopic bladder is rare and may be looked upon as a more severe degree of the epispadias described above. The epispadiac urethra leads to a bladder laid open on the abdominal wall and bounded laterally by diverging rectus muscles. The pubic symphysis is widely separated. A fibrous bar extends between the bodies of the pubis and the epispadiac urethra runs above and anterior to this. This course suggests that it may not represent the true urethra, as does its course on the upper surface of the phallus. The embryological accident is earlier and more extensive than in hypospadias. Lateral mesoderm has failed to migrate into the subumbilical ventral abdominal wall and the genital tubercle is displaced relative to the urogenital sinus.

Ectopic bladder is a severe deformity. The child is constantly wet with urine and sore from the exposed and irritated bladder mucosa. The separation of the pubes weakens the levator support of the pelvic floor, so that the straining consequent on their discomfort often results in rectal prolapse. The outward rotation of the pelvic bones gives the child a widebased waddling gait with the feet turned out (the longshoreman's gait). But there is no instability of the pelvic ring, as might be expected, for the inter-pubic fibrous bar becomes perfectly firm.

Standard treatment for many years has been the transplantation of the ureters into the lower colon so that urine and fæces are voided together under the control of the rectal sphincter. This has to be left until 2 or 3 years of age, when the tendency to rectal prolapse is likely to settle and the child can be trained to control the urine and fæces mixture. Later the ectopic bladder mucosa is removed and the abdominal wall closed by suitable flaps. The epispadiac phallus is reconstructed in the male, and the ejaculatory ducts will enter the urethra so formed.

Ninety per cent are continent but ascending infection renders the long-term results of ureteric transplant into the colon unreliable, with about 30 per cent mortality from renal failure, so, in recent years, most surgeons transplant into an isolated loop of ileum, of which one end is brought on to the surface of the abdomen as an ileostomy. Modern bags make such an orifice relatively easy to manage. But a lifetime with an artifical orifice cannot be regarded as fully satisfactory.

The usual case of ectopic bladder retains much of the normal structures—they are merely split and gaping ventrally. Reconstruction should therefore be feasible. In the past, results have been very poor. The wide skeletal defect made anatomical repair unpractical. Recently it has been found practical to close the pelvic gap by iliac osteotomies, and this makes closure of the bladder and abdominal wall more satisfactory. The closure of the bladder is not unduly difficult and the approximated rectus muscles form a good abdominal wall. But the formation of a continent sphincter has been achieved as yet only on rare occasions.

One of the authors prefers neonatal closure of the defect, when osteotomies are not required. The results as to continence are no better.

GENITAL ANOMALIES IN GIRLS

IMPERFORATE HYMEN

Thc hymen may have a very small opening or it may be quite closed. In the latter case the condition is probably more accurately described as a lower vaginal atresia and the block is often a fibrous cylinder of some length rather than a diaphragm.

HYDROMETROCOLPOS. Imperforate hymen usually presents clinically in the neonatal or early infant period as hydrometrocolpos or mucocolpos. Retention of the mucous secretions which are caused by transplacental passage of hormones dilates the vagina until it forms a large lower abdominal mass. Back pressure opens the cervix and secretions may pass back through the tubes to cause an irritative lower abdominal peritonitis. Infection is a serious complication. The mass may interfere with micturition and defæcation by its sheer size.

The mass behind the imperforate hymen can be aspirated and replaced by radio-opaque dye before definitive surgery. The X-ray will be of considerable assistance in planning the procedure. Frequently cruciate incision of the hymen with subsequent excision of the quadrants is adequate for free drainage and complete cure. In other patients it may be necessary to do a laparotomy, at which the vagina is opened and a sound passed down to the imperforate area. Then incisions from below can usually be made on to the sound. A drain from below will be required until the vagina has had time to evacuate its contents and contract down again. It contracts down to normal size in a remarkable fashion over a few months. In a few cases with a long atretic segment of lower vagina more elaborate measures may be required.

HÆMATOCOLPOS. Sometimes an atretic or stenotic hymen presents at puberty when menstruation begins. The flow is dammed back producing hæmatocolpos. Again there is a leak back into the lower abdominal cavity producing an irritant peritonitis. The condition may be mistaken for appendicitis unless there is a careful history and examination. The periodicity of the symptoms should lead one to suspect the condition.

ABSENT VAGINA

This may be complete or there may be a small short vagina bearing an often rudimentary uterus at its apex. Later in childhood a vagina can be constructed by opening a track and inserting skin grafts on a former. Some surgeons prefer a bowel transplant to give a cavity with a mucous lining. The best results of these operations are sad substitutes.

Adherent Labia Minora

This is happily a much commoner condition (Fig. 45). The baby or child appears to have only a urethral orifice and no vaginal orifice can be seen. The urinary stream may be directed forwards. But the epithelial floor behind this orifice will be seen on closer inspection to have a longitudinal fusion mark in the midline. It consists only of the labia minora adherent to each other (rather similarly to the adherence of prepuce to glans in the newborn male).

If a probe is inserted anteriorly and pressed backwards the labia separate easily, usually leaving a raw surface in parts. The mother is instructed to apply petroleum jelly (Vaseline) to the surface daily for a

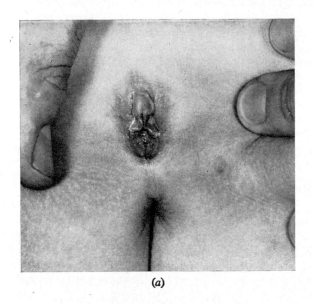

(a)

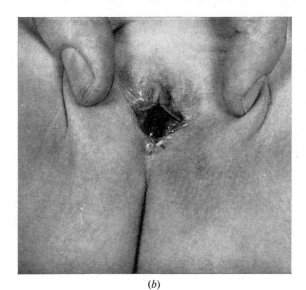

(b)

FIG. 52 (a) and (b). Adherent labia before and after division.

fortnight to keep the edges apart until healing is complete. Readherence readily occurs before œstrogenization takes place at puberty but this is not serious.

These children are otherwise normal. It is important to recognize this minor condition promptly for much anxiety is aroused when doubt as to the child's genital development is expressed, and particularly if delay and observation is recommended. True vaginal atresia is extremely rare.

REFERENCES

Browne, Denis (1949) Hypospadias, *Postgrad. med. J.*, **25**, 367.

Dennison, W. M. & Bacsich, P. (1961) Imperforate vagina in the newborn, *Arch. Dis. Childh.*, **36**, 186,156.

Dewhurst, C. J. (1963) *Gynæcological Disorders of Infants and Children*, Cassell, London.

Williams, D. I. (1961) Ectopia Vesicæ, in *Progress in Clinical Surgery*, Series II, Churchill, London.

CHAPTER 27

INTERSEX

THE term *intersex* is preferred to hermaphrodite in discussions on patients whose sex characteristics are incompletely differentiated. This incomplete differentiation is far the commonest problem met in practice. It is the problem of the patient who carries the gonads of one sex but whose body form, either in part or completely, does not conform to this sex. True hermaphroditism where male and female gonadal tissue are both present in the one individual is extremely rare.

The most important point in managing an intersex problem is to reach an *early and firm decision. This will take all the factors into account, but once given is final, binding and without appeal.* Once the decision has been made then whatever medical or surgical means necessary must be used to assist the patient to conform to the agreed sex.

The decision must be made as soon after birth as possible. This is because a person's attitude to sex depends almost entirely on upbringing rather than on the other clinical and laboratory information. It has been said that the sex of a patient should never be changed after the age of 2 years, and in some cases this may be too late.

The Factors in Sex Determination

It has become recognized that sex is no longer a matter of gonads only, but is a summation of many factors. The chromosomal and hormonal patterns, the gonad type, the sex organ anatomy as well as the psychic environment are all to be considered. But when all available information is obtained there are few difficult decisions.

The *chromosomal pattern* of each cell determines the chromosomal sex of the individual. Human cells normally contain 46 chromosomes of which 2 are concerned with sex. These two may be similar in which case they are labelled XX (the female endowment) or dissimilar and labelled XY (male). In practice cells from buccal or vaginal smears, skin biopsy or leucocytes may be used to determine this point. The presence of sex chromatin aggregations in the nuclei of a proportion of the cells is a readily available indirect guide to the presence of two X chromosomes (female). This sex chromatin body is absent in normal males. More specialized techniques allow the visualization of the chromosomes themselves. Some intersex states have a mixture of chromosomal patterns—"mosaics".

The *hormonal pattern* comes from both gonadal and extra-gonadal sources. Gonadal sources are normally quiescent in childhood and it is the secretions of the adrenal which cause most disturbances. Individual secretions can now be suppressed or augmented by endocrine preparations so that the hormonal environment can be controlled.

The *gonad sex* is revealed by a study of the histology of the gonads. Biopsy is not necessary in every case, however.

The *somatic sex* covers the general body type and in particular the internal and external genital organs. The character and development of the sex organs, particularly the copulatory organs, govern the potential adaptability of the individual and are of immense practical importance.

The importance of the *psychic aspect*, the sex of rearing has been referred to and cannot be overstressed.

CLINICAL TYPES

The principal types are:

1. **Female Intersex**
2. **Male Intersex**
3. **True Hermaphroditism**
4. **Sex Chromosome Variations** (e.g. Turner's and Klinefelter's Syndromes)
5. **Local Genital Defect**

Female Intersex. This is the commonest group. The sex chromosomes are XX (female) and the gonads are ovaries, but a masculinizing influence during fœtal life has interfered with the development of the genitalia. There is usually only a urethral opening in the perineum instead of vaginal and urethral openings. The vagina opens instead into

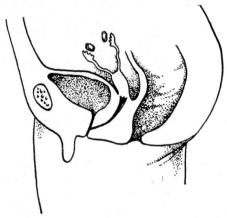

FIG. 53. The usual anatomy of the female intersex or female pseudohermaphrodite resulting from intra-uterine adrenal hyperplasia. The phallus looks like a hypospadiac penis. Urethroscopy reveals an opening at the site where the verumontanum would be expected in a male. This is the orifice of the vagina.

the wide posterior urethra. The clitoris is large but does not carry a urethra. If the masculinizing agent begins unusually early in pregnancy then the infant may be altered to the extent of having a penile urethra. A lesser degree of alteration may allow two normal perineal openings with an enlarged phallus.

The usual cause of this condition is *congenital adrenal hyperplasia*. This can be confirmed by the estimation of the 17-ketosteroids and the pregnanetriol. (Normal values are less than 1 mg./24 hours and nil respectively.) Both are raised in adrenal hyperplasia, as high as 80 mg. and 15 mg./24 hours. Some patients develop severe electrolyte disturbances because of interference with the production of other adrenal hormones, the mineralocorticoids.

Management. In the past this condition was treated by repairing the hypospadiac phallus and the individual lived more easily as a sterile male rather than as a masculinized and hirsute woman. Now cortisone and its derivatives can suppress the adrenal hyperplasia and the output of the masculinizing hormones. When these children are recognized in infancy they should be put on continuous steroid and allowed to develop as females. The dosage of steroid can be assessed from the depression of the urinary 17-ketosteroids produced. This is preferable not only because this is their gonadal sex but because it also allows control of the electrolyte disturbances which may otherwise become a serious hazard to the health and even the life of a considerable proportion of these children. Surgery is confined to clitoridectomy (its size is not a reliable guide to steroid dosage) and later vaginoplasty.

Recently a number of infants have been recognized who present a similar picture to adrenal female intersex, but in whom the adrenal hormone output is normal. These children have been masculinized by *progestin* with which the mother was treated in early pregnancy. The risk of androgenic side effects of progestin therapy in early pregnancy is now recognized. As the cause of abnormality is not continuing the only treatment required is surgical. The large clitoris is reduced and the vagina opened on to the surface.

With the above exception non-adrenal causes of female intersex are extremely rare.

Male Intersex. In these conditions the gonads are testes but the external genitalia are not completely masculine. This category has been subdivided into

(*a*) Male Intersex with Equivocal External Genitalia

(*b*) Male Intersex with Purely Female External Genitalia

(*a*) The diagnosis is made in the presence of equivocal external genitalia when the sex chromatin pattern is male, when the 17-ketosteroid level is normal and when urethroscopy shows a normal verumontanum. Testes will be found in the inguinal region or the posterior abdominal wall. Gonadal biopsy may be necessary to confirm the diagnosis.

The child is brought up as a male and when the invariable hypo-spadias is being repaired a hysterectomy is performed. Orchidopexy is performed if possible. These testes have the reputation of being prone to malignancy.

(*b*) This group have sometimes been called Testicular Feminiza-tion Syndrome. The external genitalia and bodily form are entirely female. The vagina is extremely short and the testicles may be in the posterior abdominal wall or inguinal region. Cases may present as simple inguinal herniæ in a girl during childhood: the sac is found to contain a testis. Or the discovery may be made at puberty when amen-orrhœ calls for investigation. The sex chromatin is male.

Many of these patients have married but they are inevitably sterile. Their life as a girl is quite satisfactory and there is no immediate indication for intervention. However, early orchidectomy and œstrogen substitution at puberty have been advised because some develop an intense female libido and may become seriously disturbed by the frustration of inadequate gratification, for the vagina usually remains short and small. Orchidectomy removes this libido.

True Hermaphroditism. In this extremely rare condition ovarian and testicular tissue is present. There may be an ovary and a testis or more often an ovotestis in which male and female elements intermingle. The patient cannot become pregnant though fertilization is possible. The anatomy of the genitalia varies widely, but there is usually phallus, uterus, vagina and scrotum. The scrotum may contain a testis or an ovotestis or the gonads may be internal in the usual ovarian position. The sex chromatin is equivocal. The diagnosis is made on biopsy.

The decision which shall be the sex of rearing must be taken early on and when biopsy has confirmed the diagnosis of true hermaphroditism the choice depends on the adaptability of the external genitalia. This is more often to male than female. The unnecessary gonadal tissue is excised together with the "conflicting" organs (vagina, uterus, uterine tubes and breasts; or phallus). Plastic repair of the hypospadias or vagina follows.

Sex Chromosomal Aberrations. Two types are *Turner's syndrome* and *Klinefelter's syndrome*

In *Turner's syndrome* the patient is a stunted girl with webbing of the neck, a low hair line, cubitus valgus and other anatomical abnor-malities. It was the finding that these patients often have coarctation of the aorta (a disease preponderantly of the male) that led to the discovery that they did not have the XX chromosome structure. In fact they only have one sex chromosome—XO. There is a failure in gonadal differentiation or gonadal agenesis and they have amenorrhœa. No surgery on the genitalia is necessary.

The much rarer *Klinefelter's syndrome* appears as a mirror image of Turner's syndrome. At puberty there is eunuchoidism and gynæcomastia in apparent males. The chromosome constitution is XXY—an extra chromosome being present as a result of non-disjunction. However, substitution therapy at puberty enables these patients to live as sterile males.

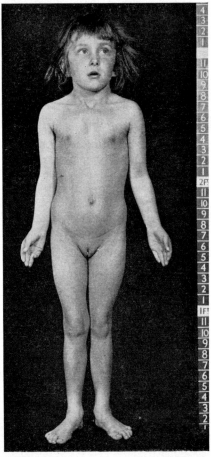

FIG. 54. Turner's syndrome showing webbed neck, deformity of right fifth finger and cubitus valgus. (Case of Dr. R. Bonham Carter.)

Local Genital Defect. This group is not really an intersex problem but the defective formation of the genital organs may be mistaken for such. Severe hypospadias with bilateral undescended testes may be mistaken for female pseudohermaphroditism. There is no hormonal disturbance in the former, though the outlook for fertility in any bilateral cryptorchid is dubious.

Conclusion

Clearly, the important thing is to reach an early decision in each case and then make every effort to bring the environment, anatomy and hormone balance into line. Laboratory findings are almost always helpful but should not be permitted to dominate diagnosis or dogmatically prescribe treatment. A buccal smear for nuclear sexing, urethroscopy to visualize the normal male verumontanum or in its place a hole representing the internal opening of a vagina, and exploratory laparotomy and gonadal biopsy should, if necessary, all be undertaken at a single hospital admission—the first.

REFERENCES

Gordon, R. R. and Dewhurst, G. J. (1962) Ambiguous sex in the newborn, *Lancet*, *ii*, 872.

Wilkins, L. *Diagnosis and Treatment of Endocrine Disorders in Childhood and Adolescence*, Thomas, Springfield, Ill.

Williams, D. Innes (1958) *Encyclopædia of Urology: Urology in Childhood*, Vol. XV, Springer & Verlag, Berlin.

CHAPTER 28

UNDESCENDED TESTICLES

IMPERFECT DESCENT OF THE TESTIS

ABOUT one in every two hundred adult males has unilateral or bilateral undescended testes. Unilateral imperfect descent is about four times as common as bilateral.

There is no evidence of endocrine insufficiency in the vast majority of cases. Undescended testis is usually a local defect of development. Indeed the organ is often ill-formed as well as imperfectly descended. The body of the abnormally situated testis may be hypoplastic, the epididymis may be completely separated from the body of the testis or the vasa efferentia may be absent. *It appears likely that in many cases pre-existing imperfect development of the testis interferes with the descent.*

Classification

Imperfect descent of the testis may be classified into two main groups. *Incomplete descent* of the testis occurs when the organ is found somewhere along the normal line of descent. *Ectopic testis* means that the testis has left the normal line of descent.

Retractile testis. This is a normal variation, not an abnormality. The testis enters the scrotum but is retracted to the superficial inguinal pouch most of the time. If it reaches the bottom of the scrotum it is called low retractile and if only the upper scrotum high retractile.

Examination

In describing the type of imperfect descent found it is necessary to describe not a position but a *range of movement*. Examination of normal children will soon make it obvious that the testis is freely mobile along its track from the bottom of the scrotum to the superficial inguinal pouch which lies in front of the inguinal canal. Cold weather or careless handling producing cremaster contraction will also demonstrate this movement easily.

Determining the exact position of a testis can be quite difficult. It requires a certain amount of practice and the following of some definite routine to discover the range of movement present.

The child should first of all be examined standing up when his body configuration can be examined, the size of the penis noted and the type of the scrotum, whether lax and deeply rugose or of small shallow but rugose and equally normal type. The presence of any inguinal bulge suggestive of a testis or a hernia either at rest or on coughing should also be noted. The child should next be examined lying down. Before handling the scrotum the fingers of the examiner's warmed hand should be placed above the inguinal ligament lateral to the inguinal canal. The fingers should be stroked gently down the line of the inguinal canal, passing over the external inguinal ring to reach the pubic tubercle. The fingers are pressed gently against the external inguinal ring to prevent the testis riding up again. Then the fingers of

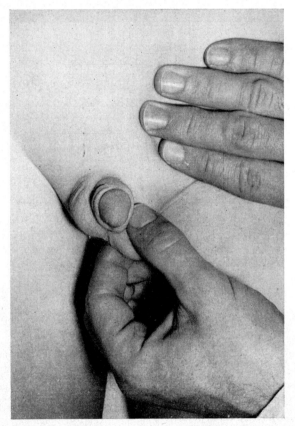

FIG. 55. Examining for undescended testis as described in text.

the other hand are cupped around the scrotum to palpate the testis. It may be felt within the scrotum or it may be palpable higher up over the pubis or in the region of the superficial inguinal pouch. If it is not present in any of these situations the testis is probably in the inguinal canal. It may be higher still on the posterior abdominal wall. Search must also be made in rarer ectopic positions such as the perineum or femoral triangle.

Retractile Testis

From this description of the three variations of the normal testicular descent it will be recognized that for practical purposes, if manipulation along the line of the inguinal canal can coax the testicle into the scrotum, whether to the upper part or to the bottom of the sac, then the child can be considered normal and the parents reassured confidently of his normal development. This retractile variant of the normal is the commonest single type seen for advice and treatment in consultant practice. There may occasionally be some discomfort at puberty when the organ develops but it will attain the normal position.

If the testis cannot be manipulated into any part of the scrotum then descent is abnormal in one of the following ways.

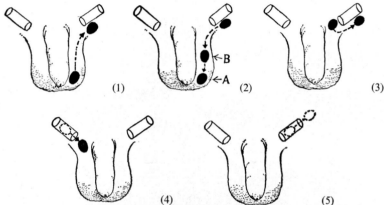

Fig. 56. Common situations of the testicle. In each case a range of movement must be described.

(1) Normal. Testis at bottom of scrotum—can be pushed up to inguinal pouch in front of the canal.

(2) (*a*) Normal low retractile. Same range as (1), but the testis lies at the upper end of the range in the inguinal pouch, and can be manipulated to the bottom of the scrotum.
(*b*) Normal high retractile. Testis lies in the pouch and can be manipulated into the scrotum, but not to the bottom of it. Although the range is incomplete, so long as the testis enters the scrotum at all it can be predicted that it will reach the usual position spontaneously with development at puberty.

(3) Superficial inguinal ectopic testis. Testis lies in the pouch in front of the canal, but a fascial "hammock" prevents it being pushed into the scrotum; on making the attempt it may pass over the pubis if the pouch is large, but it goes alongside the neck of the scrotum and not into it. Differentiation of (2) (*b*) and (3) may need repeated examination.

(4) Emergent inguinal testis. Testis impalpable in the canal, but can be coaxed out to become palpable outside the external ring along the normal line of descent.

(5) Retention in the canal. Testis impalpable and cord too short to allow it to be coaxed out through the ring. Impalpable. Outlook for operative correction of position poor compared with ectopia. Clinically indistinguishable from abdominal retention.

Incomplete Descent

Emergent Inguinal Testis. In this type the testis lies within the inguinal canal, but on manipulation can be felt to pop out of the external ring, although it will not go over the rim of the pubis into the scrotum. These testes feel more fusiform than the testis which has left the canal. Dennison has called this the "undecided" testis.

Testis in the Inguinal Canal. If the testis is retained within the inguinal canal the overlying tense external oblique aponeurosis makes it impossible to palpate the testis. It is therefore clinically indistinguishable from the intra-abdominal type. In a few cases, however, when the child is slim and relaxes well it is possible to feel vaguely that there is something within the canal, and the discomfort felt on pressure may lead one to suspect that this is the testis. However, it can be categorically stated that if the testis is easily palpable in the inguinal region and if it feels discrete and of a normal testicular shape then it is not within the canal, but is lying in front of the external oblique muscle in the superficial inguinal pouch.

Abdominal Testis. In this type the organ is arrested in its descent somewhere along the line from the lumbar region where it first develops down to the internal ring. This type is the least common form of incomplete descent.

Superficial Inguinal Ectopic Testis

The commonest form of ectopia is the *superficial inguinal ectopic testis*. The organ is easily palpable in the superficial inguinal pouch; it can be pushed from one end to the other of the pouch but will not go over the brim of the pubis into the scrotum because there is a fascial hammock blocking the outlet from the pouch.

Scorer has pointed out that this is strictly on the normal line of descent, for the pouch is a normal structure, and this is really an *obstructed* descent. However, this usage is so widespread that change at present would be confusing, particularly as Browne has used the term "obstructed testis" for a rare type in which a well formed organ is retained impalpable in the canal by a closed external ring.

The important point is that the inguinal ectopic testis is usually a better formed organ than the emergent or canal retained testis.

A less common form of ectopia is the *perineal ectopic testis*. The organ is palpable in the anterior part of the perineum and is usually a well-formed, normal testis. However, in this position it is likely to give rise to considerable discomfort, for example, on riding a bicycle, and is therefore usual to advise transplantation to the normal site.

Other ectopic positions are found on rare occasions; for example, in the femoral triangle, or in a pre-penile scrotum.

Age of Descent

Although the testis is usually in the scrotum at birth it is quite common for the descent to occur at some time later during the first few months of life. There need therefore be no alarm at the absence of a testis from the scrotum in the newborn, although observation is clearly indicated. It does not seem that descent is likely to take place after the first year of life if the diagnostic criteria used above are followed. The disparity in the incidence of the condition between infants and adults has been greatly exaggerated by vague criteria of diagnosis. It seems likely that most, if not all, of the cases of spontaneous descent at puberty are in fact cases which would here be classified as normal high or low retractile testicles from the beginning. This is a matter of some practical importance because it has been shown that if the testis is not brought down to the scrotal position with its lower temperature before the hormonal changes which precede puberty begin, then its chances of spermatogenesis are negligible. This means that any policy based on waiting to see what happens at puberty will reduce orchidopexy to a largely cosmetic procedure. A decision must be made before puberty whether the testis is of a type which requires treatment or not.

Size

The testis does not grow steadily during childhood as the body does. It grows very little until the prepubertal enlargement begins. Between the ages of 2 and 10 years the average testis only enlarges from about 0·8 cm. long to 1·2 cm. long. Lack of appreciation of this differential growth pattern may give rise to considerable alarm. When a mother notices that her big 10-year-old has testes virtually the same size as her baby she may feel that something serious is wrong, and it may be the reason for bringing the boy to the doctor.

Hernia

The majority of cases of undescended testis are accompanied by a congenital hernial sac. In only a minority of these cases does abdominal content enter the sac to produce a clinical hernia during childhood.

Undescended Testis with Endocrine Defect

Certain rare forms of bilateral cryptorchidism (impalpable testes) do show other signs of endocrine defect. The true case of Fröhlich syndrome (dystrophia adiposo genitalis) falls into this category. This is a serious condition and fortunately it is excessively rare. Unfortunately it has become a fairly common practice to refer to a particular type of prepubertal obesity as a "Fröhlich type" of child. These children are obese and they are tall for their age, whereas a true pituitary dystrophy would be expected to produce stunting. The penis, although within the normal range, is on the small side in this constitutional type and is made to look even smaller by the presence of a large pre-pubic fat pad in which it tends to be hidden. If the pubic fat is pressed back against the bone a considerable length of buried penile shaft appears. Such a demonstration may reassure the anxious parents. The testes, although normal for a prepubertal child, do seem small in relation to their large frame and the scrotum, although rugose, is of the shallow type. This is a recognized constitutional type, but there is no evidence of any endocrine defect, and enquiry will often show that other members of the family have been of similar build, and indeed the father himself may be of this type. These children usually grow more rapidly than the average for their age, and they develop puberty at the normal time, and require nothing but reassurance.

TREATMENT

Treatment is mainly indicated on cosmetic and psychological grounds in the unilateral case, because the outlook for fertility is almost normal. But, the possibility of damage to the normal testis does exist and the concomitant hernial sac is dealt with during the procedure. The incompletely descended testis is also more prone to torsion and may be damaged if the concomitant hernia incarcerates. Although it is more prone to develop a malignant tumour than the normally descended organ, such tumours are too rare to influence treatment (and orchidopexy does not appear to influence the risk).

Untreated bilateral undescended testes cause sterility and treatment is essential.

Except in the rare endocrine type described above treatment is by *surgery*. It must be stressed again that the above *classification* of types of imperfect descent should be used and that the *high and low retractile testes be considered as normal and left without treatment of any kind*.

The Place of Hormones. In true hypogonadism associated with endocrine defect a dosage of 500 units of Prolan twice a week for 6 weeks is a suitable course to use. It is dangerous to use large doses or prolonged therapy, because a normal testis may be damaged by overdosage which can produce a hyalinization of the tubules and inhibit spermatogenesis. It may seem to be a glimpse of the obvious to suggest that unilateral maldescent of the testis cannot be due to inadequacy of circulating hormone, but the number of cases in which it is still "given a trial" seem to justify making the point.

There is one situation in which a diagnostic trial of hormones may be useful. It is sometimes possible to manipulate a testis from the superficial inguinal region over the pubic bone, but it is difficult to be sure whether it is actually entering the upper scrotum or whether it is being pushed down in the fat of the region into the base of a large superficial inguinal pouch alongside the neck of the scrotum. If it is really entering the upper scrotum then, of course, it can be left alone as a normal high retractile testis. If it is merely entering the depths of a large inguinal pouch lateral to the scrotum then it is ectopic and requires treatment before puberty. It is therefore important to make the diagnosis by the time the child is 9 years old. If repeated *clinical* examinations have failed to enable one to make a confident differential diagnosis, then the exhibition of prolan as described above should solve the problem. In the case of a retractile testis the testis will enter the scrotum as it would have done later at puberty, whereas in the case of an ectopic testis this will enlarge somewhat but will still fail to enter the scrotum. One then knows that operation is required.

The retractile testis may resume its inguinal site again during the interval between hormone treatment and puberty, but can be expected to descend again when the natural hormones are produced.

The Operation

This should be carried out by the tenth year of life so that the testis will be given a reasonable chance to develop with puberty. There are some grounds for thinking that the chances of development are even better if it is brought down earlier and some surgeons suggest that 3 years of age is a wiser time. It seems that there is so little difference that the later and more usual time for operation is justifiable, though there is little point in delay when a typical inguinal ectopic testis is recognized earlier. If there is a clinical hernia, this itself merits operation and orchidopexy should be performed at the same time, however young, or the testis will become fixed in the postoperative scar tissue. The operation consists basically of mobilizing the cord. The cremaster muscle is removed. The hernial sac which tends to tether it and prevent lengthening is removed. There is an extension of the deep fascia of the posterior abdominal wall which runs into the cord as the so-called internal spermatic fascia, and this tethering band requires to be divided. One is then left with the testis suspended by the vessels and the vas. The limiting agent is almost always the vessels. It is futile to pick at the cord any further and may be dangerous by interfering with the blood supply to the testis. Orderly freeing of the cord as described above will enable the ectopic testis which has a relatively long cord to be replaced easily in the scrotum, and will enable the majority of emergent inguinal and a considerable proportion of the canal-placed testes to be brought down similarly.

If the testis is merely laid in the scrotum then postoperative œdema is likely to squeeze the testis back up to the inguinal region where it adheres to the operation scar. Some lock is needed to keep it down. In the Denis Browne operation this is achieved by drawing the testis and cord down through a tunnel made behind the pre-pubic fascia. In the Ombredanne operation it is achieved by drawing the testis through the scrotal septum. The skin and all layers of the scrotum should be divided for $\frac{1}{2}$ in. and the testis laid subcutaneously as the intact dartos and coverings also tend to push the mobilized testis up towards the neck of the scrotum. In the Bevan operation the lock is achieved by making a loose purse-string suture around the region of the scrotal neck.

All these procedures have the same object of providing a lock to prevent the testis slipping out of the scrotum in the early postoperative period. It cannot be stressed too strongly that they are not there to hold down the testis under tension. If the testis will not come down without tension it is better to fix it at the external ring, wait 2 years and carry out a second stage operation. Then it will usually come down to the scrotum without tension. To apply tension to any vascular pedicle is to invite spasm of the vessels and ischæmia of the structure. The Keetley-Thorek operation in which the scrotum and testis are stitched to the thigh is an example of this kind of misguided effort to lengthen the cord, and biopsy of the testis at the second stage to free the scrotum from the thigh usually demonstrates the expected atrophy. However, many continue to use a form of traction to the thigh with strapping and an intervening elastic band. Much depends on how much traction is put on the elastic, but with a small band and little pull it tides the patient over the first 3 or 4 days, when riding up most often occurs. Real traction will be harmful, but when slackly applied the method amounts to an alternative form of lock.

At least 3 months should elapse after surgery before passing an opinion on the result of the operation. Then the shape, size, consistence and sensitivity of the organ should be taken into account, together with its position.

There is in fact a serious dearth of good functional follow-ups of the treatment of undescended testis. It is not an easy thing to do because clearly only the bilateral cases can be used as valid in paternity studies. Postpubertal biopsies or sperm counts have not been widely performed, and as a general rule may be unwise as likely to encourage psychological impotence. Enquiries into the frequency of paternity in men operated some years ago in childhood are vitiated by doubts as to diagnostic criteria and operative technique. All that can be said is that some boys operated for bilateral undescended testes have produced children; that there is at present no preferable alternative treatment, and that further follow-up studies of accurately diagnosed cases are badly needed.

REFERENCES

Browne, Denis (1938) Diagnosis of undescended testicle, *Brit. med. J.*, *ii*, 168.
Gross, R. E. and Jewett, T. C. (1956) Surgical Experiences from 1222 operations for undescended testes. *J. A. M. A.* **160**, 634.
Johnston, J. H. (1965) Review Article: the undescended testis, *Arch. Dis. Childh.*, **40**, 210, 113.
Scorer, C. G. (1964) The Descent of the Testis. *Arch. Dis. Childh.*, **39**, 605.

Footnote

Van Essen, W. (1966). The Retractile Testis, *Postgrad. Med. J.*, **42**, 270. Discusses the "chair test" which one of the authors has recently found an invaluable screening test for the retractile group. The boy sits on a chair with his feet on the seat and hugs his knees to his chest so as to flex his thighs against the abdomen. In this posture the cremaster relaxes and the testis can be seen to descend and then be palpated. The descent without manipulation by the doctor is particularly convincing to the boy and parents that all is well.

CHAPTER 29

FRACTURES

IT is not proposed to discuss fractures systematically, as this subject is well covered in orthopædic texts. It is our intention to discuss only some lesions and trends of special interest in childhood fractures.

It is well known that in the early years of childhood the resilient bones are likely to have that incomplete form of break called the "*greenstick*" fracture. Because it retains its own internal fixation by continuity of connective tissue fibres it may present with minor symptoms, and indeed a fracture sustained during infancy may only be brought to light because of the resultant deformity. Treatment is simple because the bone heals well with some degree of protection. It is important to remember, however, that such trauma in an infant may give rise to a considerable fever with local swelling and tenderness. This may give rise to an erroneous diagnosis of osteitis.

When a child falls on its outstretched hand it is likely to suffer not the typical Colles fracture of an adult, but a *slipped epiphysis* at the lower end of the radius. In this lesion the less firmly attached epiphysis of the young child slides across the bone end to produce a similar deformity to the Colles fracture. It is a benign lesion. The epiphysis is easily replaced and unites firmly in about 3 weeks. If it is not replaced it becomes immovable within a week or 10 days and will heal with deformity, although over the next few years a considerable improvement by modelling will take place. Whilst a slipped epiphysis is an innocent lesion it should be noted that a *crushed* epiphysis resulting from a blow in the long axis of the limb, e.g. an awkward fall from a height onto a foot, may produce a potentially serious lesion. The crushed epiphysis may fail to grow and result in late shortening of the limb; or more commonly, part of it may fail to grow resulting in angulation of the end of the limb as growth takes place.

Supracondylar Fracture of the Elbow

The supracondylar fracture of the elbow is an important childhood injury. The humerus breaks across above the elbow as a result of a hyperextension strain and the lower fragment tends to be driven posteriorly. The main danger is the risk of *damage to the brachial artery* which runs in front of the elbow joint. Injury to it may cause the so-called Volkmann's ischæmic contracture in the flexor muscles of the forearm. Ischæmia of nerves may cause sensory loss in some cases. Furthermore, if the fracture is not well reduced awkward late angulation of the elbow (cubitus varus) develops as growth proceeds. Every case of the supracondylar fracture with displacement should be admitted to hospital.

The manipulation of a typical displaced supracondylar fracture is carried out as follows. If the left elbow is involved the manipulator

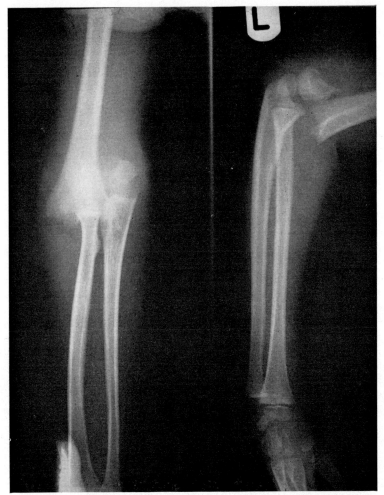

Fig. 57. Supracondylar fracture of humerus with typical displacement.

grips the child's forearm with his left hand and exerts steady traction in the long axis of the arm for a minute or two, whilst an assistant steadies the child by a hand in the axilla. When relaxation and disimpaction are achieved the fingers of the right hand are placed across the front of the lower end of the humerus with the thumb at the back over the olecranon. The thumb pushes the lower fragment forward as the left arm flexes the elbow to 45° and pulls it round the corner. A lateral pressure may then be required to correct any lateral displacement. The reduction should be stable with the arm held in flexion. A control X-ray should be taken immediately to confirm reduction and then a protective slab of plaster of Paris and a collar and cuff sling applied for 3 weeks.

This principle of preliminary disimpaction followed by correction of the deformity is a basic one in fracture manipulation. It is facilitated by good anæsthesia allowing muscular relaxation and can be hindered by the muscular tension frequent with simple gas and oxygen.

The typical supracondylar fracture in which the lower fragment is displaced backwards on the shaft of the humerus is stable when the elbow is fixed at 45°. But it is not stable at 90° and displacement will tend to recur. If there is gross swelling around the elbow the pressure caused by flexion may interfere with circulation and obliterate the radial pulse. It may then be impossible to obtain a stable degree of flexion immediately after manipulation. In *all* cases it is important to check by repeated radiography on the next day that no slipping has occurred. If it has occurred, then it should be possible to correct by a further manipulation when the swelling is less tense. It must be remembered that, like all fractures in children, and particularly juxta-articular fractures, healing will be rapid and the lesion may become immovable within 10 days. If, therefore, repeated manipulation does not produce a stable correction of the fracture it may be necessary to insert a pin through a small skin incision over each epicondyle, driving the pin obliquely upwards through the lower fragment across the fracture line and into the upper fragment so as to enter the cortex. This enables one to obtain internal fixation without the necessity of potentially harmful dissection around the joint. Dissection of the joint is to be avoided whenever possible, as it is likely to produce persistent stiffness. The less common supracondylar fracture in which the lower fragment is displaced forward should be treated on similar lines, and if it is unstable it should be pinned in position and the elbow flexed. This method of treatment is preferable to immobilization in extension.

After manipulative correction of the displacement under anæsthesia the limb must be observed half-hourly for the first day to see that there are no signs of vascular damage in the forearm. These are looked for by palpating for a radial pulse, by examining the colour of the hand, and by testing for flushing of the nail bed after pressure. Extension of the fingers is also a useful test. If contracture is occurring extension will be limited and painful. If there is any such ischæmic damage then the structures in front of the elbow must be widely exposed and clots evacuated. If the artery is exposed and then covered with a warm saline swab the spasm will usually relax. Adjuvants such as the application of

papaverine sulphate 1 per cent saline solution to the artery are probably less important than complete exposure.

Displacement of the External Condylar Epiphysis of the Humerus

Displacement of the external condylar epiphysis is an important
elbow injury in the 5 to 15 age group. The epiphysis is semicircular;
flat above and curved below. A fall on the outstretched hand may

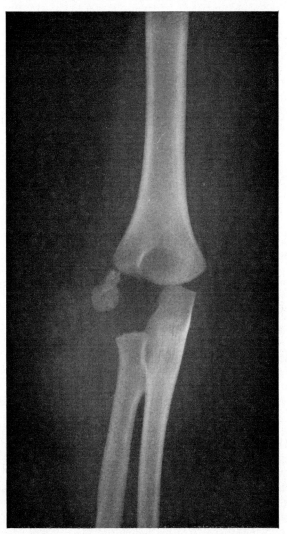

FIG. 58. Fracture of external condyle of humerus with typical rotational
displacement in two planes.

displace the epiphysis with the attached common origin of the extensor muscle group. If displacement is slight manipulative reduction is satisfactory and a collar and cuff or sling is sufficient treatment. If the tear is complete the muscles avulse the fragment and rotate it out of the joint, so that its fractured surface is directed outwards and its articular surface directed inwards. It is also rotated on a vertical axis. In this type of injury, which is more common than the partial tear, operative reduction is necessary and should not be postponed.

The fragment is sutured or screwed into the correct position and the elbow immobilized for 4 weeks. It will take the best part of 6 months for the range of movement of the elbow to return to normal. Failure to operate causes an ununited fracture. This is about the only unreduced fracture in childhood which consistently fails to unite. The late complications of the non-union include ulnar nerve palsy, which is due to trauma and stretching of the nerve when the elbow deformity (cubitus valgus) develops.

Displaced Capitellum

Another elbow injury should be mentioned because it is so easily missed. This is the displaced capitellum resulting from a fall on the point of the elbow. The epiphysis of the capitellum is tilted forward. Unless the angle of the epiphysis to the shaft in the lateral X-ray is compared with that of the normal side it is not very obvious. But correction is important or the lesion will heal with a persistent limitation of extension of the elbow.

It is a lesion which illustrates particularly well the value of *comparison of films with pictures of the good side* in doubtful injuries— especially with growing and incompletely ossified bone ends.

It is difficult to recognize the anatomical limitation of movement on early clinical examination because the acute synovitis of the injury prevents full passive movement. If it is suspected a true lateral radiograph will decide the issue and correction is simple. The elbow is fully extended under general anæsthesia and the moving ulna draws its articulating capitellum into the anatomical position.

This description of the trials and tribulations in the treatment of fractures at the lower end of the humerus makes one realize that they are not to be looked upon lightly, although the great majority merely need manipulation if they are displaced, then application of a collar and cuff sling around the wrist and neck to hold the limb at 45° flexion, with the use of a back slab to give some protection over the tender area. Such fixation needs to be maintained only for about 3 weeks and afterwards the child is allowed active use of the elbow. Physiotherapy is not necessary and if it includes passive movement it can be positively harmful. It is important to stress to the parents of these children that time and natural use will mobilize the joint well enough, though it may take several months, but any attempt to hurry matters by carrying weights or lifting heavy objects will produce increasing stiffness of the joint and can produce permanent fixation with only a few degrees of residual mobility. Fortunately children are usually anxious to do all they can. Therefore they carry out the most valuable form of physiotherapy after trauma, that of active use within the limits of pain, without any need for attendance in a department.

Pulled Elbow

In this condition the child complains of pain over the head of the radius and holds the arm in a semi-flexed position resenting movement beyond a few degrees. The typical story is of a mother hurrying over her shopping and giving the trailing child a tug by the arm to get him to follow. Pain and limitation of movement occur quickly. They are caused by dragging of the radial head through the ring formed by the fibres of the orbicular ligament. If the forearm is flexed on the arm and rotated into full supination one may obtain immediate relief of the condition. If not, one should not persist in painful manipulations but proceed to a general anæsthetic and repeat the procedure. Manipulation results in the head slipping back through the orbicular ligament in the great majority of cases.

Spiral Fractures of the Femur

Another common fracture in childhood is the spiral fracture of the femur following indirect violence. A common story of the fracture is the child who falls from a tree, his wedged foot twisting free as he goes. A fall from a bicycle with one foot trapped by the machine is another cause.

Fracture of the femur of a child under the age of 2 years can be treated simply by attaching extension strapping to both legs and hanging the limbs from an overhead beam so that the child is suspended in bed with his buttocks just off the bed. His own body-weight will pull out the fracture to full length. Healing occurs rapidly. This form of *gallows traction*, however, should not be used in older children because then the height of the leg above the heart is such that dangerous ischæmic lesions of the feet may occur from prolonged extension in this position. In older children it is satisfactory to set the fracture under anæsthesia using strapping extension on an ordinary Thomas splint and pulling out the limb to full length. In transverse fracture exact apposition of the bone ends is not important, for healing is sound with massive callus formation. After some fractures of the femur in which there is much periosteal stripping the rate of bone growth may be increased for some time after the fracture and some lengthening of the limb is produced.

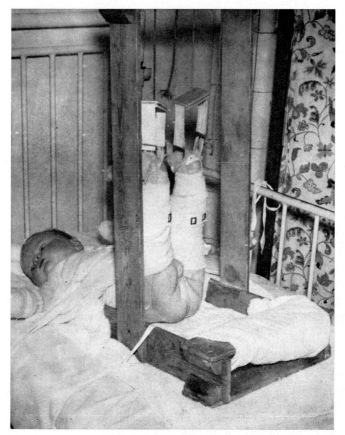

FIG. 59. Gallows traction for fractured femur.

REFERENCES

Blount, W. P. (1954) *Fractures in Children*, Williams & Wilkins Co., Baltimore.

Brady G. (1964) Fractures about the elbow joint in children (A Review of 342 Cases), *J. Irish med. Ass.* **55**, 327, 67.

Broadhurst, B. W. and Buhr, A. J. (1959) The pulled elbow, *Brit. med. J.*, *i*, 1018.

Ferguson, A. B. (1964) *Orthopædic Surgery in Infancy and Childhood*, 2nd Edition, Baillière, Tindall & Cox, (London).

CHAPTER 30

OSTEOMYELITIS

OSTEOMYELITIS was, until recently, an important cause of death in childhood, and those who survived the initial stages frequently went on to a lifetime of suffering and deformity from chronic infection. It is much less common than it used to be, but is nevertheless an important condition. The discovery of penicillin appeared to have solved the problem. It seemed that one had only to diagnose the disease early enough and treat it long enough to complete a cure in every case. Recently, however, there has been a recrudescence of the disease and in particular of infections which do not respond fully to antibiotics and aspiration of abscesses.

Pathology. Osteomyelitis of the long bones starts with a blood-stream infection which lodges in the end arteries of the metaphysis. It is always a secondary lesion, even though the primary may be quite trivial; for example a boil, or even a little pustule in the newborn baby. The infection spreads from the metaphysis up the medullary cavity and into the sub-periosteal region where it may strip up the periosteum over a wide area, forming an abscess. From there it may burst through into the superficial tissues. It may also break through into the neighbouring joint and may involve the epiphysis. The epiphysis is particularly vulnerable in young babies.

The organism is almost always a *staphylococcus*, although the streptococcus may cause a similar condition, and occasionally cases are seen from bizarre organisms such as *Bacillus ærtrycke*, Pasteurella or the typhoid group. A considerable proportion of the staphylococci are nowadays resistant to penicillin.

CLINICAL CLASSIFICATION

Clinically the condition is best considered in three separate groups. Firstly, the condition in *infancy*; secondly, the *typical acute hæmatogenous osteomyelitis of the long bones between the ages of* 2 *and* 12 *years*; and thirdly, a miscellaneous group of bone infections secondary to various other lesions such as open fractures, sinusitis and dental infections.

INFANCY

Hæmatogenous Osteitis of Infancy

The disease in infancy shows a remarkable tendency to follow one of two differing clinical courses, though the organisms may appear to be the same in both groups. In one group the bone infection is accompanied by a fulminant septicæmia which may indeed be so rapidly fatal that the local lesion is overlooked. At the other end of the scale the local lesion may cause so little in the way of general symptoms and local pain as to be recognized late for this reason. The condition may be brought to the notice of the doctor because of a pseudo-paralysis, the baby being apparently well, but not using a limb. On examination, local swelling

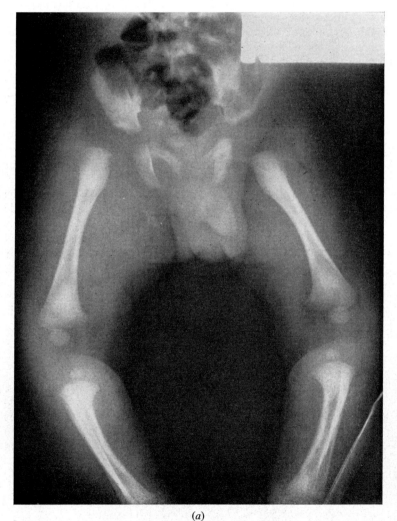

(a)

FIG. 60. Suppurative arthritis of the hip joint.

(a) Early picture—only shows a widened joint space on the right on careful examination.

and heat will be detected and the child will have a fever, and in the blood a typical polymorphonuclear leucocytosis will be found. In some cases it is only the formation of a superficial abscess which brings the patient to the notice of the doctor, and one must be on guard against missing the underlying bone infection in the kind of case where the general upset is minimal.

The organism is often acquired in hospital during the first ten days of life and the condition frequently presents at the age of three to six weeks. Every soft tissue abscess in the newborn should be treated with suspicion; "pure" soft tissue abscess is rare and many have an underlying infection. Radiological bone changes are unlikely to be seen before the end of the second week of disease but soft tissue swelling may be suggestive.

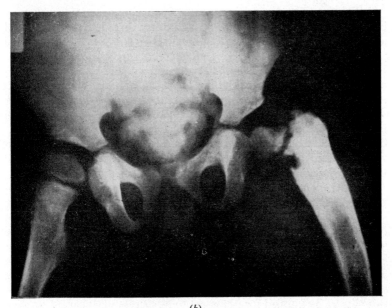

(*b*)

Fig. 60. Suppurative arthritis (Case of Mr. G. Lloyd Roberts).
(*b*) The result of delayed treatment.

Acute suppurative arthritis is a similar blood-spread infection which reaches the joint directly or by extension from neighbouring osteo-myelitis. For example, its only clinical sign in a small baby may be limitation of movement, particularly abduction and extension, in an involved hip. It is particularly important to diagnose this condition early when the hip joint is involved because the epiphysis may be destroyed within a day or two and the resultant pathological dislocation produce a serious deformity for which little can be done later. It is important throughout the management of these babies repeatedly to examine them for the development of other foci in other bones and joints and in the soft tissues such as the lungs and peritoneal cavity. It is not uncommon for a multiplicity of lesions to occur. Radiological investigation will show soft tissue swelling and capsular distortion, which occurs earlier in the infant than in the older child, though frank subluxation and bone changes show later. The bone destruction in young babies may be astonishingly gross in a child with minimal external signs. Happily, with vigorous treatment the ability to regenerate is equally astonishing in this age group. Destruction of the epiphysis of the hip will, however, give rise to an irremediable dislocation.

Treatment

Antibiotics. The basis of treatment is thorough antibiotic therapy begun as soon as the diagnosis is suspected. A blood culture should always be set up *before* starting treatment. The treatment must be prolonged for at least 2 weeks after complete clinical recovery and radiological quiescence. Shorter courses of treatment mean recrudescences of the disease. *It is therefore important to make a firm diagnosis at the outset, because a short course of treatment of a cellulitis may mask an underlying osteitis* and allow it to reach a subacute or chronic stage in which a permanent cure may be difficult to obtain.

It is best to start with a combination of methicillin or cloxacillin with streptomycin in full dosage as these bactericidal drugs cover all the likely invading organisms.

Aspiration and Exploration. A large bore needle passed into the subperiosteal space, or if a joint is involved into the joint, may produce some pus for bacteriological examination and the antibiotic can then be altered in the light of the findings. Some clinics recommend deliberate aspiration of the medullary bone for bacteriological examination in each case, but this is not a commonly accepted procedure even though it seems safe and rational. When there is a marked local swelling it can be assumed that there is a subperiosteal abscess, and it is essential that this abscess be emptied for treatment to be successful. It can be emptied by aspiration, but it is probably more effective to make a small incision, evacuate the abscess and then close the incision to avoid the risk of secondary infection. If there is joint swelling and limitation of movement suggesting involvement of the joint, then this should also be aspirated. In the case of the hip joint we have found prompt and repeated aspiration satisfactory, but the dangers of delayed treatment are so great that some clinics advise operative evacuation of the joint in every case, and this should certainly be carried out if there is any delay in the resolution of a clinical picture. Unfortunately, there are cases in which damage has occurred to the head of the femur so early that it is irreparable at the time of diagnosis.

Course. If the case is responding well to the therapy, the temperature and clinical signs improve within 24 hours and should settle within the first 5 days after beginning treatment. Any delay requires further search for abscesses, adjacent joint involvement, foci in other bones and joints or other hæmatogenous staphylococcal lesions such as staphylococcal pneumonia.

ACUTE HÆMATOGENOUS OSTEOMYELITIS OF THE LONG BONES ARISING BETWEEN THE AGES OF 2 AND 12 YEARS

Presentation. The onset is typically acute and the complaint is of severe pain. If the child is old enough he will describe it as a deep boring pain, perhaps like a bad toothache. It is characteristic of the pain that it is so bad that it prevents the child sleeping. The child will lie apprehensive in bed because he fears the pain caused by handling or moving the limb. Examination must be circumspect to avoid this. Local heat and swelling will be present over the lesion. The *localized tenderness over the bone* is intense. There is a high pyrexia and a rapid pulse. In several cases there may be rigors or convulsions with the septicæmia. In a fulminating case these general signs and symptoms may be so severe as to overshadow the local lesion and it is not unknown for these children to arrive in a fever hospital with the diagnosis of septicæmia query meningitis.

In a few cases the onset is only subacute and here the general symptoms are naturally less severe. The lower end of the femur is a relatively frequent site for this subacute osteitis.

Management. Chronic osteomyelitis of the long bones is the result of *delayed* or *inadequate* primary treatment of an acute lesion. It is therefore vital to make a confident diagnosis and to make this within the shortest possible time. It has been estimated that one should reach the diagnosis within 48 hours of the onset of acute osteitis, and if there is still really doubt at that stage one should take blood for culture and begin a full course of methicillin or cloxacillin and streptomycin to avoid the dangers of delay.

Splinting. Splinting the affected bone, in plaster if necessary, is a most useful adjunct.

Radiology in the early stage is not much help, because there has not been time for the bone changes to occur. However, it should always be carried out, if only as a base line for studying the further changes in the bone. Even with prompt treatment some changes will almost always occur in the third week of the disease. Perhaps it may be only a local rarified area at the metaphysis or a little laying down of sub-periosteal bone. This will clinch the diagnosis in retrospect. With modern anti-biotic therapy it is not uncommon for the appearance of a sequestrum to arise at the end of a long bone, and on further follow-up for this condition to disappear. If the clinical course is satisfactory then such an appearance can be safely watched in the expectation of resolution. Presumably this means that if the lesion is completely sterilized the dead bone is reincorporated as a bone graft would be.

Course. Again, the clinical signs and symptoms with fever should improve in 24 hours and settle within the first 5 days. If there is any superficial swelling suggesting subperiosteal or subcutaneous abscess this should be aspirated or evacuated without delay. If there is delay in resolution of the fever or signs, an incision should be made to locate and evacuate the subperiosteal abscess which is likely to be present. It is often advised to drill the cortex of the bone to allow release of pus under pressure within the bone end; although safe, it seems doubtful whether this is necessary, at least when an abscess has been found and evacuated. Certainly anything in the nature of a guttering operation is not wise.

Indications for Surgery. In a case which has not gone well owing to inadequate or delayed primary treatment it may be necessary to give a further course of chemotherapy for a flare up. Surgery may be necessary under certain conditions. First, if chronic disease arises in a bone such as the clavicle or fibula which can be removed without important disability, it may be wise to remove the bone. Secondly, if a sequestrum arises it will be necessary to remove the dead bone under a cover of antibiotic treatment when it has separated to obtain resolution. Thirdly, surgery may be necessary to empty an abscess, and finally, surgery may be necessary to explore a persistent sinus, excise the scarred avascular tissue and sclerosed bone. Usually a sequestrum will be found at the bottom of the sinus and it requires removal. If such a saucerized chronic lesion is going to leave a hollow space of any size it may be necessary to fill this with a muscle flap, fat or bone chips, depending on the conditions prevailing.

ATYPICAL LESIONS. In a case of atypical onset of a subacute or chronic nature it is always necessary to remember the possibility of a tuberculous or more rarely a syphilitic origin of the osteitis. In a chronic case the development of a Brodie's abscess must be considered. This is a condition in which the infection has become encysted and it is necessary to open and saucerize the lesion and fill the cavity in some way so as to allow bony healing. Staphylococcal osteitis of the vertebræ is particularly difficult to diagnose and must be suspected in unexplained back pains in childhood with minimal signs. Classical angular kyphosis and radiological changes are delayed in its usually subacute course.

Finally, a look-out must be kept for acute leukæmia in children which can give rise to bone pain, tenderness and swelling, and may be associated with some fever. It can therefore imitate osteitis clinically. Radiologically also it can produce a somewhat similar picture in that there may be rarefaction of the metaphyseal bone, and there may be some new bone laid down under the periosteum which has been lifted by leukæmic deposits.

SECONDARY OSTEITIS

In the third group of osteitis, that secondary to some other lesion such as an open fracture, or paranasal sinusitis, there is a particular lesion of infancy worth special mention. This is the *osteitis of the maxilla* in babies which results from blood-stream infection of a tooth germ spreading to the surrounding bone. It presents as an orbital cellulitis and swelling of the cheek with some fever and constitutional upset. On examination inside the mouth one may recognize the swollen gum, and indeed there may be a sinus from the tooth germ. These babies require prolonged antibiotic treatment and are prone to the same troubles if treatment is delayed or inadequate. In particular, sinuses may form from which small spicules of sequestrated bone discharge along the infra-orbital margin, and sinuses may discharge into the nasal cavity or through the hard palate. If there is an abscess under the muco-periosteum of the palate this should be evacuated to avoid further damage to developing tooth elements. An abscess in the cheek can usually be best evacuated by an horizontal incision beneath the lower eyelid. But in general the treatment is by antibiotics and surgery is avoided if possible. An analogous condition can arise in the mandible from infection of one of the lower tooth germs.

REFERENCES

Cavanagh, F. (1960) Osteomyelitis of the superior maxilla in infants, *Brit. med. J.*, *i*, 468.

Mann, T. S. (1963) Some aspects of acute hæmatogenous osteitis in children, *Brit. med. J.*, *ii*, 1561.

CHAPTER 31

DISORDERS OF THE SKELETAL SYSTEM

CONGENITAL DEFORMITIES

Talipes

THERE are three main kinds of talipes. The most important is that usually called *congenital talipes equinovarus* or clubfoot. Denis Browne has preferred to call it talipes *total varus* to stress the fact that this is a disorder involving the entire foot which is twisted in an inward direction. The usual case is indeed in equinovarus, in that the heel is in the equinus position, the forefoot and heel are also turned into varus and there is adduction of the forefoot on the tarsus. However, in the most severe cases the inward twisting of the foot is so marked that the heel seems to come down from the equinus position and the toes may point upwards parallel with the tibia.

The difficulty of management does not depend entirely on the severity of the deformity. It also depends on the state of development of the parts. There is some wasting of the calf muscles in association with all cases. In some this muscular wasting is so severe as to make treatment much more difficult. Furthermore some of the more difficult cases have a short stubby foot, and these are always more difficult to correct than the foot which although similarly twisted is of longer and more slender proportions.

Untreated clubfoot is a serious disability. One may still see adults about the streets who have had inadequate treatment or none. They walk with the feet pointing medially stepping one foot over the other and bearing their weight on the outer border of the foot or even on the dorsum.

The other types of talipes are much less serious. *Metatarsal varus* is a varus deformity of the forefoot and the tarsus is normal. Untreated it causes little disability, but it is extraordinarily difficult to shoe a patient, particularly a female, with untreated metatarsal varus. In severe metatarsal varus, owing to the oblique direction of the mid-tarsal joints, there is some limitation of dorsiflexion of the foot and this has led to their being described in some clinics as mild cases of talipes equinovarus. The prognosis, however, is completely different. The key to diagnosis of the condition is to look not only at the front of the foot but to examine the heel from behind. It will be seen that in metatarsal varus whether mild or severe the heel has a normal range of movement from varus to valgus.

Talipes valgus is the third type. Again it is not a serious disability

even if untreated, although it gives the patient an awkward slapping
gait and an increased tendency to foot strain as well as a somewhat odd
appearance. In this condition the most obvious part of the deformity is
the valgus of the forefoot so that when the patient walks the head of

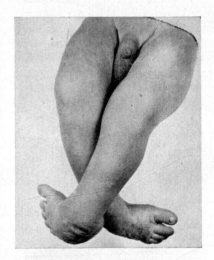

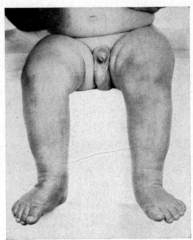

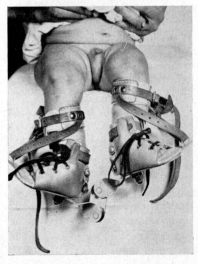

FIG. 61. Total varus (talipes equinovarus). Bilateral. Before and after
treatment and wearing the hobbled
night splints to maintain correction.

the talus pokes out medially and tends to come down towards the
ground. Examination from behind reveals that the valgus affects not
only the forefoot, but also the tarsus so that the heel goes into excessive
valgus and cannot be turned into the normal varus range.
     A less common but troublesome deformity is the *"boat-foot"*, or

rocker-foot, in which the heel remains in equinus which is masked by calcaneus of the forefoot. The head of the talus protrudes from the medial border. This is one form of "congenital flat foot" and is sometimes called "congenital vertical talus".

Denis Browne has produced convincing arguments that these conditions result from malposition *in utero*. Apart from the fact that the feet do indeed take up the positions one would expect if they were compressed against the uterine wall, these children frequently show the pressure dimples over the convexities around the knee which one would expect in such a situation. It is also interesting to notice that the feet may show the so-called mutual deformities. For example, one foot

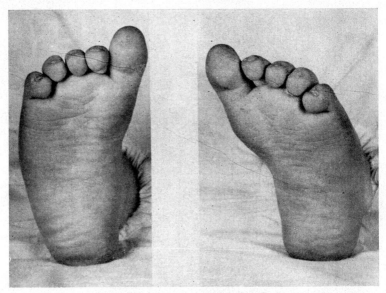

FIG. 62. Metatarsal varus of left foot.

in metatarsal varus and one in valgus so that the two feet can be fitted one curve against the other when the child is put back into its assumed uterine position. When a child has bilateral clubfoot the condition is never of equal severity in the two feet. Denis Browne explains this as the result of the cross-legged position which causes clubfoot allowing the outer leg of the pair to get the greater pressure and hence the more severe deformity.

In all talipes there is an *abnormal range of movement*, not merely a foot held in an unusual position. This distinguishes true deformity from the unusual postures seen in normal feet soon after birth which can be moved to the opposite extent of the normal range by gentle pressure (see Chapter 33–inversion spasm).

Frank neurological disorders may produce similarly deformed feet, but, having a different ætiology, they need different treatment (see Chapter 33). Arthrogryposis multiplex congenita, characterized by multiple rigid joint deformities and ill developed muscles may also include similar deformities.

TREATMENT

The treatment of talipes is one of the *acute emergencies of infancy*. If the treatment is begun within a few days of birth it has been possible to correct over 80 per cent of these deformities by accurate manipulation. It is necessary to maintain the correction and we have used Denis Browne's splints. These are L-shaped metal splints which are applied fixing one part to the foot and then using the other arm of the splint as a lever to twist the foot into the over-corrected position before fixing it. They are attached with adhesive strapping and allow the child considerably more freedom than plaster casts and fit very much better. It is therefore more easy to control the child's deformity whilst allowing desirable movement. In the case of talipes total varus it is necessary to attach the two splints to a hobble bar between the feet so as to maintain the externally rotated position. In spite of this fixation of the feet, kicking is freely possible in these splints so that the ankles are manipulated by the child's activities and he is frustrated as little as possible. The splints are changed and the manipulation repeated fortnightly. This method of treatment is simple, but it must not be thought that this means that it is easy. It is important to manipulate accurately and to get one's thrust under the lateral border of the tarsus so as to correct the deformity of the heel and not merely of the forefoot. However good the foot may look from the front while the child is standing on it, relapse is inevitable unless the heel has been manipulated into valgus. An unskilful manipulation exerting pressure on the forefoot can weaken the foot across the mid-tarsal joint and by producing the so-called rocker-bottom foot will prevent any later attempts at manipulation from being successful. Having obtained correction in this way, it is necessary to maintain the over-corrected position whilst the child is in bed at night for the next 5 years until the child's muscle balance has been corrected and the early growth period is over. This is achieved by night splints working on the same lever principle. A lateral wedge to the bootees worn is given by day so that he walks in valgus. Any reduction of this period of treatment may again lead to relapse in the condition.

It is thus a prolonged management. If it is carried out properly there is no need for general anæsthesia or hospital admission at any time. The treatment is so regulated that the child's feet are in the position he requires before he is old enough to want to walk on them. He is not restricted in his day-time activity in any way. It produces a corrected and supple foot and this method is well worth the persistence and perseverance necessary on the part both of the surgeon and of the parents. Other methods may be successful but the key to success is that *any* method must be supervised by *one person throughout*. If there is any delay in treatment then it is much more difficult to correct the condition by manipulation. It may be possible to maintain a reasonable foot during the growing period by manipulation followed by transplantation of the tibialis anterior tendon to the outer side of the foot so as to help redress the muscle balance. Lengthening the Achilles tendon improves the heel posture only at the cost of weakening the calf to a degree that may diminish function. But the majority of these children who have had delayed treatment will finish up needing a bone operation. In this case the operation must be more than the old-fashioned wedge tarsectomy which merely pointed the forefoot in the right direction and left the heel inverted. Relapse always occurred. Os calcis osteotomy to correct the varus of the heel promises well and avoids the stiffening of the foot inherent in the triple arthrodesis group of operations.

Metatarsal varsus and talipes valgus are much easier to treat. A few weeks of splinting in the over-corrected position is sufficient to achieve correction and the mother can be taught manipulations to maintain this until the child is walking. When walking begins the child who has had talipes valgus will require a medial wedge and stiffening to the shoe for a period. Unfortunately the less serious nature of these conditions and their less impressive appearance in the newborn has frequently led to their being neglected until the child is older. Often the parents do not worry until the child starts to walk, when they realize that he is awkward in his appearance. Even if the parents have worried earlier, it is likely that a doctor will have reassured them without treatment. This is a great pity, because although the lesions are simply treated in the infant they are very stubborn to treat after walking has begun. Anæsthesia is required to manipulate the metatarsal varus; correction of these feet which are usually short and stubby is difficult, and afterwards support by means of a shaped night-boot is necessary. Severe talipes valgus can probably never be corrected fully except by some bone operation, if treatment begins after walking has commenced. This is only justified in the severest cases, but in these few it may be well worth while.

Congenital Dislocation of the Hip

Congenital dislocation of the hip is a condition with genetic and environmental factors in its ætiology. It is commoner in girls than boys. The baby is usually born with a dislocatable rather than a persistently dislocated joint. Maternal hormones stimulate the production of relaxin from the uterus of the female fœtus and the effect takes some time to wear off. Delayed progress of the normal transition during fœtal life from an extended breech position of the legs to the flexed antepartum position encourages dislocation of a relaxed joint.

A hereditary primary acetabular dysplasia is also present in most bilateral cases but only in a minority of the unilateral. Familial joint laxity inherited as a dominant characteristic, is of more importance in the male cases. The dislocation is first in a posterior direction. Muscle contraction and later weight bearing cause the head to ride up higher on the pelvis with contracture of the Y shaped and other ligaments and increasing shortening of the limb.

EARLY DIAGNOSIS. There is a simple test which can be applied to the newborn which will pick out all the dislocatable hips—about one in a hundred babies of which about one tenth could be expected to proceed

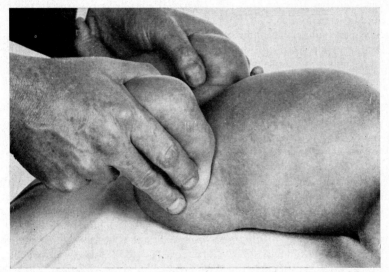

FIG. 63. The abduction test for dislocatable or dislocated hip in the newborn.

to persistent dislocation. Maintenance of abduction for two months by a simple appliance is sufficient at this stage to prevent dislocation, so that prophylactic treatment of the babies at risk can, for practical purposes, eliminate the condition.

The Abduction Test. The baby's legs are flexed 90° at knees and hips and held with the thumbs over the medial side of the thighs and the fingers on the lateral sides of the thighs so that the middle fingers come over the greater trochanters. Gentle pressure backwards will dislocate a lax hip and then, on attempted abduction, a resistance followed by a jerk of reduction will be recognized in the middle of the range. The normal hip abducts about 80°. (Fig. 63.)

Other signs are described including the presence of extra or unequal skin creases on the thighs. It should be realized that although these are present in unilateral dislocations they are also present in many normal babies. They are unnecessary because the abduction test—repeated at intervals throughout infancy—is reliable and universally applicable.

Unfortunately cases are still missed in this country and may not come to light until asymmetry of the legs in unilateral cases or a wide perineum in bilateral cases noticed. Later the characteristic dipping gait (unilateral) or waddle (bilateral) are seen. The abduction test is again reliable and at this stage the frank dislocation causes limitation at about 45°. Radiology confirms the dislocation or demonstrates the other, rarer causes of limitation such as infantile coxa vara.

Radiology. In the new-born period the high slope of the acetabulum is recognizable. The line of the shaft of the femur runs up to meet the pelvis farther laterally and the trochanter may be recognizably higher up. But the absence of a visible capital epiphysis makes the interpretation more subtle than later on, when the dislocation is directly demonstrable. Andren's position—internal rotation and 45° abduction of the hips—makes diagnosis clearer.

Treatment. Treatment should be prophylactic by maintaining abduction of all dislocatable hips in the newborn for two months.

When frank dislocation is recognized later reduction by gentle manipulation or traction in increasing abduction is required. It is followed by maintenance of abduction by an appliance such as the Denis Browne harness which allows more activity around the joint than a plaster cast for about nine months.

Bilateral cases in particular may also require an acetabuloplasty to bring down the upper lip of the undeveloped acetabulum to form a deeper and more stable hip.

RESULTS. Neonatal treatment probably gives complete elimination of frank dislocation though the usually bilateral cases with a primary factor of dysplasia may still be more prone to osteo-arthritis in middle life. Conservative treatment in the second year of life gives good early results in unilateral cases though redislocation is common in bilateral cases and may merit acetabuloplasty. Arthritis in middle life is common. After the age of four years, conservative reduction is probably better not attempted and operative measures for unilateral cases afford the best salvage.

The Trendelenburg test is of considerable use, particularly in assessing the effectiveness of treatment. The child is asked to stand on one leg. If its hip is stable the opposite buttock is raised as the child balances on one leg. If the hip is unstable the opposite buttock drops because the abductors of the involved hip are unable to support the pelvis. In assessing results it must always be remembered that the child is a very adaptable creature and will make extraordinarily good use of the most incongruous and unstable looking hip, even to the extent of playing football. This is not a high enough criterion and one must aim at a hip which will go through adult life without prematurely developing pain, stiffness and weakness. This will only be obtained reliably by treatment in early infancy.

Scoliosis

This is the condition of curvature of the spine. Hunchbacks are severe cases. The most obvious part of the deformity is the lateral flexion of the spine, but there is also an element of rotation which is of importance in treatment.

Scolioses are usually classified as *Postural, Paralytic* and *Structural.* The last term means that there is an alteration in shape of the spine which cannot be corrected by passive means. Perhaps a fourth group of *Infant scoliosis* should be considered separately.

POSTURAL SCOLIOSIS. *Postural scoliosis* is most often recognized in the adolescent girl and may amount to little more than a transient poor stance. Gymnastics will correct most cases which merit treatment. Congenital shortness of one limb will inevitably cause a slight scoliosis to correct for the pelvic obliquity. This can be looked on as a useful adaptive mechanism and there seems no real evidence that such a curve progresses. A raised shoe is likely to be more disabling and unsightly than the original condition and is only to be used when marked shortening of the leg justifies it for the greater ease in walking it may give.

PARALYTIC SCOLIOSIS. A serious cause is acute anterior poliomyelitis. Jacket support may be needed, then spinal bone grafts when growth has ceased. There may be severe disability due to interference with respiration, the respiratory cage being twisted and narrowed. Breathing exercises with emphasis on the use of the diaphragm are important.

STRUCTURAL SCOLIOSIS. There are two main types. *Congenital hemivertebræ* may clearly cause scoliosis. The baby soon produces compensatory curves in the opposite direction above and below the lesion and deformity is usually surprisingly slight. When many vertebræ are involved, however, severe progressive deformity may result from the instability.

More serious are the cases where a curve and rotation is noticed in the presence of apparently normally formed vertebræ and with no signs of muscular weakness. The condition progresses insidiously and the vertebræ become wedge shaped as it goes on. Those arising in the thoracolumbar region have the worst outlook and those arising earlier progress further. It has been shown that of those occurring before the age of 3 years 90 per cent will finish with a curve of 90° or more. No treatment has yet been evolved which will prevent this inexorable progress. Physiotherapy is of value in keeping the respiratory system as efficient as possible. When spinal growth is ceasing forced correction by jackets followed by spinal grafts will help the severe cases. The cause is unknown, so that the label *idiopathic* has inevitably been attached.

This inability to cure an established case of idiopathic scoliosis gives importance to the study of *scoliosis in infancy*. Denis Browne has devised a simple frame which holds the spine in the over-corrected position but allows the baby most other movements. It is much more easily tolerated and managed than a plaster bed.

A good many infants have a mild scoliosis and the great majority correct themselves. It seems probable that the remainder progress to idiopathic scoliosis and that the shorter, sharper curves are more likely to persist than longer, gentle curves. It would seem much more hopeful to correct the deformity before weight-bearing begins. It would be better to treat some babies unnecessarily than to miss a progressive case until the weight-bearing stage rendered it incurable. We therefore use physiotherapy and the frame in cases of persisting infant scoliosis in the present incomplete state of our knowledge.

The mother may bring the baby because he "always lies on one side". In examining an infant for scoliosis it is useless to rely on a single X-ray. The baby should be played with in the prone position. It will curl to the side it prefers and then it must be coaxed to the other side until the skin creases under its ribs show contralateral flexion of the spine. One is demonstrating not a preferred position but a *limited range of movement*. The curve is usually to the right. Associated asymmetry of the head (plagiocephaly) and slight limitation of abduction of the hips are common. If this is found radiographs should be taken at both extremes of lateral flexion. This will avoid unnecessary treatment of squirming but healthy babies.

Lever Splints and Controlled Movements

Denis Browne has made a number of valuable contributions to orthopædics and it will be seen that two principles underlie his methods of treatment. One is the use of *lever splints*. The part is not merely encased in the splint. These are so constructed that one part of the splint is attached to the deformed member and another part of the splint used as a lever to direct the member into the desired position. It is clearly seen in the application of the L-shaped splint to a clubfoot. The foot is strapped to the sole plate and the other arm of the L is drawn against the leg and strapped to it so as to twist the foot into valgus. Similarly the splint for congenital dislocation of the hip holds the femur in abduction with a fulcrum on the lumbosacral spine.

The second principle is that of *controlled movement* in contradistinction to immobilization. Many orthopædic devices developed at a period when much of the work consisted of the treatment of chronic infections such as tuberculosis. Rest is good for an inflamed part. Immobilization was the aim.

But much more of modern orthopædics involves the treatment of congenital deformities. There is no direct need for immobilization here. It can be harmful because muscle weakness follows and because unused joint surfaces degenerate and deform. Articular cartilage degenerates if not brought into contact with its opposing surface and in the absence of the stimulus of movement there is for example no stimulus to growth and deepening of the acetabulum of the developing hip. Such potential ill-effects of rest had to be accepted in treating infections, but they can be largely avoided when treating other lesions. Clearly movement in the direction of the deformity must be prevented, but the more other movements can be encouraged the better will be the development of the part. Thus the club foot is regulated in valgus but the baby is allowed to kick his hobbled feet as he wishes. The congenital dislocation of the hip is prevented from recurrence by holding the joint in abduction by rings around the thigh connected by a bar behind the body. But all other movements are encouraged and the child is able to crawl and climb in the apparatus, grinding the head of the femur into its socket and stimulating concentric development of the joint.

DISTURBANCES OF OSSIFICATION

CRANIOSYNOSTOSIS. Craniosynostosis is a condition in which the sutures of the vault of the skull close prematurely. The condition begins in fœtal life. It may affect the sagittal suture or the coronal sutures or it may involve all the sutures of the skull. It is usually a symmetrical condition, but occasionally only one side of the head may be affected producing one form of asymmetry or plagiocephaly.

If the sagittal suture is fused prematurely compensatory overgrowth takes place at the coronal suture producing a long head in the antero-posterior direction, the condition called scaphocephaly. If the coronal suture is fused brachycephaly ensues. If both sutures fuse early most of the growth takes place in an upward and transverse direction from the base of the cranium producing the towering but short head of oxycephaly or acrocephaly. Oxycephaly is sometimes associated with abnormalities of the development of the facial bones so that the face has an ugly flat-cheeked appearance with apparent exophthalmos. Cleft palate may coexist. In severe cases the limbs may also be affected with syndactyly of the fingers and toes (Apert's syndrome—Acrocephalo-syndactyly). In spite of the grotesque appearance of a severe case craniosynostotic children are usually mentally normal and grow up to be capable adults.

However, operation on the vault may be justified in many for the sake of the cosmetic effect, and because if the fusion involves all the sutures of the skull there would seem to be a real risk that the normal expansion of the brain will be prevented, resulting in an increased intracranial pressure. In cases of oxycephaly the abnormality of the bones around the optic foramina may produce local pressure on the optic nerves and blindness. Operation may be necessary to relieve or prevent such an occurrence.

It is important to realize that although, as has been said, the majority

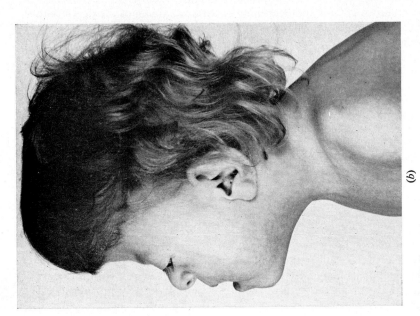

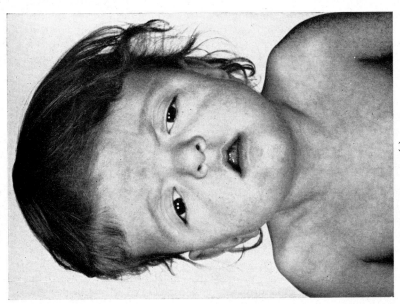

Fig. 64. Craniosynostosis (acrocephalic type).

of these children grow up mentally normal, yet if operation is required it is required early. Most of the growth of the calvarium is completed by the twelfth month of life. Operation should be carried out within the first 6 months of life and preferably within the first weeks. It will then be possible to obtain the greatest cosmetic improvement as well as allowing most freely the expansion of the brain. The operations consist in principle of making artificial sutures and it is necessary to put in some substance such as polythene film to delay recurrence of fusion. Even with such aids refusion may occur rapidly enough to necessitate repeated operation. In each individual case therefore the decision as to whether treatment is justified or not must be reached promptly.

OSTEOGENESIS IMPERFECTA (FRAGILITAS OSSIUM). This condition affects all the bones of the body. They are weak and fracture easily because they have a thin cortex with sparse and slender trabeculæ, even though they are normally calcified. There does not appear to be any abnormality of calcium or phosphorus metabolism in these children. The condition is inherited and its severity varies considerably. The child may be stillborn with multiple fractures or survive only a short while. Others may only be recognized after infancy due to their prone-ness to recurring fractures. The fractures heal quite normally, but as the result of their multiplicity grotesque deformities may develop as the child grows. As the patient gets older there is a diminished liability to fracture easily. The condition is usually associated with persistent blue scleræ and with a tendency to develop deafness in adult life.

POLYOSTOTIC FIBROUS DYSPLASIA. This is a condition affecting mainly the long bones. Islands of fibrous tissue are incorporated in the growing bones and these weak areas may allow a fracture to occur with minimal trauma. Radiography of the bone shows translucent areas in the fibrous regions so that these have been mistakenly believed to be bone cysts. The condition is often associated with pigmented patches (café-au-lait) on the skin. There is often some asymmetry in the length of the bones and precocious puberty may occur in affected girls. The bones them-selves are normal apart from the islands of fibrous tissue. Fibrous dysplasia is also seen in the facial region usually affecting the jaws.

CRANIO-CLEIDAL DYSOSTOSIS. This is a disturbance which only affects bones formed in membrane. The bones of the vault of the skull are under-developed so that wide gaps can be palpated between them. The clavicles are not properly ossified, so that these patients are able to perform the parlour trick of bringing their two arms together so that the heads of the humeri meet under the chin. The disability due to this condition is remarkably slight. There is frequently an associated defect of dentition.

DISTURBANCES OF CHONDRIFICATION

Failure of Maturation of the Cartilage

ACHONDROPLASIA. The cartilage of the long bones fails to mature properly and growth in length is therefore markedly reduced although the growth in breadth due to subperiosteal bone formation proceeds normally. This is the type of dwarfism seen in the typical circus dwarf who has a normal sized body and a large head but short yet strong limbs. The condition is compatible with an active life and as these dwarfs may grow and marry it is not uncommon to see hereditary cases.

OSTEOCHONDRODYSTROPHY (MORQUIO'S DISEASE). The Morquio type of dwarf has limb lesions just as the achondroplastic but also has a severe affection of the vertebral column with wedging of the vertebral bodies so that there is a gross kyphosis and the chest is pushed forward into pigeon-breasted appearance.

GARGOYLISM. In this condition the skeletal lesions are similar to those of osteochondrodystrophy. The name is derived from the typical coarse facies, blank expression and a flat and broad root of the nose. In these children there is also a metabolic defect. The liver and spleen are usually palpably enlarged due to mucopolysaccharide deposits and there is mental defect and a tendency to clouding of the cornea.

Displacement of Cartilage

DIAPHYSEAL ACLASIS (MULTIPLE CARTILAGINOUS EXOSTOSES). At the ends of the long bones islands of cartilage become displaced and with continued growth they develop into spurs of bone each with a cartilaginous growing cap, growing in a direction away from the joint. They may be symptomless or may cause annoyance by their protuberance or by pressure on a nerve in the region. In this case they may need to be removed although many can be left untreated.

OLLIER'S DISEASE (MULTIPLE ENCHONDROSIS). In these children islands of cartilage are also sequestrated from the epiphyseal region, but the continued growth of cartilage takes place within the bone. The bone is expanded so that unsightly knobs appear near the ends of the long bones, including the phalanges. The bones may be distorted in an angular fashion as the result of this uneven growth. Ollier's disease, unlike diaphyseal aclasis, tends to be asymmetrical in its distribution. There is also frequently a tendency to dwarfism.

POST-NATAL DISORDERS OF OSSIFICATION

CAFFEY'S SYNDROME. This disease, also called infantile cortical hyperostosis, is of unknown ætiology. It arises in infancy. Several bones may be involved at a time by a progressive thickening of the cortex, the appearance simulating that of osteomyelitis. As well as the long bones, thickening is typically seen in the maxillæ or mandible distorting the face. There is often pyrexia along with the condition and the child may be irritable. All this adds to the clinical similarity to osteomyelitis. However, no infective agent can be found. The condition is one which tends to spontaneous regression after a period and it seems that cortisone may encourage such regression.

RICKETS. Nutritional rickets due to lack of vitamin D in the diet has about disappeared in these countries. It is occasionally seen, usually amongst the children of food-faddists. Clinics' enthusiasm in offering vitamin supplements seems to be diminishing as a result of recent appreciation of the possibility of illness due to hypervitaminosis D, so that we may perhaps see more again. A few cases are still seen in which the underlying factor is a renal lesion or a resistance to normal doses of vitamin D causing the interference with calcium metabolism.

The classical rickety baby is miserable and hypotonic with a pot belly, cranial bossing, beading of the costal cartilages and non-tender swelling of the ends of the long bones best seen in the wrists, knees and ankles. The legs are usually bowed and weight-bearing and muscle pull may lead to further deformities if treatment is delayed. The ligaments are lax. Radiography of the swollen bone ends shows a wide cupped metaphysis and a broad gap representing failure of calcification. In a simple nutritional case clinical and radiological resolution begins after a week or two on vitamin D.

The local appearances in vitamin-resistant rickets may be similar, but the child's general health good. Renal rickets presents a less typical picture and osteoporotic changes may predominate.

SCURVY. This is a bleeding tendency due to lack of vitamin C. It is still seen occasionally and may be caused by boiling the orange juice or vitamin drops with the baby's milk, so destroying the vitamin C. It may be associated with rickets in a multiple deficiency. The child is fretful and has tender limbs which may be swollen. Unwillingness to move them accounts for the pseudo-paralysis. The gums may be swollen and bleed easily. The child bruises easily. Radiography shows sub-periosteal new bone forming along the shafts of the morbid bone, the periosteum having been raised by hæmorrhage. More important diagnostically is the wide dense line at the epiphysis—the zone of provisional calcification. The defect seems to be in transition from this stage to osteogenesis.

REFERENCES

Barlow, T. G. (1962) Congenital Dislocation of the Hip. *J. Bone Jt. Surg.*, **44B**, 292.
Browne, Denis (1956) Splinting for Controlled Movement, *Clinical Orthopædics*, No. 8, 91. J. B. Lippincott Co.
Browne, Denis (1965) Congenital postural scoliosis, *Brit. med. J.*, **2**, 565.
Mackenzie, D. Y. (1959) Arthrogryposis Multiplex Congenita. *Proc. roy. Soc. Med.*, **52**, 1101.
Wilkinson, J. A. (1963) Prime factors in the Etiology of Congenital Dislocation of the Hip. *J. Bone Jt. Surg.*, **45B**, 268.

CHAPTER 32

LIMB MALFORMATIONS AND PARALYSES

THIS chapter will bring together a number of congenital abnormalities involving the limbs and a discussion of the management of certain forms of paralysis. A number of lesions involving the limbs have already been discussed in other chapters.

Malformations of the Upper Limb

Congenital Shortening and Congenital Amputations. A group of malformations of the limbs exists in which segments of the limb are shortened or absent. There may be for example an absent or shortened arm and yet there may be a well-formed hand at the end of the limb ("phocomelia"—seal flipper). Or a normal arm may stop short at the carpus which may bear little spherical lobes of skin-covered flesh representing the digits. It is commoner for the distal end of the limb to be lacking with the proximal end remaining normal These are the lesions called congenital amputations. A common level for congenital amputation is at the wrist and another is about 2 inches below the elbow. The end of the limb may be small and covered with normal skin. In other cases there is a congenital scar as though the result of some intra-uterine accident. The scar may even be incompletely healed at birth leaving a granulating area to heal after birth. In another group, one border of the limb is affected. Thus reduction of the radial ray may produce the typical "club hand" swung off the end of the ulna and with absence of the thumb. Function is astonishingly good.

There are often amniotic adhesions to the site of such an accident, and this in the past led to the assumption that the bands caused strangulation. However, it appears that the superficially apparent cause was misleading. It has been demonstrated clearly in experimental work how the application of some noxious agent to the growing limb bud will produce first of all a blister which then bursts leaving an ulcerated area, followed by a necrosis at the site which may result in a constriction ring or complete loss of the distal part of the limb. This fœtal dysplasia is apparently the cause of some lesions and the amniotic adhesions are secondary, the result of adherence of the amnion to the raw healing surfaces.

In spite of many ingenious attempts, surgery has little to offer these children and usually they require a prosthesis to aid their function. It is possible when the child has reached a co-operative age to fit him with a so-called working hand attached to an artificial arm. Various instruments and utensils such as knife and fork can be clipped on and used.

248

Quite separately he can have a "dress hand" in order to give a normal appearance in public. "Powered" prostheses worked by shoulder movements or even from the currents produced by nerve action are being developed. They suffer from absence of sensation in the artificial hand, so that movement has to be controlled by vision.

It is surprising how much a child will do with the incomplete stump of an arm. The most important thing to be done at this stage is to encourage him to try to use the limb as much as possible; above all to encourage him to let it be seen so that he may become accustomed to the attention it will inevitably excite among his playfellows, and thus avoid any development of shyness and feeling of inferiority as a result of the deformity. At 2 years of age the child may be given a light prosthesis to wear in order to become accustomed to the management of such an appliance rather than in the expectation that he will wear it regularly and appreciate it at that time.

If the child has been properly encouraged to use his limb, then at this age he will usually in fact take off the prosthesis when he really wants to use the limb. The early fitting of the limb is a help, however, in getting him accustomed to the feel of the prosthesis, which will then come less strangely to him later on when he wishes to use it to develop further skills. The development of pride in appearance will itself decide when he wishes to use a dress arm.

Thalidomide Induced Deformities. The recent introduction of the tranquillizer thalidomide produced a tragic outbreak of severe symmetrical limb deformities—typically a bilateral phocomelia and gross reduction of the lower limbs. Other deformities, including anal stenosis, may coexist. The syndrome arose following the use of thalidomide in the early weeks of pregnancy when the limbs were developing.

This has underlined the importance of testing new drugs for possible teratogenic effects.

Syndactyly. Congenital deformities of the hand are not uncommon and the commonest of these is the condition of syndactyly, in which there has been a failure to separate the fingers. Syndactyly can be divided into two types. In one type there are normally developed digits, apart from the fusion of their skin. The application of full thickness skin grafts to the raw surfaces left by separating the fingers will give a completely normal functioning hand of good appearance. The operation is usually carried out at about 3 years of age. It may be stressed that the minor procedures which are sometimes tempting in the presence of a wide web of skin—i.e. division of the web and suture of its edges, or the rolling of one surface of the split web around each of the fingers—are not only valueless, but by producing contractures may interfere seriously with the function of the digits. There is never enough skin present locally to give adequate cover without the use of free grafts.

The other type of syndactyly is that in which the fingers are not only fused but ill-formed to some degree. They may be merely shorter than

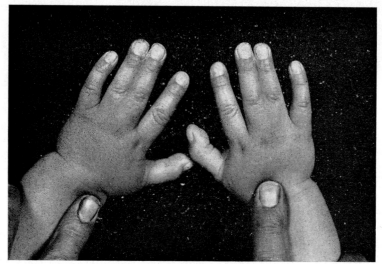

FIG. 65. Syndactyly. Well-formed fingers. (Case of Dr. G. H. Newns.)

normal, or they may be distorted, and there may be fusion between the bones of two digits. In this case separation may still produce a functionally normal hand in some cases, but in others, when the joints are ill-formed, function may better be served by leaving two fingers fused together to act as one more stable digit. In this type of syndactyly the development of the thenar eminence may be incomplete, so that the

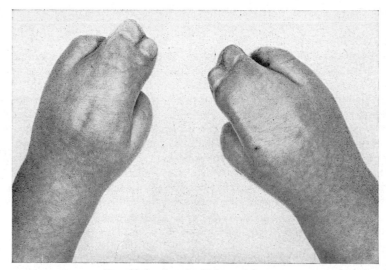

FIG. 66. Syndactyly. Ill-formed fingers.

thumb is unable to perform its essential function of opposition to the fingers in grasping. It has been said that the thumb forms 50 per cent of the hand because without a thumb the pincer type of grip is impossible. If there is no properly formed thumb, pollicization of the radial digit may improve function. This means a surgical procedure to widen the web between the radial digit and the next, and a rotation of its metacarpal and fixation so that it can be used to grasp in the manner of a thumb. In contemplating any elaborate reconstructive surgery it must be remembered that unless a digit has good sensation and tactile discrimination it will be much more trouble than it is worth, and cause annoyance to the patient without being of any real functional use. In fact one finds again and again in considering these deformed hands that one is astonished by the extremely good use to which the children are able to put the malformed hand in its natural state. Apart from the separation of skin webs, surgery has a small part to play and one must have very good reasons for contemplating anything beyond this.

SUPERNUMERARY DIGITS. Certain of the fingers may be grossly reduced in development or absent, either as a separate deformity or in association with syndactyly; or, alternatively, there may be extra digits. The extra digit is usually on the ulnar side of the hand and is often so rudimentary as to be of no practical value. It is best removed as a potential annoyance from the inability to control it. In many cases it is possible to cope with the vestigial sixth digit on the ulnar side of the hand by tying a stout ligature around it at birth and leaving it to drop off. Following this simple procedure, the development of a bony prominence at the site as a result of the development of the retained rudimentary metacarpal may require further surgery later. When supernumerary digits are removed by formal surgery care is taken to core out any such metacarpal rudiment.

Malformations of the Lower Limbs

Congenital Shortening and Congenital Malformation. Similar lesions occur in the lower limbs. Whereas the upper limb is used for fine and skilful actions, the lower limb in general performs heavier but simpler functions and its most important one is that of supporting the body in standing and walking. This means that the treatment of a congenitally short leg by the application of prosthesis can be much more effective. Indeed, the modern lower limb prostheses have developed to a stage where it is possible not only to walk and run, but to ride a horse and to go ski-ing with *two* below-knee prostheses. A short leg may have a deformed foot at the end and this may be a useless encumbrance which interferes with the fitting of a good limb. In this case it may be wise to amputate the foot. When carrying out such procedures in children it is important to realize that the type of operation preferable is not that which has been found most suitable for amputations when necessary for acquired lesions or accidents in adult life. If the classical mid-thigh or below-knee amputations are carried out in children the bone soon grows out to stretch the tip of the stump, producing a painful conical stump and eventually skin necrosis, requiring repeated reamputations during the growing period. It is preferable in children to perform a disarticulation either through the ankle joint or the knee joint, depending on the deformity. The broad end of the bone then seems able to carry the skin and soft tissues ahead of it so that the remaining stump grows with the child and remains comfortable throughout growth.

Syndactyly. Syndactyly occurs in the toes just as it does in the hands. It is, however, of much less importance because of the differing function of the toes. It is usually not necessary to separate fused toes. In a few cases there may be fusion by a bridge of skin at the tip of crumpled toes with a window through the cleft proximal to this. This kind of window may be difficult to keep clean and it may then be worth separating the digits. Also, the fusion particularly of the great toe to the next one may cause buckling of the great toe as growth proceeds, and separation with skin grafting will then again be useful. A supernumerary toe will be annoying because of the increased breadth of the foot. It makes the foot difficult to shoe. Such a toe is usually associated with at least a rudimentary supernumerary metatarsal which broadens the whole foot. In order usefully to narrow the foot it is necessary to remove this metatarsal along with the toe.

The Toes. A common deformity of the fifth toe is the so-called *cocked-up toe*. The toe is elevated and medially deviated so that it lies on top of the fourth toe. This causes no disability to the infant, but again becomes annoying when shoes are worn. It is therefore well worth treating this minor deformity. A useful method is by tenotomy of the extensor tendon and capsulotomy of the joint, rotating a flap of skin from the plantar to the dorsal surface, so as to bring the toe downwards and laterally. The toe should be strapped in full flexion to the sole of the foot for 3 weeks after the operation.

Another common congenital deformity which causes anxiety to the mother is that which is perhaps best called *curly toes*. The toes affected are usually the second and third and they curve towards each other, and also in a downward direction. The appearance is slightly abnormal but they give rise to no disability and no treatment is needed. If, however, the second toe has a marked flexion deformity of the interphalangeal joints, which is usually associated with extension of the metatarsophalangeal joint, so-called *hammer toe*, then treatment is usually justified. Again trouble does not arise until shoes are worn, but if the deformity is sufficient a painful corn then develops on the dorsum over the distal joint. It is most easily corrected by tenotomy of the extensor tendon and excision of the corn with an ellipse of skin over the proximal joint, and excising the bone ends so as to fuse the joint in a straight position. The hammer toe is usually a long one which tends to project in front of the first toe, and some shortening as a result of the operation is therefore beneficial and prevents it jamming into the toe of a shoe, causing pressure and discomfort.

HALLUX VALGUS. *Hallux valgus* is a much more serious deformity of the great toe. It is, as the name implies, a deviation of the toe laterally. The result is a prominence of the metatarsal head which becomes painful as a result of pressure and the later development of the classical bunion on it. The deformed joint is also prone to early osteoarthritic changes. Much has been said about the atavistic nature of the first metatarsal in these cases. It has been suggested that it is in varus and that this is why the compensatory valgus of the toe arises as the result of the pull of the tendons. Others have attributed the majority of cases to modern forms of civilized footwear. There is no doubt that trouble from hallux valgus is much commoner in women than in men and that ill-fitting footwear exacerbates the condition and causes it to produce symptoms. However, it is common to see hallux valgus at a stage when the foot has never been compressed by footwear. Perhaps in some cases it may even have been compressed *in utero*. It is not uncommon to notice that the fifth toe is incurved in these cases, looking as though the end of the foot had been squeezed. There is a tendency for the curling of the other toes to work out in the first few months of life, but there is unfortunately no tendency for hallux valgus to improve, but rather the reverse. Fifteen degrees seems to be the critical angle beyond which further deterioration can be expected.

In view of the trouble this condition gives in adult life various forms of operation have been considered in an attempt to improve the mechanics of the foot in later childhood. The abductor hallucis tendon may be transplanted from the first phalanx of the great toe to the metatarsal, or an osteotomy of the bone will make the metatarsal take up a more usual position. It is doubtful whether any of these operations can yet be considered as fully established, or their use justified except in extreme cases. The Royal National Orthopædic Hospital, London, have designed a very simple night splint which goes along the medial border of the foot and is attached with straps around the foot and toe, so as to hold the great toe in the varus position. This night splint is comfortable to wear and at least prevents secondary contractures and further development of the condition during childhood. It does seem, however, that one's attempts to control this deformity in girls (and in recent years boys also!) are largely doomed to failure when adolescence comes along and the desire for smart shoes outweighs all other considerations.

It is important to distinguish the condition of *phalanx valgus* from that of hallux valgus. A number of children are born with the distal phalanx of the great toe in a valgus position, although the first phalanx and metatarsal are normal in their alignment. This is a trivial deformity which does not progress and does not give trouble. Sometimes unnecessary alarm is raised by mistaking it for hallux valgus.

PARALYSES

There are three important causes of limb paralysis at the present time. One is acquired, one congenital and one may be congenital or early acquired, with a multiple ætiology. The first is anterior poliomyelitis (infantile paralysis), the second is spina bifida and the third is the so-called cerebral palsy of which the spastic child is the commonest example, although athetoid and flaccid types also occur.

POLIOMYELITIS. Happily the introduction of effective vaccination is rendering this a disease of the past, but the lessons learnt in its management are proving of value in the similar paralyses in the growing problem of spina bifida. Briefly the principles were rest during the stage of onset followed by passive movements to prevent contractures and then active movements and physiotherapy to develop the residual muscle potential. "Trick" movements could overcome certain weaknesses. However, physiotherapy could not alter the abnormal balance around a joint so that late contracture was a risk which could be averted by early "prophylactic" muscle transplantations—such as the movement of tibialis anterior tendon to the outer border of the foot when the peronei were weak and the foot tending to varus. Whilst appliances were sometimes needed to control flail joints, when growth had ceased fusion of the joint might enable these to be discarded.

SPINA BIFIDA. Spina bifida has been discussed in its own chapter. The paralysis is basically a lower motor neurone paralysis involving the lower limbs. The type of paralysis tends to fit into one of several groups of muscle involvements just as do the cases of anterior poliomyelitis, where muscle groups with their centres in neighbouring parts of the cord tend to be involved together producing various typical palsies as an end result. The deformities in spina bifida may be much more severe than in poliomyelitis because the lesion occurs earlier in growth and hence severe deformity and contracture may be present even before birth. Furthermore, the additional factor of uterine pressure on the abnormal limb may add its quota to the bizarre deformity which may result. It seems likely that much more can be done for these children by adopting similar attitudes of earlier physiotherapy and operations, including muscle transplantation, in the same way as one would for infantile paralysis. This work is in its early stages but the results are promising.

CEREBRAL PALSY. Much publicity has recently been given to what has unfortunately become known to the lay public as the new treatment of spastics. Certainly great strides have been made in the management of cerebral palsy by the hard work of devoted and skilled physiotherapists, as well as by medical research. But there is still no cure for spasticity and the best that this treatment can do is to teach the child how to use his disabled limbs better. The subject is a large one, but perhaps it would be fair to describe it as simply training the child in the various motor activities from the beginning as one would a normal child, but going slowly and with extra patience to allow him time to develop the skills in spite of his inco-ordinate and stiffly unmanageable limbs. The child is taught first to lie flat and then sit up and then to walk rather than trying to train him straightaway to the latter goal. It is this appreciation of the need to look on the child as a whole and help him to develop his pathways of control at all levels which has resulted in the improved outlook for these children.

Attempts at local surgery, for example by the largely outmoded nerve sections to reduce spasticity, are of little value. Peripheral surgery on the tendons or the nerves has little to offer although it may be of occasional value. For instance, the unfortunate child with severely spastic legs producing adduction contracture and also suffering from the mental defect which occurs in a considerable proportion of these cases will be extremely difficult to nurse and manage. A bilateral obturator neurectomy will enable abduction of the limbs to take place and allow easy perineal toilet.

A fixed equinus of the foot is commonly seen and is resistant to ordinary physiotherapy. Serial plasters in the maximum obtainable dorsiflexion will usually correct this in a few weeks. A Denis Browne equinus night splint similar to that used to retain the correction of a talipes will maintain the improvement. This approach is preferable to the apparently simpler operative lengthening of the tendo Achillis. It is easy to lengthen too little or too much.

It is important to realize that these children are usually more intelligent than they appear, and indeed the majority are normally intelligent. Their inability to control their motor system, producing odd facial grimaces and so on, inevitably makes one underestimate their intelligence. Unfortunately, grimacing, drooling and such traits, which arouse only sympathy when the sufferer is a child, are not so easily accepted in adults. These traits, and a labile temperament, may increase the problems of integration into society, even though mentality is good. Their treatment, however, is largely a matter of careful training along developmental lines requiring much time and patience and skill on the part of the physiotherapist and the parents.

A completely different type of surgery may be beneficial in a few of the more severe cases. Some of these children have severe temper tantrums which make it impossible to live with them or to allow them the freedom of a normal house. In such cases it is possible by the extensive neurosurgical procedure of *hemispherectomy* to remove the tendency to such outbursts. One might imagine that such gross destruction of cerebral tissue would be so disabling as to make the procedure unjustified. However, it is being realized that the localization of brain function of the infant is in a much more plastic state than classical neurology would have led one to believe. A child who has had an early brain accident such as these children have had can develop the ability to control both limbs from one cerebral cortex. The removal of the damaged cortex may even uncover functional abilities on the other side which were not appreciable before. One does not, therefore, necessarily condemn the child to the total hemiplegia one might expect if such an operation were carried out on a normal brain later in life.

SYNOVIAL SWELLINGS

GANGLION. This is a firm discrete swelling occurring in the neighbourhood of joints and tendon sheaths, commonly on the dorsum of the carpus. It arises in the subsynovial tissues probably by degeneration and has glairy mucoid contents. It is usually symptomless and may go spontaneously. Sometimes it is associated with aching pain in the area. Firm pressure may disperse the contents, as may the insertion of a tenotome or an injection of hyaluronidase. Recurrence is frequent. Then careful *complete* dissection under a tourniquet is needed.

SEMIMEMBRANOSUS BURSA. This is a symptomless swelling in the popliteal fossa projecting from beneath the semimembranosus tendon. It arises from the capsular region but does not communicate with the joint. It may go spontaneously and one may wait a year at least. Minor symptoms may be associated with increase in size but are rarely convincing. Persistence may justify excision and this should be complete. A straight incision across the flexion crease of the knee *must* be avoided or the scar may be more troublesome than the bursa.

ARTHROGRYPOSIS CONGENITA MULTIPLEX

Also called congenital multiple articular rigidity, this is probably a syndrome with more than one ætiology. The joints of the limbs are ill formed and have a grossly limited range of movement. The muscles are weak and inelastic. On examination one typically finds hypotonia within a limited range of movement. There may be dislocation of the hips, and there may be hyperextension of the knees. Apart from the four limb type, the lower limbs alone may be involved—either in an otherwise normal baby or in association with spina bifida. Most of these children are of normal intelligence but a similar syndrome may occur with mental retardation. Denis Browne has suggested that the failure of development of the mesenchyme is the result of intrauterine pressures (Chap. 1). Abnormalities have been described in the spinal cord in some, and if these changes are primary they may represent a separate ætiological group.

Early simple physiotherapeutic measures such as manipulation and splinting of deformed feet and elastic traction on abducted hips or hyperextended knees can much improve the position. Later development of muscle control often exceeds expectations. Dislocation of the hips cannot be treated by orthodox methods. If buttock development is adequate later operative reduction may be possible.

CHAPTER 33

POSTURAL DEFECTS

A NUMBER of babies and a large number of children are seen in surgical outpatients because of postural defects most of which can be considered variations in the normal rather than real deformities. A good deal of unnecessary anxiety may be created by treating these conditions too seriously in a laudable attempt to catch deformities early and avoid crippling. The postural defects which are usually *self-limiting* or may need simple treatment should be distinguishable from important deformities from the beginning if the doctor is aware of the natural development of and variation in postures.

Inversion Spasm of the Feet. One of the postural defects seen neonatally is that called inversion spasm of the feet. The baby holds the feet in the equinovarus position. However, on examination with gentle assistance it is possible to move the feet into a full calcaneo-valgus range of movement. There is no persistent stiffness of the muscles as there is in a spastic limb and there is *no limitation of the range of movement as there is in a true talipes.* If these facts are borne in mind it will avoid the unnecessary treatment which sometimes occurs following misdiagnosis of mild talipes. The condition is one which is seen from birth and tends to pass off over about 6 or 8 weeks of life. There is no need for specific treatment, although the mother is often recommended to manipulate the feet into the calcaneo-valgus position each day when she bathes the baby, and this seems a reasonable assistance.

Stiff Hip. Another defect which may be noted from birth is that of the stiff hip often associated with an asymmetric pelvis. The mother may notice that one hip does not go out into abduction as freely as the other when she is putting on the napkins. Alternatively the condition may be noticed by the practitioner doing a routine examination of the newborn. This should always include abduction of the flexed hips in an attempt to pick up cases of congenital dislocation which will have marked limitation of this movement or a marked "jerk" in the mid range as the dislocation reduces. Other babies will be found, however, in whom the limitation of movement is present, although not so great. The baby will appear to be otherwise well and an X-ray show no evidence of displacement of the hip. The X-ray is frequently thought to be somewhat oblique until a more careful examination reveals that the vertebral column and trunk of the baby are in fact straight but that the pelvis itself is somewhat rotated inwards on the side of the stiff hip—"asymmetric pelvis". This again is a condition which tends to spontaneous correction.

257

The mother may be taught to give abduction exercises to accelerate the development of free abduction and confirm the innocent nature of the stiffness as opposed to that of true dislocation.

Bow-legs, Knock-knees and Flat-feet

Bow-legs. The majority of postural defects brought to the doctor are probably those seen a little later on when the child starts to walk. Many of them indeed are only the child's first ungainly and unco-ordinated attempts at the upright posture. They result in various awkwardnesses in the gait which will pass off in the next few months as confidence and balance improve. Many of these children are sent up with a diagnosis of knock-knees and flat-feet. To appreciate these conditions it is necessary to understand the natural development of the lower limbs as a baby becomes an upright walking creature. There has been a tendency in the past to assume that the perfect child would have anatomically straight lower limbs from birth and that they would remain so as he or she grew. Examinations of large groups of healthy children show that this is not so. The majority of infants have a *bandy* appearance. Much of this is false due to the bulging laterally of the fat calves. If the bony tibiæ are palpated through the fat it can be seen that the limbs are straight. There may in fact at this age be some true bowing of the bones, usually in a gentle curve throughout the tibiæ and perhaps the femora too, but sometimes with a sharper curve in the lower third of the tibiæ. This kind of *bow-legs* can be expected to improve spontaneously within the first year or two of life.

Rickets can cause bow-legs, but they are usually seen later as the dietary deficiency occurs, and are extremely rare in these islands now, although they are not unknown. One must also remember the possibility of metabolic disorders such as renal rickets causing bony lesions in older infants. But these are a tiny minority and the X-ray changes in the bones will lead to further investigation of their cause.

The vast majority of bandy babies are healthy babies with fat calves and perhaps a gentle curve which can be expected to correct spontaneously under observation. A little later on when the child is walking a bandy appearance may also be produced by wearing bulky napkins so that a sturdy child tries to tuck his feet in under them and produces the so-called *napkin gait* until he gets past that stage of life.

Knock-knees and-flat Feet. When the baby begins to stand his sense of balance is poor and he often tends to stand on a wide base and to sag inwards at the knees and sometimes also at the ankles. This is the stage at which the infant is likely to be referred to hospital for *knock-knees* and *flat-feet*. Examination of normal children has, however, shown that it is the usual thing for up to 2 inches or even 3 inches of separation between the malleoli to develop in the early walking period and only about 10 per cent of children maintain a straight leg at this stage. The valgus position tends to increase up to about 3 years of age, so that it is understandable that the mother may become anxious about it. However, beyond the age of 3 there is a spontaneous tendency to improvement up to the age of 6, so that by this time the vast majority of children will again have straight legs.

Rickets may also be a rare cause of knock-knees, as may true bony defects, and these rare types may be suspected from a marked asymmetry of the limbs or from other signs and symptoms in the child.

The vast majority of knock-kneed children are only immature in their sense of balance and can confidently be expected to correct themselves spontaneously. It will do no harm to prescribe the popular medial wedges to the shoes in these children, but it is not a good idea to encourage the mother unnecessarily to have the idea that there is something wrong with her child. The use of more vigorous measures such as night splints in the toddler period may upset the child considerably and indeed may produce a reaction which makes it impossible to use such measures on the occasional older child with persistent knock-knee for whom they may be necessary and helpful.

Along with valgus of the knees the child may show *valgus* at the *ankles* so that the feet roll over and the medial arch contacts the ground. This is really a rolled-over or pronated foot, rather than a truly flat one and again there is a marked tendency to spontaneous correction over the age of 3. Some of these children, however, do persist in an awkward kind of gait, and in general they tend to be rather the less athletic type of child—either the obese or the spindly hypotonic type. If there are valgus ankles associated with the knock-kneed posture, medial wedges and valgus stiffening for the shoes are prescribed. It does not seem likely that these measures could do anything useful to correct a knock-knee, but it would seem that they may protect the ankle from the extra strain thrown on it by the valgus posture and help in this way.

In medicine there is a tendency for the pendulum to swing severely from one direction to the other, and at present the pendulum has swung from enthusiastic attempts to correct the natural valgus phase of development under the false impression that these were real orthopædic defects, to one of assuring the parents somewhat sweepingly that knock-knees always get better. It does not take much observation of the adult population to realize that this is not true and to realize why some mothers become dissatisfied with this kind of advice. There are a few cases of knock-knee which appear to have no underlying metabolic or bony cause, and yet they do persist. The majority of these are not severe enough to justify treatment, nor do they incapacitate the child, but a very few are severe enough to justify treatment, and probably the only reliable treatment is by osteotomies. Such treatment is never needed before the age of 8 years. It is important to realize that although a few cases will persist and need treatment this treatment is better given at a later stage, and that large-scale attempts at prophylaxis in toddler life by wedging and splinting are not only unnecessary but futile.

Postural Scoliosis. Later, at the end of childhood, one sees more frequently another type of postural defect. This is the *postural scoliosis of the adolescent* seen more often in girls than boys. It is a slouching stance with the weight unevenly distributed between the legs and round shoulders producing a curvature of the spine. On forward flexion this curvature disappears, as it does also on suspension. This is sometimes taken unnecessarily seriously by school health authorities, who may make the girl far more self-conscious by the attention and over-enthusiastic exercises she is given. It may even encourage persistence in this awkward stance. This kind of posture is usually best treated by the ordinary physical recreation and gymnastics of school life, along with the child's schoolfellows, rather than by too much attention in isolation. It is a deformity the child can correct when she wants to and is unlikely to correct until she wants to.

POSTURAL SCOLIOSIS OF INFANCY. This has already been discussed in an earlier chapter. Browne believes that it results from intra-uterine posture, hence the name, but it is of far greater importance than adolescent postural scoliosis. It is now realized that many of these curves will resolve spontaneously, but there is a smaller proportion which appear to progress relentlessly to the so-called idiopathic structural scoliosis with its gross and disabling, life-shortening deformity. It seems that treatment by physiotherapy and the Denis Browne frame before walking begins may prevent this progression. Although the management of these infants is still under discussion this possibility is clearly one requiring serious consideration in view of the appalling deformity of the untreated progressive case, even if it does mean treating some children unnecessarily.

Torticollis

Postural torticollis may be noticed from birth. The child tends to hold his head to one side and on attempts at turning in the other direction there is limitation of the range of movement. The head is often asymmetric (plagiocephaly) and the baby may also be noted to have some stiffness of the corresponding hip. A few may also be noticed to have associated scoliosis. These facts suggest that the condition may be due to the posture of the child *in utero*. This postural torticollis is a benign condition; it tends to get better in the first few months of life and no more treatment is needed than teaching the mother manipulations to encourage the child to turn its head in the other direction.

It does not have the serious prognosis of the sternomastoid torticollis which is not merely postural and which tends to come on some time after birth, although it may be preceded by a sternomastoid tumour palpable in the belly of the sternomastoid muscle from soon after birth. Probably all sternomastoid torticollis are preceded by a sternomastoid tumour (though not always recognized) but by no means all sternomastoid tumours go on to sternomastoid torticollis. The condition is frequently associated with *breech presentation* but is *not caused* by breech delivery.

Treatment. Firm manipulations are carried out daily by the parents. The tumour resolves after a few months and there may be no sequelæ. In some, however, torticollis (and increasing facial asymmetry) may be seen as the child grows around the fibrosed sternomastoid. Division of the muscle is then usually needed. In practice division is advisable if the condition is still noticeable at a year of age.

CHAPTER 34

THE LIMPING CHILD

THE limping child is a problem frequently seen in the family doctor's surgery and the hospital outpatient department. The cause of the trouble may lie anywhere from the sole of the foot to the cerebral cortex, but it is the region of the hip that causes most worry in differential diagnosis and management.

Nevertheless, it is important to consider and examine the whole child. The whole *limb* is examined for the local tenderness or limitation of movement in injury or infection, or the swelling of a neoplasm. The *spine* is examined for tenderness, deformity or muscle spasm. These may be the result of a congenital lesion such as spondylolisthesis (a congenital weakness of the intervertebral ligaments causing strain and fracture of the pedicles and hence allowing a vertebra to slip forward on its neighbour endangering the spinal cord), an infection such as osteitis, or an injury. The *abdomen* is examined because a lesion such as appendicitis or external iliac adenitis may cause spasm of the adjacent psoas muscle and hence a limp. The *nervous system* is examined to detect weakness or spasm of muscle or altered reflexes resulting from a space-occupying lesion of cranium or spinal canal. *Hæmatological* examination may be required as mentioned later in the chapter.

When the child arrives with a limp, there is almost always a history of slight trauma which is so common in the youngster's everyday life. There may be a complaint of pain in the hip or down a thigh to the knee. It is important to remember that when a child with or without a limp complains of a pain around the knee that the pain may be referred from the hip and that this joint must be examined carefully. Limb pains, usually without a limp, commonly have a psychological basis.

To examine a hip the child must be stripped completely below the waist as even a bathing triangle may be misleading. The first thing to do is to observe the gait approaching and going from the examiner. The active movements of the joint are tested at first freely and then against resistance. Finally passive movements are tried and limitations noted. It is useful to test with the child prone as well as supine and the lower spine should be examined at the same time. If the hip is affected there is usually protective muscle spasm particularly in abduction and external rotation. Muscle wasting and alterations in the tendon reflexes are looked for. X-rays are rarely helpful in the absence of physical signs. A Mantoux test, E.S.R. and white cell count should be done.

DIFFERENTIAL DIAGNOSIS

The commonest disorder of the hip in childhood is a transient synovitis which may be due to some unobserved trauma or be a reaction to mild infection. As the cause is often not definitely known the term *irritable hip* is used to cover this definite clinical entity. The three other conditions which must be looked for are:

1. **Tuberculosis of the Hip**
2. **Osteochondritis of the Femoral Head (Perthes' Disease)**
3. **Slipped Capital Epiphysis**

All three are more rare than irritable hip but the differential diagnosis may be extremely difficult in early cases.

Tuberculosis of the Hip

Tuberculosis of the hip, the most serious condition, is now a rare lesion in these islands and though it can occur at any age it is generally seen in the first 5 years of life. The Mantoux test will be positive and there may be evidence of disease in the chest, mesenteric glands or urinary system. Bony disease is always secondary to a focus elsewhere but the primary lesion is frequently silent. There may be signs of constitutional upset with loss of weight and appetite, night sweats, and a tender swelling around the joint with limitation of all movements. More often the generalized effects of the disease are negligible.

In the early stages radiological signs in bone are minimal and a lymph node or synovial biopsy may be necessary to establish the diagnosis. Later the moth-eaten bony erosions or narrowing of the joint space due to destruction of cartilage will make the condition clear. It should be made plain to the parents that the condition goes through a cycle of destruction and repair which is modified rather than halted by treatment.

Treatment must be directed to the whole patient. Management begins in a hospital with the special facilities for long-stay patients. Traction is applied to the limb to relieve muscle spasm and the resulting pain and compression of the affected surfaces. Skilled nursing is important. Frequent changes of position are necessary to avoid recumbency calculus in the kidneys, pressure sores and constipation. Interesting activities and schooling are important as well as rest, fresh air and good food.

Drugs have considerably improved the outlook. Triple chemotherapy is usually used at the outset to avoid the emergence of resistant strains. Streptomycin, para-aminosalicylic sulphate and iso-nicotinic acid hydrazide are begun in combination and courses will continue for 12 to 24 months. With late diagnosis the end result is often a fibrous ankylosis of the hip joint which has to be stabilized later by surgery, but in purely synovial infection a return to normality may be achieved. Cases which have progressed to the stage of bony destruction or abscess formation can now be safely operated on to evacuate pus and debris under the antibiotic cover. This has meant a great reduction in the period of incapacity and improvement in the end results.

Perthes' Disease

Osteochondritis of the femoral head (Perthes' disease) is the most common serious lesion between the ages of 5 and 10 years. In this lesion, the head of the femur undergoes demineralizing changes and eventually remineralizes with a varying degree of collapse together with shortening and broadening of the femoral neck. The cycle of changes takes 2 to 3 years to complete. The cause is not known.

The condition presents with limitation of hip movement in an otherwise healthy child. Pain is usually mild or may be absent. The limitation chiefly affects abduction, extension and external rotation. Radiology of the hip may show the typical early changes of mottled decalcification of

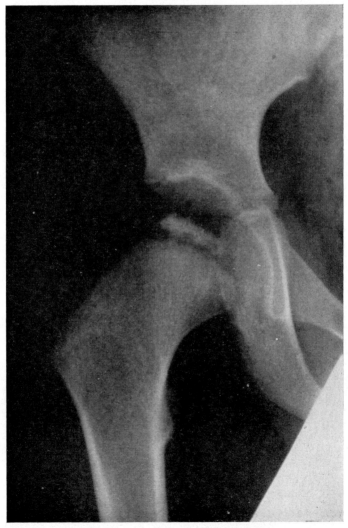

FIG. 67. The typical changes of Perthes' disease.

the femoral head. But these radiological changes may be delayed as long as 3 months after the onset of clinical symptoms.

The head of the femur goes through a cycle of changes and little can be done to modify its course. It would seem reasonable to assume that it will be weakened during this cycle and that bed rest, and even continuous traction to avoid the compression of muscle pull, would minimize the collapse (coxa plana) which ensues. Experience has not substantiated this. The point is laboured because two years during childhood in a hospital, however good, is a serious matter which may have lasting effects on the child's manner of life far beyond those of a slight limp or the increased risk of osteo-arthritis.

Rest is necessary in the treatment of an infection, but Perthes' disease is not infective. Rest may, in fact, be harmful, and there is good evidence that immobilization of a joint itself leads to degeneration of the disused areas of cartilage.

Once the early stage of muscle spasm has passed there is no need seriously to restrict the activity of a child with Perthes' disease. It is reasonable to prevent weight-bearing by a simple method such as the Snyder sling. This is like a Sam Browne belt with a shoulder strap and another strap hanging down to form a sling around the ankle. This holds the leg flexed at the knee while the child gets about on crutches. It is easily discarded when sitting, or on going to bed. Prolonged immobilization or traction are without effect on the natural history of the disease.

Prognosis. The outlook for Perthes' disease is good, and only about 10 per cent of patients are seriously troubled in later life. The one clear factor in prognosis is the age of onset. The younger the child, the better the outlook.

Slipped Epiphysis

This condition usually occurs between 10 and 15 years of age. Boys, particularly fat boys, are affected more than girls. There is a limp and limitation of movements, particularly abduction. Radiology shows a massive slip clearly, but at an early stage the neck slides back before the upward shift is marked. Hence the usual view may be misleading. An antero-posterior X-ray in internal rotation is required.

When there has been an acute slip, it may be possible to restore the epiphysis to a good position by manipulation or traction, and then fix the bone with multiple pins. These will give stability and hasten fusion of the epiphysis. If, as is more usual, the slip is gradual, forced correction is unwise and may result in aseptic necrosis of the head of the femur following damage to its blood supply. A moderate degree of slipping is acceptable, and pinning in that position will fix the epiphysis with minimal residual deformity and no real disability. A severe slip may justify osteotomy of the femur to correct coxa vara.

Conclusion

Most children with a couple of weeks' limp do not have any of these conditions. They will have *irritable hip*. However, the early differential diagnosis is difficult, and if X-ray and blood investigations are normal, the therapeutic test of three weeks *complete* bed rest must be insisted on. This can be done at home, but it must be full rest. To temporize with less will only prolong confusion. After three weeks in bed, the hip will have regained a normal range of movement in the great majority of cases and pain will be absent. Activity is then recommenced and the patient is again examined to see that signs and symptoms do not recur. The large proportion who remain well are presumed to have had a transient synovitis. If signs or symptoms persist or recur, then further observation and investigation is required to find which of the above lesions is the cause.

Irritable hip may also be due to intracapsular hæmorrhage from a blood dycrasia. Leukæmia is perhaps the most important to keep in mind.

Rheumatoid arthritis produces an irritable hip and aching pains. Usually the stiffness is out of proportion to the symptoms and the involvement of other joints makes the diagnosis straightforward. But the occasional case of mono-articular non-specific arthritis can be puzzling. It may only be distinguished from tuberculosis by biopsy of the joint synovia.

CHAPTER 35

THE HEAD AND NECK

IN this chapter a miscellaneous group of conditions will be discussed on a regional basis. Many important conditions in the head and neck have been treated elsewhere in the book along with the systems in which they arise.

THE HEAD

Harelip and cleft palate are such important conditions that they have already been discussed in a separate chapter. Craniosynostosis has been discussed in the chapter on Diseases of the Skeletal System. Hydrocephalus has been discussed along with spina bifida, a condition with which it is frequently associated. Birthmarks have also been discussed in a separate chapter.

CONGENITAL PTOSIS

Congenital ptosis is due to incomplete development of the levator palpebræ superioris muscle. It may be unilateral or bilateral. It usually becomes noticeable during infancy when the child is seen to throw its head back and wrinkle its forehead in an attempt to look upwards, or, in the more severe cases, when trying to look straight ahead. The upper eyelid itself is incapable of being lifted. Clearly a severe case will require early operation in order to allow satisfactory development of vision, whereas a milder case may come to treatment later when the ptosis becomes more obvious and annoying.

It is corrected by an operation. Blascovics' is the usual one. The upper lid is everted, and working from the conjunctival surface the levator muscle is freed and shortened and the tarsal plate is narrowed by excision of a strip. Several other operations exist and may produce good results.

Epicanthic Folds. At the medial angle of the eye there may be a fold of skin between the upper and lower lids similar to that seen in the Mongolian races and also in Mongolian idiocy. It may arise as an isolated phenomenon, when it is merely of cosmetic importance. It can be corrected simply by a small Z-plasty transposing the two little triangles of skin formed, so that they lie flat against the edge of the nose.

EXTERNAL ANGULAR DERMOID

The lateral end of the eyebrow is a common site for the development off a small dermoid cyst arising by separation of epidermal cells during fusion of the embryologic lines in the face. It presents as a little pea-sized discrete swelling, somewhat mobile under the skin but sometimes fixed firmly to the underlying bone in which it may indeed lie in a saucer-shaped depression. Apart from the slightly unsightly appearance the only danger of this external angular dermoid is that with infection it may form an abscess and then recurrent infections and a sinus may follow. It is therefore usual to excise the lesion through an incision placed suitably in the line of the eyebrow. The eyebrow should not be shaved for this procedure.

An occasional dermoid has a deep communication extending through the skull and communicating with a dermoid cyst in the anterior fossa of the skull. Such a dumb-bell type of lesion, though rare, is clearly of great importance, for the cyst inside the anterior fossa will act as a space-occupying lesion in its pressure effects on the brain, and infection would also lead to meningitis. It is therefore important when removing these small structures to observe the base lest such a communication be present even though it is very rare.

Deformed Ears

The commonest form of deformity of the ears is that popularly known as *bat ears*. In this condition the antihelix ridge has failed to form so that the ears project unduly. There may also be overgrowth of the conchal cartilage which adds to the projection. The condition is of purely cosmetic importance but is often sufficiently noticeable to justify operation. As in many of these minor cosmetic conditions the child's attitude to his abnormality is very much affected by that of his parents. They may lead him to accept the condition happily or may by their own anxiety encourage him to be so affected by the condition as to justify surgery even in a mild case. If operation is to be performed it should clearly be done before the child goes to school where he is most likely to meet unkind teasing at a stage when he is most likely to be affected by it.

The condition may be unilateral or bilateral. Operation is carried out by an incision on the back of the ear removing an ellipse of excess skin and then dividing the cartilage along the line of the antihelix ridge so that this can be folded back in a natural position. The older operations which excise much of the retro-auricular fold do not produce such a natural appearance and furthermore may be of considerable annoyance if the child needs to wear spectacles later and has lost his fold.

More severe defects of the ears exist. The *lop ear* is characterized by a small pinna with inadequate cartilage particularly in its upper part, which hangs away from the side of the head. This condition is often associated with small size or absence of a part of the external ear and there is a tendency for the ear to be lower than normal. These more severe types of abnormality of the external ear are characterized by absence of tissue as well as a mis-shapen pinna and they require elaborate surgery for their correction. The results of such elaborate plastic surgery are not beautiful, but nevertheless they may be greatly preferred to a prosthesis which can be perfect to look at. The patient may naturally be anxious about an organ which could get accidentally knocked off at an embarrassing time. In the case of a girl it may often be the wisest course merely to encourage the patient to accept the deformity and wear a hair style which hides the ear, but in the case of a boy this will not be practical. This is one of the rare conditions in which cosmetic surgery is of more importance to the male than the female.

Some cases of total absence of the external ear have been caused by maternal rubella during early pregnancy and by thalidomide.

PRE-AURICULAR SINUS

During the formation of the ear from the tubercles a congenital sinus may arise with a pinpoint opening just on or just in front of the ear. It is genetically determined and several members of the family may be affected. The track may ramify considerably around the region of the cartilage of the tragus and into the cheek under the zygoma. The congenital sinus orifice itself is scarcely visible, but the track is prone to infection and these patients are frequently seen at a stage when acute staphylococcal infection has already produced an acquired sinus opening on and scarring the skin in front of the ear. Treatment is by tedious surgical excision of the entire tract as soon as the acute infection has settled down.

ACCESSARY AURICLES

Little buttons of skin may be present just in front of the ear, perhaps along with a pre-auricular sinus, and they may also occur down on the neck roughly along the line of the anterior border of the sterno-mastoid. There may be little islets of cartilage at their base. They simply need excision for cosmetic reasons and it is important to get out the little cartilaginous rest with them.

Parotitis

Acute parotitis is rarely seen except as a complication of some seriously debilitating disease. Chronic or recurrent subacute parotitis is not uncommon. The story is of recurrent swellings in one or both cheeks in the parotid area. The swelling is tender and there is discomfort on opening the mouth caused by pressure on that part of the gland which extends behind the mandible. The gland feels firm and has a rather irregular surface and it is possible to express drops of pus or turbid salivary fluid from the orifice of the parotid duct inside the cheek. The organism is quite frequently the *Streptococcus viridans*, although other organisms such as the pneumococcus may be the cause. It is possible that in a number of cases it starts as a virus infection. When the condition first arises it is not uncommon for it to be mistaken for an attack of mumps and it is only when it recurs that the true nature of the lesion becomes apparent. The differential diagnosis of parotitis is mainly from mumps and from infection of the lymphatic glands within the parotid sheath. These may be infected from a lesion in their drainage territory such as the scalp and will produce a similar tender swelling in the cheek. There will not, however, be any purulent efflux from the parotid duct. A much rarer cause of parotid enlargement is the so-called uveo-parotid syndrome in which the uveal tract of the eye, the lacrimal glands and the parotid glands may enlarge together.

The treatment of recurrent parotitis is systemic chemotherapy based on the sensitivity of the causative organism, perhaps with instillations of the antibiotic into the parotid duct. If treated early and vigorously the results may be good. But most have a long and tedious course before finally settling down. However, eventual resolution is the rule and it very rarely persists into adult life. The major operation of parotidectomy is very rarely to be considered.

It is interesting to note that the parotid gland very rarely develops a calculus whereas the submandibular salivary gland quite frequently develops one either in the duct or in the anterior part of the gland itself causing recurrent obstruction, or infection behind it.

Parotid Hæmangioma. The parotid region is a not uncommon site for the development of an *angioma* which may be entirely under the skin or may be associated with a capillary strawberry mark element on the surface. These lesions have been treated vigorously by surgery and radiotherapy, but it is probable that most would follow the natural history of angiomas if given the chance and the authors prefer to control their growth with injections of saturated saline as a sclerosant fluid and temporize in this manner. In some cases, however, the lesion spreading into the cheek is likely to produce a considerable cosmetic defect even if later regression takes place, and skilled plastic surgery may be required. One need hardly stress the hazards in the surgery of a highly vascular lesion in this region of the facial nerve.

The Frænum

A frænum is a tethering band of tissue and there are two within the mouth which have probably given rise to a lot of unnecessary anxiety and surgery. The first is the *frænum linguæ*. It runs from the under-surface of the tongue to the floor of the mouth as a fold of mucous membrane over a fibrous cord. The frænum is present in every person, but when it attaches far forward or even to the tip of the tongue and is short then it may interfere with the ability to protrude the tongue. When protrusion is attempted the tongue rubs over the gums and when the incisor teeth erupt it may rub on them and produce an ulcer. It appears that severe degree of tongue tie may also interfere with the natural use of the tongue in sucking. The great majority of cases of so-called tongue tie are cases in which the normal frænum has been noticed by an anxious mother or perhaps more often by an enthusiastic welfare clinic nurse. No treatment is needed beyond reassurance. It is pointed out that the infant's tongue grows mainly at the tip and that the present square appearance is quite normal. However, there are some cases in which the tongue cannot be protruded beyond the gums or elevated at its tip and in these cases the frænum should be divided and the mucosa properly sutured under a general anæsthetic.

The other frænum is that attaching the centre of the upper lip to the region of the upper alveolus. A tight mucous fold in this region may tether the central part of the lip producing a curious appearance on smiling in a few cases. Perhaps more important is the fact that the fibrous cord running back from this frænum between the roots of the upper medial incisor teeth may produce a separation of these teeth and lead in later life to the Terry Thomas smile. For this reason it may sometimes be justified to excise such a frænum. A mere snip of the scissors is no use because the fold will re-form, and furthermore the tendency to separate the incisor teeth will not be affected. It is necessary to divide the fold and suture it properly under general anæsthetic having excised the cord running back between the two halves of the alveolus.

Ranula

In the floor of the mouth a cystic swelling may arise usually to one side or the other of the midline under the anterior part of the tongue. Sometimes the swelling spreads across the midline. It is a cystic dilatation of a mucous gland of the floor of the mouth, the so-called ranula. Occasionally ranulas plunge deeply under the muscle of the floor of the mouth. They are annoying by their size and may, by irritating the child, produce a lot of drooling. They are simply treated by uncapping the lesion and placing hæmostatic sutures around its edge. This is preferable to an attempt to excise it completely and close the wound which is not uncommonly followed by recurrence; for if the lesion is uncapped one exposes a normal mucous lining such as covers the remainder of the floor of the mouth and a natural condition ensues.

THE MIXED SALIVARY TUMOUR

The so-called mixed salivary tumour may arise in childhood just as in adult life. It is most common in the parotid gland, but may also occur from any of the similar small glands scattered in the buccal cavity. Its course and treatment are no different from that of the adult.

THE NECK

There are two important congenital tracts which may arise in the neck. The thyroglossal tract is a midline structure which usually gives rise to a cyst but may form a sinus. The lateral cervical sinus or branchial sinus is lateral and an incomplete remnant may also form a cyst anywhere along its track.

Thyroglossal Cyst and Sinus. The thyroglossal tract runs from the foramen cæcum down to the region of the hyoid bone and just below it, along the track of the developing thyroid gland. It is quite common for a cystic remnant to occur and it usually lies on the hyoid bone or just below it, in the midline or slipping just to one side of it. It is a firm, discrete cyst, but it is prone to infection. It is often noticed that with

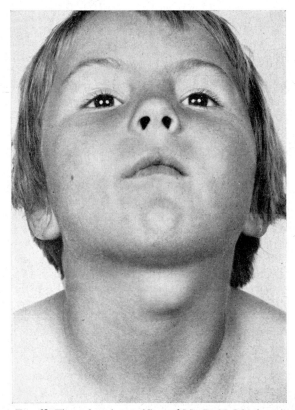

FIG. 68. Thyroglossal cyst. (Case of Mr. D. N. Matthews.)

upper respiratory infections, when the cervical lymph glands enlarge so a thyroglossal cyst will swell temporarily. Sooner or later acute infection with suppuration takes place. If it bursts spontaneously or the abscess is incised then a chronic thyroglossal sinus will arise in the midline.

Less commonly the thyroglossal cyst will be further back, when it presents as a swelling in the base of the tongue and can on occasion, although rarely, become dangerous as a possible obstruction to the respiratory tract. From the diagnostic point of view it is also important to realize that ectopic thyroid tissue may be left in the same way along this tract and may on clinical examination feel similar to the tense cyst. This is of great practical importance because the ectopic tissue may be the only thyroid tissue in the body so that its inadvertent removal would render the patient myxœdematous.

Treatment is by Sistrunk's operation. The cyst is excised along with the central centimetre of the hyoid bone and a core of muscular tissue extending up to the mucosa in the region of the foramen cæcum of the tongue. Only by such a block excision is it possible to avoid leaving remnants behind which give rise to recurrence. Once a recurrence has taken place in the thyroglossal tract further treatment becomes very tedious and difficult. The actual tract is so delicate that an attempt to dissect it out is likely to be incomplete and therefore a block of muscle is excised including the expected course of such a tract. The results following such treatment are excellent and the transverse skin incision in the crease line of the neck heals well.

Branchial Fistula. The lesion commonly called a branchial fistula is a persistent tract of the second branchial cleft of which the outer end is covered by the operculum to form the *cervical sinus*. The typical fistula shows an insignificant pinpoint orifice in the lower third of the neck at the anterior border of the sternomastoid muscle and then tracks up under the skin as a firm cord up to 3 mm. or 4 mm. in diameter until it reaches the level of the bifurcation of the carotid artery. Here it plunges deeply to its internal opening in the region of the fossa of Rosenmüller alongside the tonsil. At first it may be dry or there may be a little mucus discharge. Later the track becomes infected and an unpleasant yellow or green purulent discharge takes place. This is a considerable annoyance and the usual complaint of a man with this lesion is of constantly getting a stain on the collar which is an embarassment to him. It is therefore usual to excise these tracts. The tract is so long that in the older person it is not practicable to excise it completely from a single transverse incision at the level of the external orifice. An incision in any other direction is too unsightly on the neck and it is therefore usual to make a tiny incision around the orifice of the track to mobilize it and then make a second incision halfway up the neck from which the track is identified and then dissected upwards and downwards to remove it completely.

Occasionally there is only a short track leading perhaps half an inch up the neck from the external orifice and ending in a blind pouch. It is not uncommon for the orifice of such a sinus to be overhung by a little tag of skin which may have a piece of cartilage in its base (accessory auricle).

Instead of the persistence of the complete track occasionally only a section of it persists as a branchial cyst. The typical branchial cyst presents as a swelling under the angle of the jaw extending in front of and under the sternomastoid muscle and it has a typical soft feeling and fluctuation. It has been well described as feeling like a half-full hot-water bottle. These cysts being slack and not unsightly until they become large are more commonly seen in adolescence and young adult life than earlier in childhood in spite of their congenital nature. They usually have a mucous lining and contain a fluid which typically contains cholesterol crystals. Treatment is by excision.

Less common is the sinus or cyst of the *first branchial cleft*. A sub-mandibular swelling is usually mistaken for an infected lymph gland and incised—leading to recurrent infection and discharge. Complete excision is necessary and the tract, if complete, leads back adjacent to the facial nerve to open in the depth of the external auditory meatus.

FACIAL SINUSES OF DENTAL ORIGIN. In any persistent sinus in the region of the mandible, a dental cause should be suspected and radiographs taken. The sinuses will close without treatment if the dental causes are treated.

CLASSIFICATION OF SWELLINGS OF THE NECK

It will be useful to consider the differential diagnosis of swellings in the neck. It is usual to divide them first of all into those swellings in the midline and those arising laterally in the neck.

Midline Swellings

The most important *congenital* swelling in the midline of the neck is the thyroglossal cyst described above. Because of its attachments it is typical that the cyst moves up when the tongue is protruded. Ectopic thyroid tissue may present a similar picture, but will not give the story of varying size with infections sometimes obtained in the case of the cysts.

The commonest *neoplastic* swelling in the midline of the neck is the sublingual dermoid cyst. This is a smooth-walled discrete swelling in the floor of the mouth the edge of which may be masked by the mylohyoid muscle stretched over it. It usually has a characteristic doughy consistency.

The commonest *inflammatory* lesion in the midline of the neck again arises in the sublingual region and is an acute pyogenic lymphadenitis resulting from infection around the roots of the lower incisor teeth. Tuberculosis may arise in these glands as a result of an intra-oral primary focus, but this type of chronic lymphadenitis is rare.

Swellings of the thyroid gland are uncommon in childhood though, of course, of great importance in discussing midline swellings of the neck in adults. However, the swelling of the thyroid gland due to subacute thyroiditis is not unduly rare in childhood and a thyroid adenoma may arise as a nodular swelling in the gland. One may also see an enlargement of the whole gland, either smooth or somewhat nodular in the condition of goitrous cretinism in which enlargement of the gland is associated with signs of endocrine hypofunction. Exophthalmic goitre or primary thyrotoxicosis also occurs on occasion in childhood and is associated with a smooth enlargement of moderate degree in the whole gland and signs of endocrine excess and malfunction. The thyroid nature of the swelling is recognized by its position and shape and by the movement of the swelling along with the thyroid cartilage on swallowing.

Lateral Swellings in the Neck

The commonest swellings of *congenital* origin are the branchial cyst described above; angiomata (this is not an uncommon site for the subcutaneous angioma), and cystic hygroma. The side of the neck is the commonest site for a cystic hygroma.

Cystic Hygroma

Cystic hygroma is a multilocular malformation of the lymphatic trunks and is most commonly found in the neck though it occurs in the axilla and rarely the groins, buttock and elsewhere.

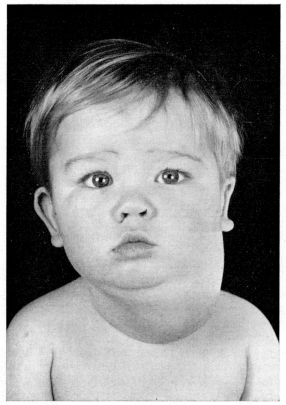

Fig. 69. Cystic hygroma. (Case of Mr. G. H. Macnab.)

The lymphatic vessels become distended and form a soft swelling which is brilliantly translucent. There is no tenderness or even discomfort in all but the biggest masses. The mass increases slowly in size though an infection in the pharynx may cause it to develop rapidly. The swelling is often thought at first to be a lipoma, but its progressive enlargement and brilliant translucency rule this out.

It is invariably treated conservatively when small in the hope that it will go away, but it very rarely does. The gradual increase in size may cause pressure on the carotid sheath or even the trachea and œsophagus and intervention should be undertaken before this occurs.

The injection of boiling water or saturated saline is practised by many with varying success. No other sclerosants should be used as they too readily enter the blood stream.

The most reliable approach is a painstaking dissection of the hygroma. As many cysts as possible are excised and the remainder opened. Suction drainage is invaluable. The ramifications in the neck are usually extensive and the operation should not be undertaken without time, patience and blood for transfusion. The occasional but important extension into the mediastinum must be sought.

NEOPLASTIC SWELLINGS

The commonest *neoplastic* swelling to be found in the side of the neck is the enlargement of the lymph glands associated with Hodgkin's disease and the allied reticuloses. A mass of glands, usually in the lower part of the neck in the posterior triangle, may become apparent in Hodgkin's disease and may precede any other symptoms or signs. The glands are firm with a discrete margin and an elastic consistency and they tend to be matted together into a group. Excision of the mass may be the most satisfactory form of biopsy, but if it appears that important structures are involved in the mass it will probably be wise merely to remove a peripheral gland for section. The condition is almost always fatal though antimetabolite drugs have some effect in palliation and radiotherapy can also produce very satisfactory remissions. The life span after diagnosis of Hodgkin's disease averages about 3 years.

INFLAMMATORY SWELLINGS

Inflammatory swellings in the side of the neck are common since the lymph glands in the region drain the pharynx which is so often involved in upper respiratory infections. The commonest site of an acute inflammatory swelling is the region of the tonsillar or jugulodigastric gland. It presents as a firm tender swelling proceeding to reddening of the overlying skin and later to fluctuation as an abscess forms in the gland. The commonest cause is tonsillar or pharyngeal infection by the streptococcus. It is important, however, to remember that infection at this site may be secondary to osteitis of the mandible or to an infection of a tooth root. If the infection is the result of an osteitis the mass will be fixed to the jaw and cannot be moved upon it. However, in the acute stage of any lymphadenitis with much periadenitis, fixation may also be present due to the tenseness of the fasciæ in the region. It may be necessary to take X-rays to exclude a bone infection around a tooth root, and in the hope of finding evidence of osteitis after the first 10 days or so. It must also be remembered that tuberculous infection of these glands may present relatively acutely, especially when the child gets a superimposed pyogenic infection in the throat.

Tuberculosis is the most important chronic inflammatory lesion, but is becoming much less common. The usual story is of swelling which may have been present for several weeks and is only just becoming tender or may still not be tender in spite of its considerable size. There may be reddening of the overlying skin if it is proceeding to abscess formation.

Nowadays one sometimes sees a chronic inflammatory swelling of the upper cervical lymph glands giving a very good imitation of tuberculosis as a result of the persistent use of antibiotics in an attempt to abort a pyogenic infection of glands after pus has already formed centrally in them. This iatrogenic condition can give rise to a good deal of anxiety. Beyond the infant period when the dangers of blood spread infection overrule local considerations it is often wiser to treat acute pyogenic adenitis of the neck by simple local heat and await events. Many will settle down and some will go on to abscess formation. They may then be treated by a small incision to evacuate the abscess. It is important not to incise too early as drainage may then be inadequate. The use of antibiotics after the pus has been let out will lead to prompt healing with a good cosmetic result. If the tender gland is small, a short course of antibiotic is justified, but a gland 2 cm. in diameter or larger can be assumed to have begun central suppuration. The use of anti-biotics before drainage may indeed shorten the course of the adenitis in a few more cases, but in others it will lead to chronic enlargement or recurrent adenitis, and on the average the invalidism is likely to be longer than by following the course just outlined.

Tuberculous Cervical Adenitis

Tuberculous cervical adenitis is not a serious condition. It is a primary tuberculous complex in a site where the regional enlarged glands happen to be much more easily visible than, for example, in the mediastinum.

MANAGEMENT. Beyond the age of infancy it can be treated expectantly as one would any other primary tuberculous complex. The source of infection is usually the tonsils and these bear tuberculous lesions within them in a large proportion of cases. The presence of tuberculosis in the tonsils cannot be recognized by external examination as can pyogenic infection of the tonsils, and it is therefore wise to remove the tonsils routinely as part of the primary treatment of tuberculosis of the glands of the neck. The glands themselves are probably best left untreated until they form an abscess. This is then evacuated through a small incision preferably by *expression* in the Denis Browne fashion.

Antituberculous drugs. There is no real evidence that treatment with antibiotics is of any value in this form of tuberculosis. Because the lesion is avascular and necrotic in the centre drugs cannot penetrate to that area. Breakdown occurs sooner or later even during prolonged anti-tuberculous therapy. Certainly streptomycin treatment over a prolonged period is not justified, for it has possible complications more serious than those of the disease itself. However, it is wise to use a short course of streptomycin to cover operative interference. It has also been shown (Miller) that if the condition is recognized early then the use of anti-tuberculous drugs, including streptomycin, for a month followed by an excision of the glands will cut short the condition and prevent the otherwise *inevitable* development of an abscess sooner or later. This is doubtless true when the disease is seen early, but usually, by the time they reach the surgeon, this chance is past and there is no doubt that local excision of the glands *later* during the course of the disease is unreliable in cutting short the condition. Recurrences are quite common and the result of the excision which is often a difficult one may be cosmetically unsatisfactory.

In order to preserve a sense of proportion in treating this disease it should be remembered that tuberculosis of the cervical glands was a condition which was self-limiting even in pre-antibiotic days. It may have gone on for 2 to 4 years and left an ugly scar in the neck after a degree of invalidism due to the presence of an unpleasant secondarily infected sinus. But it did get better and treatment is therefore only justified in order to improve the cosmetic results and any attempt to shorten the natural history of the disease must itself be free from risk.

SUBMANDIBULAR SIALADENITIS. Infection of the submandibular salivary gland causes a firm nodular swelling in front of and under the angle of the jaw. It is tender during exacerbations and the typical story is of a swelling which comes up at mealtimes. This is because the majority of cases involving the submandibular gland, unlike those in the parotid gland, are secondary to an obstruction by a calculus either in the anterior end of the gland or in the duct. The calculus may be a tiny one the size of a grain of sand blocking the papilla of the duct, or it may be a large stone the size of a hazelnut impacted in the anterior border of the gland. If the calculus is accessible in the duct it is possible by a simple incision over it, under a local anæsthetic, or in a young child under a general anæsthetic, to extract the calculus and this is all that is required. A calculus in the gland itself, however, may be impossible to remove by the intra-oral route. The gland may have suffered considerable changes so that infection may persist, and if this has occurred it is usually preferable to excise the gland itself through an external submandibular incision. There is no disability from the loss of one salivary gland.

REFERENCE

Miller, F. J. W. (1959) Peripheral tuberculous lymph adenitis in childhood. *Postgrad med. J.*, **35**, 348.

CHAPTER 36

CONGENITAL HEART DISEASE

ABOUT six in every thousand new-born infants have congenital heart disease. Of these six, three will not survive the first year of life unless they can be treated. Many of the lethal cases have complex anomalies, but simple, remediable conditions may also cause death in infancy.

Accurate pre-operative diagnosis is the most important prerequisite for a completely successful operation. Operations performed without a precise diagnosis, or where the diagnosis is in error, carry a high mortality even in the best hands.

METHODS OF DIAGNOSIS

Up to recent years the diagnosis of the various types of congenital malformation of the heart was considered a difficult problem and disagreements on interpretation were settled only at the eventual post mortem. *Morbid anatomical* studies by workers such as Maud Abbott provided a groundwork to the subject, then Dr. Helen Taussig's use of X-rays and particularly *fluoroscopy*, together with her clinical observations put it on a scientific footing.

Electrocardiography has also developed and the unipolar leads particularly have given much useful information about atrial and ventricular hypertrophies. The *phonocardiogram* has given us permanent, visual and comparable records of sounds audible only to the trained ear.

Cardiac catheterization is performed through a vein in the antecubital fossa, or the femoral vein in the groin. Under a fluorescent screen the catheter is introduced into the right atrium and thence into the right ventricle and pulmonary artery. The pressures and oxygen saturations in the various chambers are measured. Dye dilution studies are a further refinement of cardiac catheterization. The concentration of an injected dye at various points is measured and quantitative information about the size and position of vascular shunts, as well as the severity of stenoses and regurgitations, may be estimated.

The principal value of this right-heart catheterization is in the diagnosis of left-to-right shunts of blood, e.g. patent ductus arteriosis, atrial septal defect, ventricular septal defect and in pulmonary stenosis. Catheterization of the left side of the heart is mainly of use in acquired rather than congenital lesions.

In *angiocardiography* the catheter is also introduced into the right atrium and 10 to 20 ml. of 50 per cent Diodone are injected rapidly by a pressure injector. The course of the dye is followed by rapid film change or by ciné-radiography. In selective angiocardiography the dye is introduced into the particular chamber where the abnormality is suspected. Angiocardiography is principally used in cyanotic conditions, and in small children image-intensification techniques and ciné-radiology are important to reduce the dose of radiation.

The use of cardiac catheterization and angiocardiography has made the diagnosis certain in many cases, and from experience with these investigations we have learnt to rely on some clinical signs, and to discard others. These complex investigations have in fact buttressed clinical observations so that nowadays, using information first obtained by these special techniques, an accurate diagnosis can often be made without having recourse to them.

A provisional diagnosis should be reached in each case as soon as a suspicion of heart disease is aroused. On that basis any further investigations may be planned. *Severity of symptoms is not a really reliable guide to the urgency of the condition*, and too often the first symptom will indicate irreversible pulmonary hypertension or ventricular failure. In time to come most conditions will be dealt with before the child goes to school, so that development will proceed normally, and the child will require no special attention or protection.

INDIVIDUAL LESIONS

Figures on the relative frequency of the various forms of congenital heart disease vary greatly. This is due to the wide age spread and usually high average age of the patients examined. As the age at which diagnosis and treatment of the condition take place is lowered, the true pattern of incidence emerges. The first and most obvious distinction is between those who are cyanosed and those who are not. In congenital heart disease persistent cyanosis is usually due to shunting of venous blood from the right to the left side of the heart so that it passes into the systemic circulation without being oxygenated in the lungs. The acyanotic group are at least four times more common.

Acyanotic Group

Ventricular Septal Defect. Isolated ventricular septal defect is the commonest single lesion in infancy and childhood. It may be large or small. Small defects, i.e. less than half the diameter of the aorta, will give a loud systolic murmur over the third and fourth left interspaces and may or may not have a systolic thrill. The heart is not enlarged, the shunt of blood is small and surgery is not required.

With large defects there is frequently a history of pulmonary infection in the early years. The thorax often has a precordial bulge and there is a definite thrust over the pulmonary area. There is a loud systolic murmur and thrill, maximum in the fourth and fifth interspaces. On

X-ray the pulmonary artery is enlarged, the pulsation more marked than normal, and the pulmonary vascular markings increased. The electrocardiogram usually shows a left ventricular hypertrophy. A large defect with a big shunt of blood from the left side of the heart to the right may cause a change in the pulmonary arterioles which raises the pressure in the pulmonary circulation and may even cause reversal of the shunt. If this occurs (pulmonary hypertension) then cyanosis may develop and the murmur diminish.

TREATMENT. Small ventricular septal defects may safely be left alone. Up to 5 per cent of all the defects will undergo spontaneous closure, a fact which has only recently emerged and caused an "agonizing reappraisal" of the entire problem.

For those who require closure, cardiopulmonary by-pass with a heart-lung machine is necessary. The majority requiring operation need to have a patch of synthetic material stitched in the defect. The mortality of this operation is about 5 per cent.

Formal closure is performed at four years of age or more, but some infants go into failure during the first months or year of life and cannot survive to this age. They can frequently be tided over by banding the pu'monary artery with a tape, creating an artificial pulmonary stenosis which protects the lungs from pulmonary hypertension. The constriction can be removed when the defect is closed.

Patent Ductus Arteriosus. Patent ductus arteriosus is the second most common acyanotic lesion. Classically there is a continuous, machinery-like murmur, maximum over the first and second left interspaces. In young infants (in whom the systemic blood pressure more closely approximates to the pulmonary), patients with gross cardiac enlargement or pulmonary hypertension the murmur may be systolic only. There is often a thrill and usually a bounding pulse. X-ray appearances vary with the size of the ductus but there is usually an increase in the pulmonary vascular pulsations and markings. Electrocardiographic findings arc not pathognomonic but evidence of right ventricular hypertrophy excludes an uncomplicated patent ductus arteriosus.

The treatment is interruption of the ductus by division or double ligation at the age of 1 year, or as soon after this age as the diagnosis is made. An infant may go into cardiac failure with no other lesion than a patent ductus arteriosus and a few will demand operation in infancy almost as an emergency.

The operative mortality is 1–2 per cent in uncomplicated cases.

Atrial Septal Defects. When atrial septal defects are present there is a systolic murmur of moderate intensity, maximum over the second and third left interspaces with duplication of the pulmonary second sound. The electrocardiogram usually shows an incomplete right bundle branch block. Fluoroscopic findings vary with the size of the defect but there is usually cardiac enlargement, increased pulmonary pulsations and vascular markings.

One important variant is the ostium primum defect which is low down on the inter-atrial septum and is associated with a split mitral valve with possibly a ventricular septal defect. Here symptoms arise earlier, the murmur is louder, the pulmonary vascularity and cardiac enlargement more noticeable. The diagnosis between the common or ostium secundum type of septal defect and the ostium primum is of considerable importance.

TREATMENT. Ostium secundum defects are at present closed by open heart surgery under moderate hypothermia (30°C). The time limit for the procedure under these conditions is about 8 minutes. But a septum primum defect is more complex and requires cardio-pulmonary by-pass for its correction. In either type it nows seems essential that the defect should be sutured under direct vision.

Coarctation of the Aorta. The easiest and best way to diagnose coarctation of the aorta is to palpate the femoral arteries in all routine examinations. In the presence of coarctation the femoral pulsations are diminished or absent. Up to 25 per cent will have a palpable femoral pulse, but it is delayed compared to the brachial. The blood pressure is higher in the arms than in the legs. The murmurs of coarctation of the aorta are not characteristic, but a systolic murmur is usually present, particularly between the two scapulæ. In older patients collateral vessels, particularly along the scapulæ, can be palpated or seen. The electrocardiograms are not characteristic. There are two main forms of coarctation, the common short segment post-ductal variety, which is the type commonly seen in children, and the preductal variety with palpable femoral pulses and a segment of varying length, which is present in early infancy. Many of this latter type have associated cardiac anomalies, such as ventricular septal defect.

The treatment of the condition is resection of the narrowed segment of the aorta with end-to-end anastomosis. Even long gaps may be bridged by mobilization in early infancy and prompt treatment is essential. The mortality is over 50 per cent in these patients. In the more common type, with a short segment, the operation should be completed some time around the sixth year of life. Here the mortality is of the order of 5 per cent. It has been found that by operating in the first decade grafts are almost never necessary to bridge the gap left by the excised segment.

Pure Pulmonary Stenosis. The patient with isolated pulmonary stenosis is not cyanosed until in terminal cardiac failure. There is a harsh murmur and usually a thrill maximal over the pulmonary area. The intensity of the murmur may be proportional to the degree of stenosis. The heart size may be normal even in advanced cases, but the lung fields are usually clear (oligæmic) on X-ray. The electrocardiogram shows right ventricular hypertrophy. Severe cases may develop cyanosis and cardiac enlargement in early infancy, as there is a right to left shunt through the foramen ovale. Squatting is common in older children.

The treatment is valvotomy under direct vision. The operation is usually performed under hypothermia with circulatory but not cardiac arrest.

AORTIC AND SUBAORTIC STENOSIS. In aortic and subaortic stenosis there is a harsh systolic murmur maximum over the aortic area and proportional to the degree of stenosis. It is widely transmitted, particularly over the neck. There is usually a systolic thrill in the aortic area. A low pulse pressure may or may not be present. The X-ray appearances and the electrocardiogram may be within normal limits. The more severe cases get anginal pain and even an infant may suffer from it. Sudden death is not uncommon.

The treatment is valvotomy under direct vision using hypothermia. It is essentially a palliative treatment as the normal anatomy of the valve cannot be restored and aortic incompetence is a real risk.

RARE FORMS

In addition to these mentioned a residual 10 per cent of acyanotic cardiac enlargements require complete laboratory investigation for accurate diagnosis. Most of this group are individually rare and treatment is not often satisfactory at the present time.

Cyanotic Group

Tetralogy of Fallot. In this condition the septum of the developing heart forms off centre causing infundibular pulmonary stenosis, overriding aortic root, ventricular septal defect and right ventricular hypertrophy, cyanosis may not be present until the child begins to move about. Such is the mortality of the other cyanotic conditions that 75 per cent of blue babies over the age of 2 years have Fallot's tetralogy. Again, the older children tend frequently to assume the squatting position which seems to ease their discomfort.

There is usually a systolic murmur and thrill in the third left interspace. On fluoroscopy and X-ray films the heart apex is raised (cœur en sabot), pulmonary vasculature diminished and there is a concavity in the region of the pulmonary artery. The electrocardiogram shows right ventricular hypertrophy.

Surgical correction of the infundibular stenosis and the ventricular septal defect is performed under cardio-pulmonary by-pass. The procedure is a lengthy one and the technical difficulties are considerable. The mortality of the operation in patients under the age of 5 years has been considerable and patients with severe tetralogy of Fallot who cannot be nursed along to the age should have a systemic-pulmonary shunt procedure, i.e. Blalock's subclavian to pulmonary artery anastomosis or Potts' aorto-pulmonary anastomosis. The shunts divert systemic blood into the oligæmic pulmonary circulation, where it is oxygenated and hence palliate the effects of the anomalies by producing yet another. A Blalock shunt is easier to take down than a Potts should the infant be brought through to an age at which definitive repair of the tetralogy can be performed.

Complete Transposition of the Great Vessels. The aorta arises from the right ventricle and the pulmonary artery from the left ventricle. Murmurs may be absent, but the heart appears egg-shaped on X-ray. A venous angiocardiogram gives the diagnosis readily, but the condition is difficult to elucidate in the newborn infant. There are several important variants of transposition. "Uncorrected" transpositions have quite separate right and left heart circulations but, in "corrected" transposition, abnormalities of venous return allow some right to left transfer of blood. So does an associated septal defect.

TREATMENT. Most transpositions die in the first three months of life and virtually the only worth-while palliative procedure is the creation of an atrial septal defect after the manner of Blalock and Hanlon. This allows admixture of oxygenated blood with the reduced blood going to the left ventricle.

Various ingenious operations for correction have been described and performed but, although the condition is common, total corrections are numbered in dozens.

TRICUSPID ATRESIA. These cyanotic patients on first examination appear to have a dextrocardia because the right ventricle is hypoplastic, thus altering the shape of the heart on X-ray. The conclusive finding is that of left ventricular hypertrophy on the electrocardiogram.

The treatment is necessarily palliative, but good results have been obtained with both Blalock's subclavian to pulmonary artery anastomosis, or Potts' aorta-pulmonary anastomosis. Anastomosis of the superior vena cava to the right pulmonary artery gives the best results but is not satisfactory in early infancy.

Anomalous Pulmonary Venous Drainage. There are frequently no abnormal sounds in this condition and cyanosis may not occur until late in the disease. The X-ray shows a characteristic double shadow, the figure of eight, in the upper mediastinum. Cardiac catheterization and possibly angiocardiography are necessary to confirm the diagnosis. The anomalous veins should be transplanted from their entry into the cavæ or right atrium to the left atrium, using cardio-pulmonary by-pass. Not all varieties can be satisfactorily treated.

Persistent Truncus Arteriosus. There is a systolic murmur over the third or fourth interspaces. The lung fields show increased vascularity on X-ray and there is a concavity where the pulmonary artery would normally be. Truncus arteriosus is often a most difficult diagnosis to make and it is important to recognize it because no treatment is of any use, though banding of the individual pulmonary arteries will palliate those with hyperæmic lung fields.

RARER CYANOTIC CONDITIONS

There are many other malformations most of which can be greatly alleviated at the present time. If the patient is cyanotic and the heart is not enlarged but the pulmonary vascularity is diminished as shown by clear lung fields on the X-ray, then a shunt operation would probably be of benefit. The choice lies between Blalock's pulmonary-subclavian anastomosis and Potts' aorto-pulmonary anastomosis with a slight bias towards Blalock's procedure. The object is to get more blood into the lungs.

ACUTE CARDIAC ILLNESS IN INFANCY

At least 50 per cent of cases of congenital heart disease die during the first year of life. Cardiac failure is becoming increasingly recognized as a common condition in infancy, particularly in the neonatal period. The over-all prognosis is bad. Perhaps 90 per cent of patients who develop failure in the first year of life die either then or shortly afterwards. A great effort must be made to distinguish the remediable conditions which present with cardiac failure at that age.

DIAGNOSIS. The signs are basically the same as in adult life. The infant is dyspnœic and possibly cyanotic. The *liver* may be enlarged and there is frequently peripheral œdema. The neck veins are distended. Anginal and syncopal attacks may occur from myocardial or cerebral anoxia. There is usually marked tachycardia and the pulse pressure is reduced. The infant may be unable to feed and, at this age, a six-ounce bottle feed is an excellent exercise tolerance test. Murmurs, if present, are difficult to define due to the rapid heart rates, and the timing of thrills is almost impossible. The femoral pulses and blood pressure checked in arms and legs. Vomiting and regurgitation of feeds is common and may be the initial presenting symptom.

Percussion of the heart is useless because the heart is only 4 cm. long. A chest X-ray should always be taken and will almost always give useful information about the condition. It answers the questions of whether the heart is enlarged and the lung fields congested. Right-sided cardiac enlargement may cause deformity of the left chest. Electro-cardiography has severe limitations at this age, but the unipolar leads may at least help to eliminate some possibilities.

TREATMENT

General	Drugs	Surgery
Oxygen Moisture Posture Feeding Travelling	Digoxin Sedation Diuretics Antibiotics Iron	Corrective Palliative

GENERAL. *Oxygen.* A tent with 4 to 6 litres oxygen per minute is required to try to maintain a saturation of 50 per cent. Wetting agents may help breathing.

Posture. A 40 per cent tilt is essential and pillows are not adequate.

Feeding. Small, frequent feeds avoid overdistension of the stomach and respiratory embarrassment. An indwelling naso-gastric tube spares the infant the effort of feeding. Low salt milk may help if there is œdema.

Travelling. Over-heating should be avoided. These patients are more comfortable when cool, but easily drift into hypothermia.

DRUGS. *Digoxin.* 0·0625 mg. every eight hours for a newborn or double for an older child may be enough, but, if necessary, these doses may be doubled. Individual adjustment of the dose is required to obtain the effect without overdosage which, itself, can cause vomiting.

Sedation. Morphine, 0·025 mg. per lb. body weight, repeated every 4 to 6 hours, is the drug of choice. Phenobarbitone is useful when the acute stage is over and during physical examinations.

Diuretics. Mercurials are best and the dose is 0·2 to 0·5 ml. I.M. daily.

Antibiotics. It is impossible to say whether or not an infant with wet lungs has an infection and it is safer to use antibiotics from the start.

Iron. Many of these infants are anæmic due to inability to take their feeds. Cyanotic infants may be anæmic ("Picasso blue") and may require folic acid as well as iron.

SURGERY. If any improvement is to take place it will take place in under four days on this régime. With the slower heart rate and raised pulse pressure murmurs may now be audible. The heart may decrease in size and œdema subside. Diagnosis can then sometimes be made when it was impossible during congestive failure. A rapid decision about further investigation must then be taken. Perhaps the most useful single investigation is a cardiac catheterization with selective angiocardiography and ciné-radiography. These procedures are difficult and hazardous in a new-born infant. In some cases a thoracotomy may carry no greater risk than cardiac catheterization. But thoracotomy for diagnosis is of no value except when patent ductus arteriosus cannot be excluded. If patent ductus cannot be excluded then thoracotomy is advised because it is such an eminently treatable cause of failure. There is no doubt that all other methods will at times fail to show a considerable patent ductus and hence exploration is justified. However, if a patient has a thoracotomy for congenital heart disease in the neonatal period and no useful procedure can be performed the mortality is almost 100 per cent. Thus once more it is emphasized that preoperative diagnosis is crucial.

Patent ductus, coarctation of the aorta and valvular pulmonary stenosis may require curative operations in infancy. Ventricular septal defect, Fallot's tetralogy, pulmonary atresia, tricuspid atresia and transpositions of the great vessels can be satisfactorily palliated in the infant and many will survive for total correction while others will live surprisingly long and well.

REFERENCES

Goldblatt, E. (1962) The treatment of cardiac failure in infancy, *Lancet*, **2**, 212.

Keith, J. D., Rowe, R. D. and Vlad, P. (1958) *Heart Disease in Infancy and Childhood*, The Macmillan Co., New York.

Nadas, Alexandar S. (196) *Pediatric Cardiology*, W. B. Saunders Co., Philadelphia and London.

Oschner, J. L., Cooley, D. A., McNamara, D. G. and Kline, A. (1962) Surgical treatment of cardiovascular anomalies in 300 infants younger than 1 year of age, *J. Thorac. cardiov. Surg.* **43**, 2, 182.

Sabiston, D. C. (1963) Cardiovascular Surgery: Chapter in Recent Advances in Pædiatric Surgery. Ed. A. W. Wilkinson. Churchill. London.

CHAPTER 37

THE CHEST

THE CHEST WALL

PRECOCIOUS BREAST DEVELOPMENT. This may occur in the neonatal period due to transfer of maternal hormones across the placenta. The infant breasts may actually secrete and have a tendency to become infected. The management of this condition is rigidly conservative and handling or squeezing of the area should be avoided. Should an abscess nevertheless occur it may have to be opened and this should always be done from well underneath the nipple to avoid local damage as much

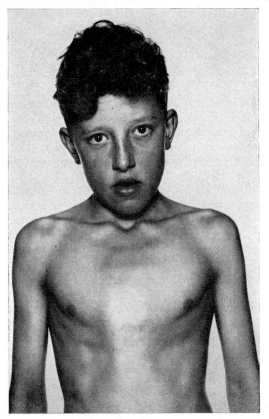

FIG. 70. Pigeon chest (*Pectus carinatum*).

289

as possible. In the absence of infection the condition usually subsides spontaneously within a month.

Precocious breast development is quite common in girls from the age of 8 years onwards and may arise earlier. More often than not one breast begins to enlarge long before the other. There is nothing to worry about when this is an isolated finding and all concerned may be reassured that the condition is common and not abnormal. The other breast always catches up in size later.

PUBERTAL "MASTITIS". A patch of chronic nodular thickening under or near the nipple is not uncommon in pubertal girls and boys. It is tender at first, but this slowly subsides and the thickening disappears or becomes lost in the developing breast in girls. It is difficult to relate all these conditions to trauma though that is the usual explanation in boys.

GYNÆCOMASTIA. Pubertal boys sometimes show considerable breast development which is more than the nodules of mastitis already mentioned. This alarming condition is usually of no importance and settles in about 6 months. Of course, a full examination should be carried out to exclude the possibility of an intersex condition (see Chapter 26). If the enlargement is persistent mastectomy may be justified to avoid embarrassment.

DEFORMITIES OF THE THORACIC CAGE

Pigeon Chest. (*Pectus Carinatum*. L. carina—a keel.) Pigeon chest is a protrusion of the sternum which presents a sharp edge particularly in its lower half. The ribs are usually flared. The condition is frequently familial and there is occasionally a history of frequent respiratory infections or asthma. Surgery is rarely advisable, but breathing exercises help the associated conditions.

Funnel Chest. (*Pectus Excavatum*.) Funnel chest is a funnel-shaped or conical depression of the anterior chest wall in which the sternum and attached costal cartilages curve backwards. The xiphoid is at the bottom of the depression and the distance between the xiphoid and the vertebral column is abnormally short. The depression is probably caused by an abnormal tethering of the xyphoid cartilage and sixth costal cartilage by the diaphragm. It appears that there is a local developmental defect of the anterior portion of the diaphragm. The deformity is most marked on inspiration when descent of the diaphragm can be shown on the X-ray screen to cause backward retraction of the sternum (paradoxical movement). The deformity is labile in infancy but becomes fixed after about 5 years of age.

The appearance of the condition upsets most parents to some extent and it does not regress spontaneously. Symptoms do occur, but genuine complaints are uncommon. The infants may be subject to respiratory infections which readily become chronic because coughing is inadequate and secretions are retained. But this tends to be outgrown as the thoracic cage becomes firmer and paradoxical movement diminishes. Respiratory indications for surgery are rare. If there are respiratory symptoms, removal of the tonsils, and particularly the adenoids, may be surprisingly beneficial. Rotation of the heart also occurs and in-

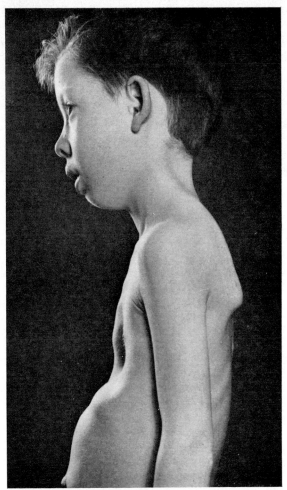

Fig. 71. Funnel chest.
Also shows the typical round shouldered posture.

complete filling of the right ventricle has been demonstrated on angio-cardiography. The heart tends to be flattened between sternum and vertebræ, rather than displaced to the side. Some believe that the untreated condition may result in diminished exercise tolerance though respiratory investigations do not usually show it. There is no doubt that, after operation, many children are more vigorous and active.

Withal, the cosmetic aspect is probably the most compelling one. Most patients with funnel chest have a normal life expectancy without symptoms, but a funnel chest may keep a boy from playing games in which communal undressing is involved. As he gets older he is unlikely to expose himself on a beach. The decision about surgery has to be taken at an age when he has little say in the matter. With girls the decision is easier as exposure is not necessarily a problem and the upper portion of the chest may benefit by the lower part being depressed and breast development will tend to mask the appearance.

The only treatment of any value is operation. Breathing exercises do not help at all. Operation should be advised if there are genuine symptoms and discussed if there are none.

The deformed costal cartilages are resected subperiosteally and the upper end of the sternum is osteotomized and pulled into a more anterior position. A metal strut may be used for temporary fixation. The pleural cavities need not be opened, but often will be. It is a major surgical procedure, but has a negligible mortality and morbidity in good hands.

The Diaphragm

Congenital Diaphragmatic Hernia. When suspected or discovered in the neonatal period this is the most urgent of all chest conditions. The patient will become asphyxiated unless the mediastinal shift and cardiac embarrassment are dealt with by reducing the hernia and repairing the defect.

The condition can, however, remain silent at first and may only be discovered accidentally on chest X-ray for other reasons—or on investigation of mild unexplained symptoms. Under these circumstances only part of the bowel will have herniated into the chest as the defect is usually smaller.

Whenever these defects are discovered they should be repaired promptly as tension syndrome or bowel strangulation may occur at any time.

Traumatic rupture of the diaphragm is rare in children as the flexible rib cage gives protective elasticity under sudden pressures.

Eventration. This is an abnormal rise of one cupola of the diaphragm without any increase in intra-abdominal pressure. It is due to a congenital weakness of the muscle. Surgery may also cause eventration by damage to the muscle or the phrenic nerve.

Respiratory embarrassment is uncommon, but the collapsed lung is prone to bronchiectasis and repair should be carried out. The chest is opened and an imbricating darn with nylon or a dacron patch restores the normal anatomy.

THORACIC CONTENTS

The basis of diagnosis in any serious intrathoracic condition is a good history and a chest radiograph. Physical signs are only of help in deciding when an X-ray is necessary and lethal conditions can progress in the absence of abnormal signs. In the severely ill infant a chest X-ray as a shot in the dark will occasionally point up the limitations of bedside examination.

Bronchiectasis

Bronchiectasis is a persistent dilatation of the bronchi and bronchioles, usually as a consequence of infection. There is an accumulation of secretions in the affected segments and further infection invariably occurs.

TREATMENT. The basis of treatment is postural drainage of the affected areas and chemotherapy. Excision of affected segments and lobes was carried out enthusiastically in the past, but the end-results have not been really satisfactory on long-term follow-up. Further development of the disease and a tendency to emphysema in the residual segments together with the reduced respiratory reserve, have made us cautious in advising surgery.

Children have a greater ability to recover from this condition than adults and repeated bronchography over a period of years often shows remarkable improvement even in severe cases. A conservative attitude is justified particularly in the young.

Surgery is most successful in well-localized disease especially where bronchiectasis follows inhalation of a foreign body or where the middle lobe alone is involved. Segmental lung resection is on the decline and in most patients requiring operation a lobectomy is necessary.

Lung Cysts

The commonest type seen in pædiatrics is the cyst following staphylococcal pneumonia in infancy. These may be treated conservatively unless they become enormous and cause severe symptoms. The subject is discussed in Chapter 6.

Congenital cysts of lung occur and are best excised as bronchiectasis may develop in association.

The Mediastinum

Tumours of the mediastinum are not rare. In the anterior mediastinum teratomas and tumours of lymphatic tissue are commonest. In the posterior mediastinum, neuroblastoma and ganglioneuroma are important. Cysts of the trachea or bronchi, duplications of the œsophagus and neuro-enteric canal remnants make up most of the remainder.

THE THYMUS

In the past enlargement of the thymus was blamed for many symptoms and treatment by irradiation was readily undertaken. Little genuine benefit followed and there have been a number of late thyroid malignancies thought to be due to "scatter" of the rays.

There are still some patients with stridor and gross enlargement of the thymic shadow whose condition improves following natural regression of the gland.

REFERENCES

Clark, N. S. (1963) Bronchiectasis in childhood, *Brit. med. J.*, *i*, 80.

Polgor, G. and Koop, C. E. (1963) Pulmonary function in pectus excavatum, *Pediatrics* (August), 209.

Ravitch, Mark M. (1958) Operation for correction of pectus excavatum, *Surg. Gynec. Obstet.*, **106,** 619.

CHAPTER 38

BURNS AND SCALDS

BURNS and scalds remain an important cause of disability, disfigurement and death in children. The matter is not a medical one only, but
is also a social problem. Many of the causes of burning such as the
frequent scalding caused by overturned coffee-pots and frying-pans,
seem easily avoidable. There is no doubt that another factor is the
overcrowded conditions in which many families have to manage. The
peak incidence of burns is in the toddler age group. It is easy to see why
this should be. The children have become mobile but have not yet the
experience to avoid danger. Recent studies in Edinburgh have shown a
remarkably greater peak for girls than boys at this age. Analysis has
shown that it is almost entirely due to the wearing of inflammable
nightdresses. This is certainly a matter which could be simply remedied.

Classification of Burns

Burns are now usually classified simply as *superficial* or *deep*. The
superficial are sometimes called partial skin loss and the deep involve
complete skin loss. The practical importance of this differentiation is
that a superficial burn, which may be defined as one which damages
only the outer layers of the skin and leaves the basal layer intact, will
heal spontaneously in 2 to 3 weeks. A deep burn, in which the basal
layer is lost, can heal only by slow granulation and ultimate scarring.
Such burns therefore need grafting procedures to accelerate healing and
prevent chronic illness, sepsis, difigurement and contracture.

A subdivision called the deep dermal burn is also of practical
importance. This is a burn in which the main part of the basal layer
has been lost, but little areas of epithelium persist in the ducts of the
skin glands which extend deeper. Epithelium spreading slowly from the
mouths of these glands will produce healing in 5 or 6 weeks in good
conditions and this may be preferable to grafting, particularly on the
face and in young toddlers.

The *depth* of the burn can often be judged by its appearance. A
superficial burn may show as an area of erythema with blistering. The
blisters may have burst, exposing a pink area with deep red spots over
it. A deep burn will have a dead white and more parchment-like
appearance. Burned tissue which is doomed by stasis to death looks
vascular and red during the first twenty-four hours and it remains so
for three to four days until the red cells lyse, indicating the boundary
of necrosis. This may be masked by the presence of charred epithelium
over the surface. On testing for sensation with a pin there is anæsthesia

in full thickness burns, but sensation will remain in partial thickness burns of the skin. These tests are not entirely reliable and sometimes it may be necessary to observe the burn over a few days before making a definite decision. If the burn is being treated by exposure the type of the primary eschar which forms may also be a guide to the depth of the burn. Partial thickness burns of the skin produce an eschar which is heaped up on the surface as a result of copious outpouring of plasma which coagulates. The eschar over a deep burn, however, tends to be thinner and to be slightly depressed below the surface of the limb presenting a hollowed appearance. It should be noticed that a scald can cause a full thickness burn and this is particularly likely to happen if the hot fluid is held in contact with the skin for some time, for example by soaking the clothing.

Most burns and scalds over 10 per cent of the body surface are a combination of partial and complete skin loss. Virtually all extensive burns and scalds have an area of complete skin loss usually centrally. It is perhaps even more important to realize that the depth of the burn can be increased during treatment. A partial thickness burn of the skin may easily become full thickness as a result of poor treatment allowing infection or poor circulation to destroy further tissue. Abrasion by loose dressings may also convert a partial skin loss into a complete one.

The Effects of Burns

The general illness of burns may be described under three headings which are time-honoured if somewhat inaccurate from the pathological point of view. The first phase is that of shock; there may also be a phase of early toxæmia and one of late toxæmia.

Shock is due to reduction of the circulating blood volume associated with the loss of protein-containing fluid from the surface of the burn. This oligæmic shock arises in the first few hours after burning and the fluid loss goes on at a diminishing rate over 36 to 48 hours. If the burn is a deep one there is also blood destruction. The *extent of the shock* is therefore proportional to the *extent* of the burn rather than of its depth. For this reason a scald which is diffuse may kill the child even though the lesion itself would be practically completely healed within a fortnight if the child could be kept alive through this early period.

An unexplained condition which has been called early toxæmia may arise about 36 hours after burning. The child has a high temperature, signs of peripheral circulatory failure, shivering and rigors. There may be pin-point pupils and a raised blood pressure.

At this stage renal failure may also occur with tubular damage. This presents as oliguria and may respond to careful management if it is noticed early whereas excessive fluid administration under these conditions might cause rapid death.

Later the child may develop the so-called chronic toxæmia which is due to protein loss from the persisting open wound of the burnt surface and a negative nitrogen balance which may be exacerbated by the presence of infection of the wound. It is also possible that a condition of adrenal exhaustion contributes to this clinical state.

The after-effects of the burn are disfigurement and the ill-effects of contractures. Contractures may limit the movement of joints directly and may cause danger to other organs; for example contracture of the eyelids by exposing the eye may render the cornea liable to late damage. In addition to these physical effects one must stress the fact that many of these children are toddlers who are not only terrified by the burn but unable to understand the sequelæ of the accident with the discomfort of treatment and separation from the family. Emotional upsets are frequent and should have more attention paid to them than has been in the past.

TREATMENT

A burn is an aseptic necrosis of tissue. The complications of this necrosis—*shock*, *sepsis* and *scarring*—are to a great extent preventable.

FIRST AID. This consists of covering the burn with the cleanest object available, usually a clean sheet or handkerchief and no further interference. It is only meddlesome to try to do more and delay in reaching hospital is serious. A burnt child will travel well in the first 3 hours after the accident. Then oligæmic shock will become manifest and movement dangerous. Any delay in getting the child to a unit with facilities for management of the severe metabolic disturbance of the first crucial 2 days may mean that the chance of survival has been missed.

A further specific point is worth mentioning here. This is the management of the child whose clothing catches fire by brushing against a fire. The flames burning around the child rise round its face and head. The natural instinct of the child is to try to pull the clothes over its head and this may result in severe burns around the face. It is well worth trying to disseminate amongst the public the importance of lying the child down immediately and damping out the flames in this position. The child should be taken to hospital as rapidly as possible. The kind of shock which is likely to kill the child will not respond to any treatment except intravenous fluid and the degree of shock which may be improved by simple first aid measures is unlikely to prove serious anyway.

Assessment and Resuscitation

When the child arrives in hospital the first duty is to assess the extent and depth of the burn. Any burn which effects more than 10 per cent of a child's body will cause shock requiring fluid replacement. Burns involving 50 per cent of the body will have a considerable mortality even with the best of attention. The immediate treatment is directed to preventing shock before it becomes manifest. It will be possible to assess by the extent of the burn the amount of fluid the child requires and this should be given promptly. There is no place for waiting to observe the child's progress; the object should be to give the fluid as it is needed and not to wait until oligæmia is established. The fluid used is usually blood plasma and it seems that the modern dextrans are a satisfactory substitute as plasma expanders. A generous sample of blood should be taken initially, particularly if the artificial plasma expanders are to be used, because they interfere with the agglutination reactions used in blood-grouping. If the burn is extensive, say more than 20 per cent, or if it is deep, then it will be necessary to give a proportion of the fluid as whole blood to allow for red cell loss. The amount of fluid required can be initially estimated by a simple formula based on body weight and percentage area burnt and then *when treatment has been started it is controlled by observation of the patient.*

Simple clinical observation of the child's appearance and pulse rate are themselves of value and the blood pressure should be repeatedly recorded. In addition any patient with extensive burns should have a catheter in the bladder so that the urine output can be measured from hour to hour. A minimum of 20 ml./hour should be achieved. Diminution in the urinary outflow is an important sign of undertreatment. If a suitable apparatus is at hand the use of serial hæmatocrit estimations which can be carried out from finger-prick blood will give an accurate assessment of the success of the treatment in maintaining the blood volume. It is usually practicable to disregard the electrolyte requirements until these are orally replaceable. It is important to realize that shivering and vomiting are unlikely to be due to the child being cold, but more probably due to inadequate fluid replacement or to infection of the open wound.

Sedation. A suitable sedative will be needed at the onset because the child will be frightened and in pain. The sedation should be carefully controlled to avoid any undue depression. Morphine is a valuable drug. It should not be given subcutaneously at this stage because in the presence of shock it may not be absorbed at the time but may be absorbed later with dangerous results. The intravenous route is safest and surest initially. (0·025 mg. per pound body weight.)

The calculations of fluid requirements are based on loss from the time of burning (*not* from the time of admission), and the earlier fluid replacement begins the more effective it will be in preventing shock. Time should not be wasted in getting advice from consultants or pathologists; the plasma drip should be put up first and other things should follow in treating a severely burnt child.

If it is calculated that such a large quantity of fluid will have to be given quickly that the collapsed peripheral veins will not accommodate the volume, an indwelling inferior vena caval catheter is justified in such serious circumstances. The metabolic requirement of fluid is also given by mouth as 5 per cent glucose 40 ml./kg./day.

After the initial shock phase of 2 days or so it is important to get the child on to a *high protein diet with ample calories,* for much protein is lost from the burns. There is an inevitable negative nitrogen balance following the trauma which limits what can be done nutritionally in the first 2 weeks or so. It is particularly important to maintain a good diet in those cases whose burns remain incompletely covered by skin after the first 2 weeks. Healing is delayed by malnutrition.

Sepsis and fear of dressings and handling are important causes of anorexia. Exposure may be invaluable in reducing toxæmia and restoring morale. It should be remembered that it is quite practical to use exposure methods after grafting as well as before.

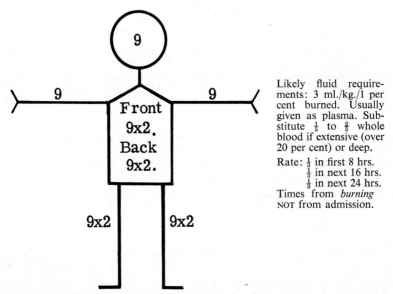

Likely fluid requirements: 3 ml./kg./1 per cent burned. Usually given as plasma. Substitute $\frac{1}{8}$ to $\frac{2}{8}$ whole blood if extensive (over 20 per cent) or deep.

Rate: $\frac{1}{3}$ in first 8 hrs.
$\frac{1}{3}$ in next 16 hrs.
$\frac{1}{3}$ in next 24 hrs.
Times from *burning* NOT from admission.

FIG. 72. Wallace's Rules of Nine. A convenient guide to percentage body surface area expressed in nines and multiples of nine.

Fortified dried milk preparations such as Complan have simplified feeding problems. It is possible to give a full diet by nasogastric drip if necessary. For the sake of morale pleasanter and varied, if more expensive, menus are also used.

Local Treatment

The object of local treatment is to produce a *dry* surface inimical to the growth of bacteria. There are two ways of doing this. The more popular way nowadays is to expose the burn by positioning the baby to suit each individual burn. The position must avoid resting on the burnt surface and must keep involved joint flexures extended. The burn is then allowed to form an eschar over the first day or two. It is no longer considered wise to apply antibacterial powders locally because these tend to make a thick crust under which infection more easily develops.

Closed Dressings. An alternative method of obtaining a dry surface is to cover the burn with a *voluminous* dressing of fluffed gauze which will absorb the secretions over a layer of wide-meshed non-adherent tulle gras. The key to the treatment is the thickness of the dressing. There should be 2 to 3 inches thickness of fluffed gauze over all the burnt areas, then cotton wool as a further absorptive. Cotton wool should be kept out of contact with the actual wound to avoid unpleasant adherence and caking. Such dressings are covered in crêpe banadages to give firm application. The crêpe bandages are kept in place by zinc oxide strapping. They used to be called pressure dressings but a little experimentation with a balloon inside the dressing will soon demonstrate the futility of attempting to maintain constant pressure in this way. They act rather by absorbing the exudate from the burn and keep the surface from becoming water-logged. They are only efficient as long as their outer surface remains dry. Once it becomes moist there is a direct route of ingress for bacteria along a plasma-sodden dressing, the best possible nidus for organisms. The dressings are changed as infrequently as possible in keeping with the policy that they must never show moisture externally. Dressings are apt to be frightening, if not painful, to children, and the repeated anæsthesia often necessary to avoid this interferes with the feeding which is so important to maintain their general condition.

Exposure. It is certainly possible with modern anæsthesia or skilled analgesia to cope with the management and dressings when they are needed, but it is frequently simpler to adopt the exposure technique. In most sites it has all the advantages of the absorptive dressing technique and is a happier one for the child who seems sooner to redevelop an interest in life when he realizes that his burns are going to be left alone. There is an important exception to the use of exposure. This is in the circumferential burns of the limbs and particularly of the fingers. Here the formation of an eschar may act as a tourniquet with serious interference to the circulation and even gangrene of the digits. Circumferentially burnt hands are therefore better nursed in a big boxing glove type of dressing, and this should be elevated to minimize the formation of œdema within the hand during the first day or two.

It is also important to apply some form of cream around the eyes, nostrils and mouth should these be burnt to avoid the formation of a tight eschar which can lead to unpleasant contractures. A burnt face swells up very easily and the sight a few hours after burning is most alarming. It may be particularly terrifying for a child to find that his eyes are shut and he is unable to see. Reassurance that this is only temporary is extremely important. Fortunately the face does in fact heal extremely well and many of these frightening-looking superficial burns of the face will settle down rapidly. The œdema resolves after the first few days to present a virtually normal end result.

Tracheotomy may be life-saving in the child suffocating following the inhalation of scorching fumes.

Blisters more than 1½ inches in diameter (half a crown) should be snipped and evacuated under strictly sterile conditions while small vesicles may safely be left to reabsorb.

An antibiotic such as tetracycline is given for the first few days to all major burns. It cannot prevent contamination of the exposed surface, but will prevent the ingress of organisms to cause clinical infection until a dry surface is obtained. Management is controlled by the findings from swabs of exudate taken for culture from the burnt surface at suitable intervals.

In spite of a trend away from the local use of antibiotics, with their risks of sensitization and of encouragement of resistant organisms, sprays of antibiotics not used systemically may be invaluable, particularly at the time of grafting (e.g. Polybactrin = polymyxin, neomycin and bacitracin). There has also been some return to favour of antiseptics, of which chlorhexidine (Hibitane) is probably the most popular. Most clinics restrict the use of antiseptics to the trivial burn being treated as an outpatient, or to the infected case.

The most important point in the management of minor hand burns is to keep them out of water, otherwise they will become infected.

If the burn has caused only partial skin loss one leaves the eschar to separate at about the end of the second week. If there are deep areas, however, these will require split skin grafting to cover the areas and avoid delayed healing with consequent scarring.

Skin Grafting

In deep burns with much tissue destruction it may be wise to perform an early excision of the damaged area and apply grafts soon after burning. In addition to producing a better local result this may avoid a good deal of the illness of trauma following the burn. In very extensive burns also it may be important to get early skin cover to reduce the plasma loss from the burnt surface, and if there is insufficient area available on the child it is possible to use homografts taken from some volunteer. Homografts from parents or siblings of the same blood group may be best. The homografts will be thrown off after a week or two as a result of the development of an antibody reaction in the host. But they will give that period of skin cover which may enable the child to be brought through the acute illness. The child's own donor areas will then have healed sufficiently for further grafts to be taken from them. With modern techniques it is possible to take skin grafts from the same area two to three times if this is necessary.

The late infected burn may benefit from a period of soaks and frequent dressings to separate sloughs. Hibitane solution 1 per cent, Edinburgh University Solution of lime (Eusol), hydrogen peroxide or trypsin preparations are useful at this stage, but such treatment should not be prolonged more than a few days. Switches from open to closed treatment or the reverse may be rewarding. The toxæmia and anorexia of an infected child will often clear miraculously when the lesion is exposed.

Aftercare

Warm baths will help the patients to "kick out" contractures. Splinting and stretching grafted areas may also be necessary. Lanolin or Anthisan cream will help to soften healed areas and grafts. An area which looks well healed one month after burning may look much worse in three months with hypertrophic scars. This is not true keloid and, after a few months, it begins to soften and flatten and continues to improve for two years or more.

When the burn is healed there may be contractures requiring late plastic procedures in spite of all care. For example, a burnt axilla may leave the child with a bridle scar preventing abduction and elevation of the arm. It may be possible to treat this by transposing skin flaps in the "Z" fashion but it is usually necessary to open up the area again and apply further skin grafts to the raw surface exposed. Burnt eyelids are replaced by full thickness grafts. It may be necessary to carry out major plastic procedures. For example, the application of pedicle flaps under the chin of a child who has been burnt by flames from a burning dress. For skin and subcutaneous fat may have to be moved to fill such a defect.

CONCLUSIONS

The severe burns present a difficult metabolic problem and there cannot be any doubt that they are best treated in specialized burns units with experience of this condition. But for each of these severe burns there are as many as 20 minor scalds and burns admitted in which the immediate problem of treatment of the shock is slight, yet careful management to minimize disfigurement and contracture are important. Many of these burnt children are toddlers, and from the point of view of the child as a whole may be better managed in the atmosphere of a general pædiatric surgical department of a children's hospital, with all its facilities for the occupation and handling of young children, rather than that of the "metabolic unit" of a specialized burns unit. Probably the best arrangement is to have the burns unit in the children's hospital so that children can graduate from the constant care of the burns unit to the general pædiatric ward as they improve.

The most difficult part of the treatment of severe burns is probably the treatment of the hypovolæmic shock. This develops over about

8 hours after burning; it is therefore also the most urgent treatment. It is therefore important that these children should go directly to the place where they are to be treated. During the first 3 hours after burning they will travel well. Later they will become shocked and it will be necessary to hold the child for 2 days in whatever unit he happens to be whilst the shock is controlled, before passing the child on for any further specialized treatment that may be required. This means that the Casualty Officer has an important duty to perform in deciding quickly whether his hospital is able to cope with the child, or whether it should be sent on to a special unit. Consultants should co-operate in making this possible by giving their Casualty Officers the authority to make such decisions without delay. It can only do the child harm to be admitted to a ward and then to be moved back to an ambulance for transfer. It is probably best for the Casualty Officer to see the child in its ambulance and decide there and then whether it comes to his hospital or goes on.

REFERENCES

Artz, C. P. and Gaston, B. H. (1960) A reappraisal of the exposure method in the treatment of burns, donor sites and skin grafts, *Ann. Surg.*, **151,** 939.

Clarkson, P. W. (1965) The Burnt Child in London, *Ann. roy. Coll. Surg. Engl.*, **37,** 207.

Muir, I. F. K. and Barclay, T. L. (1962) *Burns and their Treatment,* Lloyd-Luke (London).

CHAPTER 39

HEAD INJURIES

IT is a regrettable commentary on our civilization that injury is a commoner cause of death in childhood than any single group of diseases.

Amongst these, injuries to the head are increasing in frequency, with road accidents an important group.

BRAIN INJURIES

The important lesion in a head injury is that of the brain. A brain injury can be serious or even fatal without any fracture of the skull or laceration of the scalp.

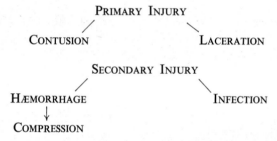

The damage to the brain may be *primary* or *secondary*. Sudden acceleration or deceleration of the head causes brain injury because the inertia of the brain in its waterbath of cerebrospinal fluid causes it to be forced against the rigid containing vault and deforms it. Thus a primary *contusion* or *laceration* may occur. This may be accompanied by a contrecoup injury to the opposite side of the brain.

Secondary injury to the brain arises after the accident. There are two important causes. Tearing of vessels may cause *hæmorrhage* in or around the brain. Such bleeding produces a space-occupying lesion within the inextensible cranium. Thus *cerebral compression* further damages the brain.

Infection may enter through the wound of an open head injury causing meningitis, cerebritis or ventriculitis and again cause further brain damage.

The secondary causes of braïn damage (compression and infection) are of particular importance to the surgeon because they are avoidable or treatable. Good surgical care should prevent infection and surgery can relieve compression by hæmorrhage. The great majority of primary insults to the brain will recover spontaneously with no more than medical management and nursing care, while many of the severe ones will die whatever is done because vital centres are destroyed. In between these extremes are cases in which special techniques may be needed to keep a patient alive long enough for the brain to recover; including tracheostomy to assist respiratory toilet, intragastric tube feeding and perhaps cooling to avoid hyperthermia of central origin, or deliberately to subnormal levels to reduce cerebral metabolic requirements.

The management of head injuries in practice then becomes a matter of skilled nursing and the repeated observation of many cases so that the small proportion needing active intervention to combat secondary effects—hæmorrhage, infection, respiratory complications—may be recognized in time.

THREE BASIC STATES FOLLOWING HEAD INJURY

CONCUSSION. This is the result of a diffuse neuronal upset causing temporary cessation of all but the vital functions. Perhaps the jarring produces a temporary circulatory stasis and anoxia. The patient is unconscious with pallor, a slow weak pulse, dilated pupils, flaccid limbs and absent tendon reflexes.

Recovery is usually prompt and complete, though the duration of unconsciousness varies from a moment to, say, a couple of days. On recovery the patient shows amnesia for events before the accident (retrograde amnesia) as well as for the period of unconsciousness (prograde amnesia). The length of this period during which memory patterns are not laid down is an index of the severity of the concussion. (Those cases with prolonged unconsciousness are likely to be associated with some degree of frank *contusion* of the brain which may heal by gliosis leaving a permanent defect of function.) The role of generalized cerebral œdema in head injuries is now thought less important than was considered in the past.

CEREBRAL IRRITATION. This is the result of contusion with loca œdema of the brain, or of subarachnoid bleeding around it. The latter produces what amounts to a chemical meningitis, blood being irritant in the cerebrospinal circulation. The child lies curled up on his side with his face covered and resents any attempt to move him. He has photophobia and a headache.

CEREBRAL COMPRESSION. Compression results typically from *subdural* or *extradural hæmorrhage* causing increased pressure on the brain. The conditions are quite commonly bilateral. The patient may have recovered consciousness following a mild head injury when consciousness begins to deteriorate again (the lucid interval), or the further effects of pressure may arise more insidiously in a patient still unconscious from concussion. The hæmorrhage commonly arises from a torn middle meningeal artery (extradural hæmorrhage) or a vein spanning the interval from parietes to the surface of the cerebrum (usually a subdural hæmorrhage). *The most important sign of compression is deterioration in the level of consciousness.* Along with this pressure on the motor cortex will produce first spasticity of the contralateral limbs and with greater pressure flaccidity of the limbs; herniation of part of the temporal lobe through the tentorium cerebelli forces the uncus against the third nerve. Irritation first produces a small pupil followed by paralysis with a dilated non-reacting pupil. By this time the contralateral pupil will have begun to contract and later will dilate. *It cannot be too strongly emphasized that fixed dilated pupils are not a sign of cerebral compression.* *They are a sign of compression neglected for so long that death is imminent within hours if relief is not forthcoming; furthermore the damage is unlikely to be completely reversible even if the pressure is relieved.* The tentorial herniation will soon lead to pressure on the brain stem with decerebrate rigidity and direct interference with vital centres. The earlier stage of *unequal pupils* is the one at which investigation for compression should take place.

Compression causes important effects on the vital centres. The pulse becomes slow and bounding. It is important that nursing staff should realize that this is one of the few conditions in which a *slowing* pulse is even more serious than a rising one. The systolic blood pressure rises but the diastolic pressure falls, giving the high pulse pressure which is so readily felt. Respiration becomes slow and deep and later it may become periodic and eventually gasping. Temperature control is upset so that the patient may have hyperpyrexia and yet be shivering.

ASSOCIATED SKULL FRACTURES

It has already been said that the important lesion is the cerebral one. But a skull fracture at least demonstrates that a blow has been sustained severe enough to cause primary or secondary brain damage and to justify observation in hospital. Absence of a fracture by no means indicates that the cerebrum is unlikely to have suffered.

LINEAR FRACTURES OF THE VAULT are unimportant in themselves. They heal by fibrous union within 3 weeks and later often achieve bony union. A fracture crossing the temporal region has special significance as it may be associated with a torn middle meningeal vessel.

FRACTURED BASE OF THE SKULL is more important. This is because anterior fossa fractures may open into the paranasal sinuses and fractures of the middle fossa into the middle ear cavity; i.e. they are open fractures in that infection may enter though their contact with the air is not on an external surface.

Fractured base of the skull can rarely be diagnosed radiologically. A clinical diagnosis is reached. Anterior fossa fractures are likely to be associated with escape of cerebrospinal fluid and/or blood from the nose. There may be a typical subconjunctival hæmorrhage. This extends as far back along the globe as can be seen for the blood is tracking out from the orbit: in contrast the hæmorrhage associated with a direct injury black eye is mainly around the pupil and fades away laterally.

Middle fossa fractures may be associated with escape of cerebrospinal fluid and/or blood from the ear. Of course, bleeding from ear or nose may also occur as a result of direct injury.

DEPRESSED FRACTURES. The direct damage to the underlying brain may be serious and healing with scar is likely to leave an irritable focus. Thus, depending on the area of brain involved, post-traumatic epilepsy may develop as long as 10 years after the injury.

OPEN FRACTURES. These are clearly serious because of the danger of infection.

Management

The patient is examined fully undressed with particular care to establish and *document:*

1. *The Level of Consciousness.* Is this normal, confused, lightly or deeply unconscious? This is assessed by ability to respond to questions, simple commands, touch, painful stimuli or tendon reflex stimulation. It is better to record the response obtained than to use phrases such as lightly comatose, stuporose, etc., which may not convey the same meaning to all.

2. The tone and reflexes of the limbs.

3. Pupil size and reactions. The fundi should be examined.

4. Whether there is any neck stiffness from cerebral irritation or concomitant cervical injury.

5. Any bleeding or discharge or cerebrospinal fluid from ears or nose.

6. Local signs of injury on the head, e.g. bruises, lacerations.

7. Other injuries. Pneumothorax, hæmothorax, ruptured intra-abdominal viscus and fractures of the long bones or vertebræ are the most important associated problems. The chest is percussed and auscultated. The thoracic cage is sprung by pressure on the sternum. Hæmothorax may present with severe shock as well as respiratory symptoms. The abdomen is palpated and auscultated for bowel sounds. The long bones are gently palpated and moved and the vertebral spinous processes tapped and their alignment observed.

There is *no* need for immediate X-ray of every head injury on admission. The routine films obtained in emergency conditions with a portable machine are unlikely to be of value in guiding treatment and the decision whether treatment is needed depends on the cerebral condition, not that of the skull. The further upset to the patient newly transported to hospital may be actively harmful. Radiology is carried out at the earliest convenience and should certainly take place before any surgical intervention.

Sedatives should be used as little as possible, but may be essential to allay restlessness. (But remember that the restless, confused patient may only have a full bladder.) Intramuscular phenobarbitone (15–45 mg.) is valuable and intramuscular paraldehyde (1 ml. per 6 kg.) is unpleasant but safe. The reaction to opiates may be excessive and may mask the progress of the lesion or prove fatal by depression of vital functions.

Prolonged or deep unconsciousness may lead to respiratory distress from inability to cough up the pulmonary secretions. Tracheostomy to allow regular bronchial toilet may be life-saving. It should be performed before cyanosis or anoxia reaches a serious degree.

Oxygen when needed should be given by tube or mask to prevent the child becoming cut off from the nursing staff in a tent.

Hypothermia induced by surface cooling or drugs such as chlorpromazine (5 to 25 mg. according to weight) and phenergan (5 to 25 mg. according to weight) reduces brain metabolism and helps to control the cortical swelling. It should be used in the more severe injuries, particularly where there is any tendency to hyperpyrexia or in the presence of the decerebrate state from which it may make recovery possible.

Antibiotics need be used only if there is an extensive wound, a clinical diagnosis of fractured base, rhinorrhœa or otorrhœa. Pulmonary hypostasis may demand antibiotic cover later.

The unconscious patient is nursed on the side with one firm pillow *taking care that the airway is clear*. The side should be changed regularly and periods prone included in the rota to reduce pulmonary hypostasis. Without special supervision to keep the head to one side the supine position is dangerous, for there is danger of tongue swallowing resulting in asphyxia and of inhalation of vomit when the cough reflex is depressed. For this reason also no attempt should ever be made to force fluid or food by mouth on an uncooperative patient. A suitable fluid diet should be fed through a nasal intragastric tube.

The nursing staff must be trained to make repeated observations and records of:

     (*a*) Level of consciousness.
     (*b*) Pupil size and reactions.
     (*c*) Limb tone and/or reflexes.
     (*d*) Pulse, respiration (rate and depth) and temperature.

At first these may be needed every quarter of an hour; later they may be made hourly, depending on the state of progress of the patient. It must be made clear that the level of consciousness should be tested even though the patient appears to be asleep lest the change from sleep to unresponsive unconsciousness be missed.

REPEATED EXAMINATION IS THE KEY TO DIAGNOSIS AND THE LEVEL OF CONSCIOUSNESS IS THE YARDSTICK TO WHICH ALL OTHER DANGER SIGNS ARE LINKED. It is on such serial examinations that treatment is based. The majority of patients will slowly and steadily improve and need no more than good nursing. Any interruption of this progress or

deterioration in the level of consciousness means *secondary* brain damage
and active measures will be needed.

If there is no improvement in 12 hours, lumbar puncture may be
performed. If a raised pressure is found (perhaps with marked bleeding)
most authorities agree that it is safe in practice to lower this by draining
the cerebrospinal fluid with a lumbar needle. This can be repeated
daily as needed. The use of dehydration to reduce cerebral œdema,
whilst it may be valuable in special circumstances, is no longer routine.
Intravenous urea may be life saving when œdema threatens the function
of the vital centres.

SURGERY

There are three indications for urgent operation:

1. Open wound
2. Cerebral compression by:
   (a) Intracranial hæmorrhage
   (b) Brain swelling following contusion.

OPEN WOUNDS. Open wounds clearly need urgent attention to avoid
the serious consequence of infection of the central nervous system.
The principle of removal of damaged tissue, cerebral as well as parietal,
and conversion to a closed wound by suture or flaps applies here as
elsewhere. But it will often be expedient to wait 12 or 24 hours to allow
the brain to get over the initial effects of the injury before subjecting it
to the further trauma of operation and anæsthesia. Clean dressings and
antibiotic protection should be used meanwhile. Oligæmic shock due to
associated injuries may need treatment by transfusion, but care is
needed to avoid over-infusion which may increase intracranial
hæmorrhage or œdema of the brain.

CEREBRAL COMPRESSION. In the presence of the signs of cerebral compression as described above the head should be shaved and burrholes
made to look for a *clot*. Extradural hæmorrhage may be suspected from
associated boggy swelling in the temporal fossa and a fracture at this
site. A local scalp bruise may be a more reliable guide to an underlying
hæmorrhage than the site of a fracture. A temporal burrhole is made
for inspection. If extradural hæmorrhage is found it can be enlarged by
removing bone in the area protected by the overlying temporalis muscle
to evacuate blood, plug the bleeding vessel and, most important, to
decompress the brain (subtemporal decompression). Subdural hæmorrhage is recognized by blue colouring showing through the dura. Dural
venous sinuses are more often a cause of bleeding than the middle meningeal artery.

If no blood is found in the subtemporal region of the explored side
then a hole should be made in the temporoparietal region. If this is also
fruitless the scalp should be sewn up and the other side explored in
similar fashion. If there is any suspicion of a subdural clot then the dura

should be incised and the clot washed out. If these four burrholes fail to reveal a hæmorrhage but the brain is tense, and if there has been a frontal blow, then it may be wise to make frontal burrholes also to exclude bleeding there.

In difficult cases much valuable information may be obtained by contrast radiography. Air encephalography or carotid angiography may enable localization of intracerebral or intraventricular hæmorrhage as well as surface lesions.

AFTERCARE

Convalescence is easy to regulate for child patients. When they feel well enough they will want to sit up and then get out of bed. Whilst they are still in an unstable post-traumatic state sudden changes of posture will induce giddiness or headache and the child will wish to be still. Common-sense supervision is needed to prevent excesses due to momentary enthusiasms, but beyond this observation the child's inclination will enable him more or less to regulate his own convalescence. There is no virtue whatsoever in the time-honoured 3 weeks flat in bed after concussion. Such a programme will induce iatrogenic weakness and postural hypotension in a normal person. The child should sit and then stand as soon as he is ready for it on an individual assessment of his progress. Romberg's test is a convenient way of inducing giddiness in one still prone to post-traumatic disturbances on sudden changes of posture.

Some authorities advise the prophylactic use of phenobarbitone for 1 or 2 years after any fairly severe head injury and many believe that penetration of the dura is an indication for prophylactic anticonvulsants. It is believed that this reduces the incidence of post-traumatic irritable (epileptogenic) foci.

REFERENCES

Alexander, G. L. (1962) Clinical assessment in the acute stage after head injury, *Lancet*, **1**, 171.

McIver, I. N., Lassmann, L. P., Thomson, C. W. and McLeod, I. (1958) Treatment of severe head injuries, *Lancet*, **2**, 544.

Potter, J. M. (1961) *The Practical Management of Head Injuries*, Lloyd-Luke (London).

Potter, J. M. (1963) Simplified Management of Head Injuries, *Lancet*, *i*, 374.

CHAPTER 40

ABDOMINAL MASSES IN INFANCY AND CHILDHOOD

ISOLATED cases of all possible tumours and malformations occur in the abdomen of children from time to time and an exhaustive tabulation would not be really useful. Because many of the conditions are of considerable urgency every effort must be made to reach a prompt clinical diagnosis, or at least a decision about what further investigations or consultations will be necessary.

Probably one-third or more of abdominal masses felt in infancy are malignant, and although benign conditions make up a greater proportion in older children the really important decision to make is whether or not a mass is malignant. It is not always possible to make a conclusive diagnosis clinically, or even with X-rays and laboratory tests. *Laparotomy is then amply justified to determine the nature of any unidentified abdominal mass.*

The age of the patient, taken together with the system to which the mass is thought to belong, will provide the most useful guide to differential diagnosis.

Straight X-ray of the abdomen is really of use only in demonstrating calcification, as in adrenal hæmatoma, nephroblastoma, neuroblastoma or old tuberculous mesenteric lymph nodes.

The intravenous pyelogram is much the most useful investigation, particularly as the two commonest malignancies are in the kidney and the adrenal and will almost always alter the X-ray picture. Barium meals and enemas are seldom much help unless there are symptoms of intestinal obstruction.

A full blood count is perhaps the only routinely worthwhile blood investigation. Moderate anæmia is almost always present in neoplasms of all kinds, and there is often a leucocytosis as well. The intravenous pyelogram is the most valuable test of renal function in practice.

An examination under heavy sedation or general anæsthesia will often give a surprising amount of additional information and help plan the next move.

The necessary tests should be carried out preferably as a group and a decision reached promptly. The only possible decision may be that a laparotomy is necessary for definite diagnosis, and if this is so it should not be delayed. Laparotomy on a mass of unknown ætiology may mean an extensive operation and blood should always be available for transfusion. It is an added precaution to give a non-absorbable chemo-

311   x 2

therapeutic agent to reduce the bowel flora in case a colonic resection becomes necessary in the course of the operation.

CLINICAL DIAGNOSIS

Some of the commoner masses will be classified under general headings of system and age group, with the inevitable reservations about all clinical diagnosis in this problem.

Alimentary Tract

APPENDIX MASS. A mass in the right iliac fossa, tender or not, with or without a temperature, at *any* age is an appendix mass until proved otherwise. It is one of the few almost certain diagnoses and can usually be treated conservatively.

FÆCAL MASSES. A mass low in the left iliac fossa is more often fæces than anything else. Extreme constipation may present with diarrhœa from overflow and an enema may produce a small result. But rectal examination is conclusive. It reveals the impacted fæcal mass and it may require many washouts to clean the bowel. The fact that fæces indents if pressed hard is diagnostic, but if a tumour is indented thus the ill effects can be imagined. Fæcal masses may not be palpable through the rectal wall in Hirschsprung's disease if the affected segment of colon is a long one, but if this is so gross gaseous distension will usually be diagnostic and indeed is usually so marked that abdominal masses of fæces cannot be felt even though present.

MESENTERIC CYSTS AND INTESTINAL DUPLICATIONS

These masses are often globular and their position in the abdomen is often disputed by different clinicians because they are so mobile. They may be moved almost anywhere in the abdomen and only come to light through complications such as reaching great size or obstruction, bleeding and volvulus.

TUBERCULOUS MESENTERIC ADENITIS. This disease may present as ascites without other cause, as a tender abdominal mass (rolled omentum) or as obstruction. It should be completely preventable by B.C.G. vaccination. The condition in the female carries a poor prognosis for fertility.

INTESTINAL OBSTRUCTION BY BANDS. If the obstruction is incomplete it may present as a mass, the palpable swelling being the chronically enlarged loop of bowel proximal to the obstruction.

INTUSSUSCEPTION. This is usually dramatic in its onset, but chronic intussusception may occur with slight symptoms, as the obstruction is frequently incomplete. *Henoch-Schönlein purpura* may cause intestinal masses (hæmatomata) as well as intussusception.

CHRONIC REGIONAL ENTERITIS (Crohn's Disease)

This condition affects older children and affected loops of bowel may form a tender mobile mass. There is usually anorexia, loss of weight, anæmia, colicky abdominal pain and intermittent diarrhœa. It is rare in childhood.

LYMPHOSARCOMA

This malignancy usually occurs at the ileocæcal angle. It spreads in the mesentery. Resection does not cure but a short circuit may palliate by relief of obstruction. Deep X-ray or chemotherapy may give a period of relief.

The Liver

Enlargements of the liver are so characteristic that they are rarely confused with any other organ. The normal infant's liver is palpable and the edge may be a finger's breadth below the costal margin, but the enlarged liver of venous congestion may be the first sign of congenital heart disease with acute cardiac illness in early infancy.

Cirrhosis may occur without a history of jaundice. There is a diffuse firm enlargement with a distinct edge and perhaps an irregular surface. Later the liver shrinks and may become impalpable.

Simple cysts of the liver occur, but are difficult to distinguish clinically from *hepatoblastoma*. The *choledochus cyst* presents most frequently in a jaundiced adolescent girl but may do so at any age. It is a mass palpable below and separate from the liver.

Pyogenic and amœbic abscesses are rare here. The liver may be palpable because it is being pushed down from above by a silent *subphrenic abscess*.

The Spleen

The spleen presents a typical swelling. Enlargement is down towards the umbilicus and if it is really large the notch is often palpable. Many diagnostic aids are described to distinguish the spleen from the kidney, but the spleen is usually much more *superficial* and is detected by the lightest touch in the right place.

In childhood splenic enlargement often means *leukæmia* or one of the *reticuloses* such as Hodgkin's disease. Enlargement may be gross in portal-hypertension, with or without an enlarged liver. It becomes moderately enlarged in acholuric jaundice (hereditary spherocytosis) and other hæmolytic anæmias and may be enlarged in thrombocytopenic purpura. It may be greatly enlarged in glycogen storage disease. Bone marrow biopsy may aid diagnosis.

Genito-urinary System

Masses in the loin are dangerous and Wilms' tumour (*nephroblastoma*) and *neuroblastoma* of the adrenal must be suspected until another diagnosis is proven.

Hydronephrosis may present as a symptomless mass—in which case the prognosis for that kidney is bad. Bilateral renal masses may be hydronephrosis, but are more likely to be *polycystic disease* and the outlook for the patient is bad. The lobulated surface of polycystic or multicystic kidney can usually be recognized. The swelling of hydro-nephrosis is more likely to be smooth and soft unlike a tumour and in the giant hydronephrosis of infancy the firmer plaque of kidney parenchyma can be felt on the mass. A renal mass usually moves on respiration—a fixed malignant tumour will not.

The ectopic kidney can be a puzzling mass. It is usually in the pelvis, and if the condition is once thought of unfortunate conclusions and precipitate action may be avoided.

A benign but worrying mass is the *calcified adrenal hæmatoma* for patches of calcification also occur in malignancies of the gland and differentiation may be impossible without exploration of the gland. A history of acute neonatal illness with collapse is suggestive of adrenal hæmorrhage.

Bladder. The bladder is an abdominal organ in infancy and even when full is not as tender as in an adult. The overflowing bladder is often missed as the child appears to be passing plenty of urine into the napkins. The observation that the napkins are *always* wet, even just after changes, is an important one. There may even be quite a good stream, but if there is residual urine making the bladder feel hard like a golf ball then further investigation is urgent. Bladder-neck or urethral obstruction are the lesions to be considered.

Ovarian cysts occur rarely in childhood and may be very mobile.

Mucocolpos may occur from imperforate hymen or vaginal atresia. This occurs in the neonatal period with an abdominal mass and in the former a bulging membrane at the vagina. At the menarche the condition presents similarly, but the retained secretion is menstrual blood—*hæmatocolpos*. At this age there is often abdominal pain presumably due to blood leaking back through the uterine (Fallopian) tubes.

Retroperitoneal Masses

These are the most varied and least classifiable group. Kidney and suprarenal masses have already been mentioned. Neuroblastoma or the simple ganglioneuroma may also arise as paravertebral swellings at any level and may have "dumb-bell" extensions within the spinal canal giving rise to neurological signs by compression. The masses cannot be moved in any direction in most cases. *Retroperitoneal sarcoma* arises from undifferentiated tissue in the region. Total excision is usually impossible and widespread deep X-ray impractical.

A *simple retroperitoneal hæmatoma* may arise in a patient with a bleeding dyscrasia with little or no history of trauma.

Presacral and *sacrococcygeal teratomas* may be palpable from the abdomen and may give bizarre X-ray pictures due to calcification or bone formation in a well-differentiated tumour. Many are malignant. (The sacrum is typically pushed back and straightened giving the duck bottom appearance in the sacrococcygeal type.)

Conclusion

Many masses will be diagnosed clinically, many more with the aid of X-rays and blood examination. But a diagnosis must be reached in *all*. The inflammatory masses are out-numbered in our experience by those requiring active intervention. Exploration, with frozen section biopsy at the operating table if possible, is a necessity and must not be thought of as a last resort.

CHAPTER 41

MALIGNANT DISEASE

MALIGNANT disease is an uncommon condition in childhood, but it is still a regrettably common cause of death, whilst the infections are now coming under the control of antibiotic therapy. It is at present the commonest single cause of death after accidental injury in children beyond infancy, yet it has been calculated that a busy general practitioner is likely to see only two children with tumours in forty years of practice.

The tumours seen in adult life are occasionally met in children. For example, adenocarcinoma of the bowel and even carcinoma of the cervix uteri have been encountered. *But the bulk are malignancies special to the child.* About half of these conditions are *acute leukæmias.* This is not a condition amenable to surgical treatment, but even these may present to the surgeon under unusual circumstances. The presenting sign may be some unexplained bruising, or there may be an acutely tender swelling over a bone involved by a leukæmic infiltration. The painful swelling may be associated with fever, and the X-ray will show raising of the periosteum and erosion of underlying bone so that there may be quite a good imitation of a subacute osteitis.

TERATOMATA

Teratomata, which may be simple or malignant, are seen in childhood. They are tumours presenting elements from all the germ layers and may be considered as arising from totipotent cells. A typical example is the sacro-coccygeal teratoma which arises in the space between the rectum and the sacrum. It may form an enormous mass which may be already present in a new-born infant. It pushes the sacrum back and straightens it to produce in the classical case a distinctive duck bottomed appearance. Some of these are simple and may progress to form a wide variety of well-differentiated structures. For example, pieces of bowel and recognizable bones may be noticed and the latter may give a distinctive picture on the X-ray. The appearance in some of the well-differentiated tumours may be akin to an included twin. The malignant tumours may contain large areas of ill-differentiated tissue with cystic spaces and necrotic areas. Hæmorrhage may arise in the tumour and produce an acute reaction giving an appearance like an abscess.

Wide excision of these tumours is well worth while and the outlook seems to be particularly hopeful in those arising in the first year of life.

316

EMBRYOMATA

The group of *embryomata*, as their name implies, are tumours arising from primitive embryonic cells.

Neuroblastoma

Neuroblastoma is one of the common ones. It may arise from the adrenal area, or anywhere up and down the paravertebral region, where autonomic nervous tissue is present. It metastasizes widely through the blood stream and then produces a marked malaise and anæmia. Other cases may be recognized at an earlier stage through observation of a symptomless mass in the abdomen. The *ganglioneuroma* is a benign well-differentiated variant. It may merely present as a symptomless mass and indeed it may not be noticed throughout life and may only be recognized as an incidental finding in post-mortem examination of the adult. These tumours not uncommonly contain areas of both ganglio-neuromatous and neuroblastomatous tissue and this may have given rise to a mistaken conception that the tumour can differentiate from one state to the other. The evidence for this change is not conclusive. Some children with this tumour have a hypertension which suggests that more differentiated cells in the tumour may actually be functional and capable of producing noradrenaline. There is frequently increased urinary excretion of homovillanic acid and hydroxymandelic acid in neuroblastoma and repeated estimations may give valuable evidence of completeness of eradication or development of secondaries.

The treatment of neuroblastoma is radical surgery followed by small doses of deep X-ray therapy. Most of the tumours are extremely radio-sensitive and doses of 1,200 to 1,500r appear adequate. Even in the presence of bony secondaries surgery and radiotherapy are often worth while.

Vitamin B_{12} has been used in the treatment of neuroblastoma (Bodian). This vitamin is needed for maturation of red cells and it was hoped that it might similarly encourage maturation of the neuroblasts so that the malignant tumour would differentiate into a simple ganglio-neuroma. Disappearance of the tumour has occurred in the first year of life using very large doses (say 1 mgm. on alternate days) but may have been coincidental. The rôle of other chemotherapy is unsettled.

Under one year the survival rate is 60 per cent. After one year the survival rate is only 16 per cent. The presence of bony metastases renders the outlook very unfavourable. Those in the chest and pelvis do better than those in the abdomen. Almost all infants with neuroblastoma who survive for fourteen months may be regarded as "cured".

Spontaneous regression has been recorded more often in neuro-blastoma than in any other form of malignant disease. The course is so unpredictable that virtually no case should be given up as hopeless.

Nephroblastoma (Wilms' Tumour)

The nephroblastoma is a tumour arising from primitive renal formative cells. Again the common presentation is as a *symptomless mass*, or the mass may be found during routine examination of a child who is merely *out of sorts and looking pale*. Too often it is the mother bathing the baby who first notices the mass. After a symptomless mass *anæmia* is the commonest presentation of this condition. A few cases present with hæmaturia and a few cases have an acute presentation with abdominal pain and fever—presumably the result of a hæmorrhage into the tumour because this type of onset is often also associated with the development of acute anæmia. This is the tumour eponymously called the Wilms' tumour. Left-sided tumours may present with constipation, due to pressure on the descending colon.

A large symptomless swelling in the side of a child's abdomen will always give rise to suspicion of either a neuroblastoma or a nephroblastoma. They are particularly prone to arise in the first years of life but may arise throughout childhood. In both tumours the prognosis seems to be better in those who present younger. The clinical differentiation of the one from the other may be difficult. Typically the nephroblastoma has a smooth surface whereas the neuroblastoma is more likely to be lobulated and is more likely to extend across the midline. On intravenous pyelography the nephroblastoma arising within the kidney substance is likely to *distort* the pyelogram on the affected side, whereas the nephroblastoma arising adjacent to the kidney is more likely to displace the pyelogram shadow *en masse*. In some cases the diagnosis can be made only at operative biopsy.

The treatment of neuroblastoma is a combination of radical surgery, chemotherapy and deep X-ray.

Actinomycin D has materially altered the immediate prognosis and it now seems indicated in every patient. 50 mcgm. is given, divided into 5 daily portions, and the operation is performed on the third day. Batches of the drug differ and it can cause leucopenia with severe skin rashes, bloody diarrhœa and wound inflammation, but it is worth while. Nephrectomy is followed by deep X-ray up to 3,000r. Pulmonary metastases may disappear radiologically on actinomycin D and there is some evidence that the drug potentiates radiotherapy.

On rare occasions a solitary metastasis, e.g. in the lung, may be successfully removed by operation.

The results are better in younger patients and the outlook is best in infants under 1 year. The statistics in the United States are better than most countries possibly because routine examination of well babies picks up the lesions at an earlier stage. The best figures for this gloomy condition are about 70 per cent survival rates in infants under 1 year, and about 40 to 50 per cent survival over that age.

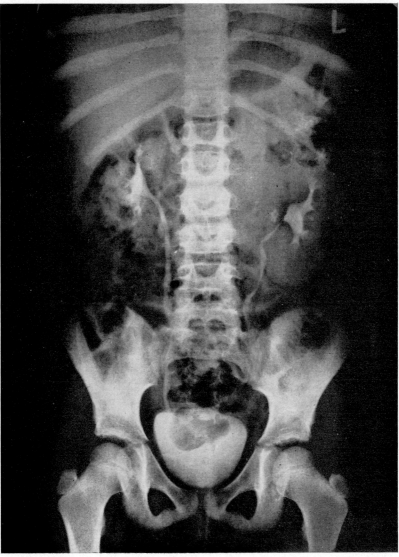

Fɪɢ. 73. Intravenous pyelogram showing left-sided neuroblastoma. The pyelogram is displaced and the tumour partly calcified.

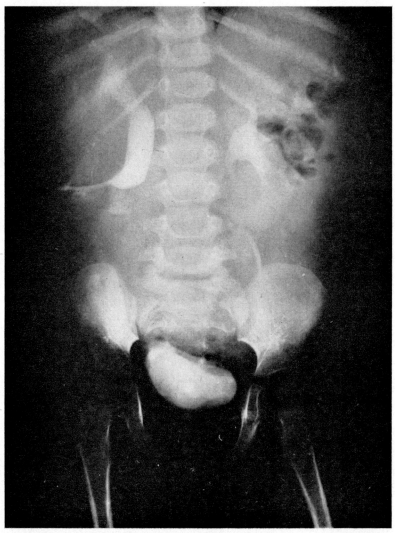

Fig. 74. Intravenous pyelogram showing right-sided nephroblastoma. The pyelogram is distorted by the tumour arising within the kidney.

RHABDOMYOSARCOMA

The rhabdomyosarcoma is a tumour of striated muscle formative cells. It is almost always found arising from the area of the urogenital sinus and the specific name urogenital sinus sarcoma may be preferred for this group. It frequently presents with interference with micturition, producing retention of urine or infection or hæmaturia. The outlook for those arising in the bladder is better than those arising in the prostatic region. They sometimes respond to excision and ureteric transplant and those of the vagina (sarcoma botryoides) may be amenable to surgery. It may less commonly arise in the heart muscle or the pharynx. There appears to be no explanation why this striated muscle type of tumour should arise in these sites rather than the large volumes of typical striated muscle distributed throughout the body. They are radioresistant tumours and chemotherapy has little yet to offer.

HEPATOBLASTOMA

Hepatoblastoma is another though less common embryoma. It is a tumour of the liver parenchyma-forming cells. It usually presents as a painless swelling of the liver in a child in poor general health. It is not usually amenable to treatment but surgical resection—lobectomy or hemihepatectomy—may be feasible when the tumour arises in one half only of the liver.

Sarcomata

Sarcomata are also seen in childhood. These are malignant tumours of the mesenchyme.

OSTEOGENIC SARCOMA. The *osteogenic sarcoma* may be seen in later childhood. It usually arises at the end of a long bone, a favourite site being the lower end of the femur. The child develops a painful swelling at the site of the tumour. On palpating the limb the bone itself is recognized to be expanded, and there may be increased vascularity over it. The tumour may be osteoblastic, laying down a good deal of new bone, or more commonly osteolytic showing the typical X-ray appearance of an expanded bone end with the remnant of the shaft still visible through the centre of the tumour. The epiphyseal line is usually preserved and not transgressed. Osteogenic sarcoma is usually treated by radiotherapy followed by amputation, but the survival rate is only about 10 per cent.

Osteoclastoma also expands the ends of long bones, but this usually benign tumour does frequently involve the epiphysis, and the shaft of the bone in the involved area is itself expanded and thinned out. Centrally trabeculæ of bone weave across the area to present a cystic appearance.

Fibrosarcomata may also be seen. These may arise from the intermuscular sheaths, and probably many arise from the sheaths of nerves as a malignant variant of the *neurilemmoma*. This latter is a not uncommon simple tumour with a typical honey-yellow appearance in the cellular soft type. A firmer type looking like fibrous tissue which tends to infiltrate between muscle fibres may thus give the false impression of a malignant tumour.

Another tumour which may be seen in childhood involving the bone is the so-called *Ewing's tumour*. Clinically the presentation is as a painful tender area usually near the middle of the bone and some swelling may be recognizable. Radiology shows rarefaction centrally in the bone and around it the laying down of onion skin layers of subperiosteal new bone. This was originally described as a tumour arising in the medulla of the bone, but it is now thought that at least the great majority of cases are in fact secondary deposits from neuroblastomas, the primary focus of which may be clinically silent.

Reticuloses

Yet another group of malignancies encountered in childhood are those of the reticulo-endothelial system. The three classically described reticuloses are as follows.

The *acute reticulosis* or *Letterer-Siwe disease*. There is an enlargement of the spleen, the liver and the lymph nodes. There is a hypoplastic anæmia and a typical dark red papular skin eruption. Localized areas of erosion may be seen in the bones. Radiography also reveals a typical diffuse mottling of the lung fields. The disease is almost uniformly fatal within a few months, although steroid treatment may delay its course.

The second classical clinical description is of the *Hand-Schüller-Christian*, or subacute type of reticulosis. The triad of exophthalmos, defects in the membranous bones and diabetes insipidus make up the syndrome. They result from granulomatous deposits in the orbit causing the exophthalmos; in the bones causing the defects and in the pituitary region causing the diabetes insipidus. The histological picture is of foam cells which are filled with lipoid droplets. It is seen in rather older children than the Letterer-Siwe disease which usually arises in infancy. Again treatment is unsatisfactory. X-ray therapy may appear to help lesions in the bone and corticosteroids may produce at least a temporary arrest of the process. However, about a third of these children recover spontaneously, although the fibrosis which remains at the site of the lesions may give residual impairment of function.

The third classical type of reticulosis is the *eosinophil granuloma* of bone. In this type, which is seen usually in later childhood, the lesion may be solitary or multiple. The skull bones are frequently affected and presentation may be as a rather soft boggy swelling of the scalp causing minor annoyance to the child. Radiology reveals a typical erosion of the bone with a fluffy edge. Histologically the granuloma contains many eosinophilic cells. The lesions are usually self-limiting and healing appears to be accelerated by radiotherapy, corticosteroids or such simple measures as curettage.

We thus have three conditions, the one almost uniformly fatal at one extreme, the eosinophil granuloma pursuing a benign course at the other extreme, and the Hand-Schüller-Christian disease in an intermediate position both as regards the seriousness of the prognosis and pathological features. It is now recognized, however, that these clinical pictures seem to be of facets of a single type of disease process. Many intermediate forms occur and one type may progress to another.

BRAIN TUMOURS

Tumours of the brain are relatively common amongst the tumours of childhood. The majority are *gliomata*, that is tumours arising from the supporting tissues of the brain. A relatively benign type consisting of well-differentiated astrocytes and often largely cystic, is frequently located in the cerebellum. Another relatively common tumour is the *medulloblastoma* which frequently arises in the roof of the fourth ventricle, and is markedly invasive. It may disseminate through the cerebrospinal spaces producing multiple lesions of the meninges. The range of cerebral tumours as found in adults may all occasionally occur in childhood. It is characteristic of the childhood brain tumours that a large proportion arise in the posterior fossa as subtentorial neoplasms. As a result of this papilloedema is a frequent sign. The general symptoms of raised pressure—headache and vomiting with a change of disposition or coma are common and may overshadow localizing symptoms of the site of the tumour which may be minimal or in some cases absent in the early stages. *The diagnosis of a suspected brain tumour may involve extensive investigation.* Lumbar puncture will usually reveal a raised cerebrospinal fluid protein but this investigation should be avoided when tumour is suspected and ventriculography should be the first investigation. The use of angiography—the injection of radio-opaque substances into the carotid and vertebral arteries—is now widely used and by visualizing the distortion of the vascular pattern may be an extremely valuable method of localizing a brain tumour. Electro-encephalography may be of great value in localizing the site of a lesion near the surface, although it is less specific in suggesting the nature of the lesion.

THE TREATMENT OF MALIGNANT DISEASE IN CHILDREN

Surgery in our present incomplete knowledge of the disease and in the absence of any reliable form of treatment still plays a considerable part. The extirpation of the mass with the organ of origin and surrounding tissues when practicable is clearly a reasonable procedure and should be associated with a monobloc dissection of the lymphatic glands draining the area when this is practicable. However, in many of the situations of the common tumours of childhood it is not practicable and their more frequent metastases through the blood stream makes the technique of less value than in the common adult carcinomata.

Biopsy may be required in the majority of cases to confirm the nature of the lesion even when this is inoperable. This will usually mean a reasonably wide exposure to examine the extent of the lesion and inspect it, and to remove pieces from suitable areas for histological study. Blind needle biopsy in which fragments only are obtained from unspecified parts of the tumour may be misleading, since it is not uncommon for the tumour to present a varying picture in different parts, and necrotic areas which are valueless for histological study are common.

Radiotherapy is of considerable palliative value and may be in some cases curative alone or in conjunction with surgery. All cells are destroyed by a sufficient dose of X-rays but growing cells are more prone to damage. Thus in suitable situations it may be practicable to give a dose which will destroy the growing tumour cells without inflicting irreparable damage on the surrounding body. The treatment of the nephroblastoma (Wilms' tumour) may be quoted as an example of reasonably successful management by these forms of treatment. The usual story will have been the recognition of a mass in one side of the abdomen, symptomless or observed during the routine examination of a child complaining of general malaise. The most likely causes of such a swelling are nephroblastoma or neuroblastoma (both malignant); hydronephrosis or multicystic or bilateral polycystic kidneys (benign, although the latter is ultimately fatal). Treatment is undertaken as an emergency and examination should only be carried out by the surgeon who is to operate on the case if the diagnosis is confirmed. The frequent palpation of such a tumour and demonstration to classes of students is likely to lead to metastasis of tumour cells through the blood stream. The only investigations required are a blood examination (because hæmorrhage into the tumour may have produced anæmia and blood will be required for transfusion during operation) and intravenous pyelography to demonstrate the typical appearances of the lesion, which have already been described, and to confirm the presence of a normal functioning second kidney. Following this examination actinomycin D is given and the tumour is removed by a wide transperitoneal approach, enabling the veins draining the tumour to be ligated before the mass itself is handled and removed. The operation is followed by radiotherapy of the tumour bed, in order to attempt to remove microscopic spread beyond the limits of the mass and to the para-aortic nodes. There is no need to await wound healing. The earlier the radiotherapy can be given the better. As a result of this aggressive policy this tumour which used to be uniformly fatal is now frequently capable of cure.

It is clear that such forms of treatment are unlikely ever to become reliable, and they are futile in the presence of distant metastasis to regional lymph nodes or in particular to blood-spread metastasis to liver or lungs or skeleton. Some systemic attack on the malignant cell holds out a far better promise of ultimate solution of the problem. Our knowledge of the physiology of the malignant cell, although growing, is still in its infancy and it seems that only through these researches are we likely to achieve our goal. Already promising new approaches are being developed.

Antimetabolites are substances which interfere with the metabolic pathways peculiar to the malignant cells. A method by which they can work is that of competitive inhibition. The substance used is closely related to one of the natural substrates of the cellular metabolism. It is sufficiently like it to become linked to the enzyme system, but still sufficiently different for the cell to be unable to use it. The enzyme pathway thus becomes blocked and the cell dies. Aminopterin (akin to folic acid) was one of the first of these substances and is being replaced by less toxic substances, such as 6-mercaptopurine, which can produce remarkable remissions in the course of leukæmia, even though cure is not yet achieved.

Hormone therapy may similarly be used to upset the metabolism of the malignant cell by altering the milieu interne. Corticosteroids produce worth-while remissions in leukæmia.

Management of the Child and Family. In malignant disease of childhood, in which only a minority of cases can be cured, the management of the child and family is of great importance. Clearly this is a matter for individual consideration in each case, and it is one for discussion with the parents and not for dogmatic pronouncements by the doctor. Different families may need very different handling. But as a general rule it can be said that in these cases where many months or perhaps even years of life may be expected one should never remove all hope. Life with the child can become intolerable for the parents if no hope is held out, and may lead to hopeless spoiling of the child which only makes it unhappier, or to fruitless searches for someone with a new treatment. An aggressive approach to treatment by every possible means is not only of value in helping the family to realize that something is being done, but in our present incomplete knowledge of the problem is fully justified by the occasional unexpected success. It is frequently wise to caution the parents that the indulging of the child's every whim will not make him happy but will only make him more demanding. The tendency to do this is, of course, most natural, but the child will be happiest with as near as possible to normal management.

REFERENCES

Bodian, M. (1963) Neuroblastoma: an evaluation of its natural history and the effects of therapy with particular reference to treatment by massive doses of vitamin B_{12}. *Arch. Dis. Childh.*, **88**, 606.

Dargeon, H. W. (1962) Neuroblastoma, *J. Pædiat.*, **61**, 3, 456.

Koop, C. E. and Hernandez, J. R. (1964) Neuroblastoma; Experience with 100 cases in Children. *Surgery*, **56**, 727.

CHAPTER 42

PRE- AND POST-OPERATIVE CARE

Admission and Investigation

THE approach to the child requires considerable variation from the normal practice in adult hospital work. To begin with, the common custom of admitting the patient on the evening before an operation is in general not a good arrangement for the child. It is better that the child should be admitted, say, 2 days before the operation to allow a day up and about in the ward to get used to the people who are going to handle him and to the place itself before the operation takes place. Frequent visiting by the mother should be an accepted routine. Many doubts were expressed before this practice became general and it was thought it would make nursing difficult and interfere too much with the work of the ward. It is now realized, particularly by the nursing staff themselves, that the mother's presence may in fact make the management of the child very much easier and that the mothers can indeed make a useful contribution by feeding their own children and doing simple nursing tasks for them. Clearly this is a matter not for strict regulations but for an individual approach to particular cases, depending on the personalities involved. In some cases it will be better to have the mother living in with the baby or child but this depends on individual personalities and family situations. Measures to reduce cross-infection are of the utmost importance, but they must be adjusted, say, to allow the child to retain a favourite toy, and be applied in an intelligent manner so as to avoid the unfortunate spectacle of a child in a cubicle in splendid isolation, like a goldfish in a bowl sitting silent and withdrawn and losing interest in all around him.

It is particularly important in children's work to see that a full history is taken from the mother when the child arrives at the hospital; both for the sake of the history itself which will be necessary, but also to give an opportunity to the mother to meet the people who will be looking after her child and establish the kind of contact which is essential in management. The child's own history may itself be extremely valuable, but the parent's story is essential and it is easy to overlook the importance of obtaining a detailed history of the child and his family in what may appear at first sight a straightforward admission for a routine procedure.

In arranging for investigations of the child particular thought must be given to the necessity for X-ray investigations in view of the additional genetic and general hazards of irradiation of the growing child. It is not always remembered that for every chest X-ray of a small toddler which appears on the ward there may be two blurred films left in the department. It is in the avoidance of such unnecessary exposure that the value is seen of the practised radiographer of the children's hospital rather than the occasional children's radiography of a busy department in a large general hospital. The advantages of having technicians in the ancillary departments who are inevitably of the type who are happy dealing with children is also seen in the management of the many biochemical tests which may be needed. In a children's hospital the routine methods will be micromethods which will allow, for example, an adequate electrolyte examination of the blood for control of intravenous therapy on a single millilitre from a pin-prick, and thus avoid any need for unpleasant repeated venepunctures.

The children should always be allowed the freedom of the ward and playroom unless there is some specific reason for keeping them in bed, rather than the reverse system of giving a particular child permission to get up.

PREPARATION FOR OPERATION

It is as a general rule preferable to arrange preoperative drugs so that the child falls asleep before going to the theatre. When intravenous therapy is needed it can often be set up more conveniently after the induction of anæsthesia. Children having abdominal operations will often need to have a per nasal gastric tube for postoperative aspiration of the stomach. In small children the tube which can be passed is inevitably a rather narrow one. The modern polyvinyl chloride tubes are very much less irritating than rubber and tend to block less easily, but nevertheless it must be remembered that the narrow bore tubes do block easily and repeated test injections of a few millilitres of water and aspiration are necessary to maintain drainage. Continuous suction removes the swallowed gas as well as the fluid, but it requires careful watching and should be supplemented by intermittent aspiration.

If the child is severely anæmic and the operation has to go on, an infusion of packed red cells may be preferable to whole blood. This can easily be prepared by decanting the supernatant plasma from a bottle of blood.

Intravenous Fluids

The management of intravenous therapy in children is even more delicate than in adults. It is remarkable how a good nursing staff can keep an intravenous drip running at a really slow rate. The quantity of fluid required has to be measured in relation to the size of the child, and it is usual to take the child's weight as a guide. Daily weighing is also of the greatest value in assessing the efficiency of one's treatment. A rapid rise in weight in a baby on intravenous therapy may be the first danger sign of overtreatment with water retention. The postoperative requirement of intravenous fluid is only about 30 ml. per pound per day for the first few days and many believe that even this is better avoided. Increased œdema at the site of an anastomosis and increased secretion into the intestines may cause more trouble than the benefit from the retained fluid. If oral feeds cannot be started within a few days, fluid is required up to 60 ml. per pound body weight per day, containing for an infant 1 g. of sodium cloride, the pre-school child up to 3 g. and the school child up to 5 g. per day. If intravenous therapy is prolonged it will be wise to add 1 g. of potassium chloride to each litre of the infused fluid. These are crude estimates of the fluid and electrolyte requirements. It is necessary to check the dosage given by observations of the child's clinical condition, the urinary output and the weight. Electrolyte determinations will provide a further check on one's therapy, but it should be remembered that the young infant's kidney will often leak chloride during the intravenous administration of a saline solution, even before the child has obtained enough sodium, so that the presence of chloride in the urine may be of little value as a guide to the adequacy of intake. However, in general terms one's anxiety about chloride administration is usually to be sure one is not giving too much rather than too little. If the child has additional losses, of which the commonest is by vomiting, then one must add to each day's requirements the amount lost in this way in the previous day. An amount of 0·9 per cent sodium chloride equal to the volume of vomit may be added. This description is of the *postoperative* requirements of the child.

Before operation it may be necessary in addition to correct pre-existing losses resulting from vomiting or loss by diarrhœa. Different levels of intestinal obstruction produce different electrolyte problems. In duodenal obstruction chloride excretion exceeds that of sodium. There is a rise in the bicarbonate due to loss of hydrogen ion and a tendency to alkalosis. In lower obstructions involving loss of intestinal secretions, acidosis is the rule.

It must be realized that *after operation* the situation is altered by the body's response to stress and that in this case the requirements are considerably less in the first day or two, at least so far as sodium and chloride are concerned. It is extremely important *during the operation* itself to replace blood loss beyond 10 per cent accurately, allowing for loss into the operated tissues as well as externally. If this replacement is adequate and the child's condition immediately after operation is good, then it is probable that for the next day or two the child will be able to take care of its own electrolyte adjustments, and need only the post-operative maintenance amount of water made isotonic with glucose to allow for the insensible loss. There is considerable doubt whether even this is beneficial in the first days. It may be considered that the metabolic response to stress is a protective mechanism and only excessive disturbances need correction. The utilization of intravenous electrolyte and glucose infusions during and after operation as "maintenance" is open to discussion. The water and salt retention diminish the need and if intake is forced it may not be properly utilized. There is no doubt about the need for prompt quantitative replacement of blood loss and for the replacement of abnormal losses. Active growth (anabolism) is the best stabilizing factor and as yet can be achieved only by oral or jejunal feeds containing adequate protein and calories. An analogy can be made to the febrile response to infections. Whilst hyperpyrexia needs urgent treatment to save life, any attempt to correct the usual degree of pyrexia is only harmful.

SEDATION. Morphine 0·025 mg. per lb. body weight should be given after major surgery and it may require to be repeated over 48 hours or more. Children cannot ask for analgesics but this does not mean they do not need them. The barbiturates and the phenothiazines are *not* analgesic and may be antianalgesic.

Care of the Newborn

The care of the newborn poses special problems. The new-born infant is particularly prone to the aspiration of vomit, is likely to be too weak to cough up any aspirate and is hence particularly prone to pulmonary complications. It is therefore especially important to nurse these babies on their side and to aspirate the throat frequently. If one waits until one hears the rattle of mucus in the throat one may indeed wait too long, because the weak sick infant may allow mucus as well as vomitus to pool there and inhale it effortlessly without a cough response. When an indwelling gastric tube is necessary for suction the use of polyvinyl chloride (PVC) is extremely valuable. When prolonged suction is likely to be necessary or on a small premature baby there should be no hesitation in doing a gastrostomy. Elective gastrostomy has been much more freely used in recent years and it certainly simplifies care.

Free use of wide spectrum antibiotics is justified in operated newborns because of their poor resistance and the risks of infection during the frequent handling they must have.

ENVIRONMENT. After operation, when the bronchial tree has been irritated by the passage of an endotracheal tube the newborn should be nursed in an atmosphere of high humidity to avoid inspissation of bronchial mucus. They should also be maintained at an equable temperature because they have difficulty in controlling their own temperature and may easily become cold when the danger of potentially fatal sclerema occurs. The simplest way of obtaining the desired conditions is to nurse the baby mainly on its side in an incubator where it can be constantly observed and attended, as necessary, with the minimum of interference. *Sclerema* is a hard change in the consistency of the subcutaneous tissues. It is seen in association with low temperature, but it is probable that infection somewhere in the body is also necessary to cause its onset and there may be a hæmorrhagic pneumonia. The exact nature of the condition is not fully understood. It used to be almost always fatal but it appears that postoperative cases may respond to cortisone and with a warm atmosphere and a wide-spectrum antibiotic the outlook is no longer hopeless. The action of the cortisone is ill-understood. Cortisone has also seemed of value in the management of the peripheral circulatory collapse which sometimes occurs, particularly in babies who have needed a reoperation in the presence of infection.

INTRAVENOUS FLUIDS. The newborn withstands starvation and dehydration well. "There are more infants drowned on the banks of the Thames than in it." Thirty ml. per pound body weight per day is adequate unless there are large fluid losses through vomiting, diarrhœa, ileostomy or a fistula. Ten per cent dextrose provides some calories, although it tends to thrombose veins.

Cardiac and Respiratory Arrest

These most urgent of emergencies occur at all ages. No apparatus is needed for immediate treatment. External cardiac massage is particularly effective in children. Put the left hand under the dorsal spine and compress the lower end of the sternum thirty times a minute with the right. Mouth to mouth breathing is far the most effective method of artificial respiration and is also almost free of complications.

Biochemical correction of the anoxic acidosis should begin promptly. The heart may not beat until this has been done.

INFECTION

Young babies have low antibody titres and may contract virulent infections with little response. The principal sources of infection are other infected patients and nasal carriers—patients, nurses and doctors. Broad spectrum antibiotics *must* be used freely in operated newborns.

Steroid Therapy

With the widespread use of steroid therapy it is important to enquire if the patient has had any of these drugs in the two previous years.

If a steroid has been given in the past two years it should be given again preoperatively and continued for three days after operation. Unless this precaution is observed circulatory collapse due to adrenal failure may occur under anæsthesia or in the postoperative phase.

RESTRAINTS AND AMBULATION

The use of restraint in bed is practised as little as possible, but it may be essential in some cases. For example, a child with a cleft palate repair may need a kind of cardboard splint loosely applied around the elbows so that he cannot get his fingers in his mouth to pick at the stitches. A child who has had a perineal urethrostomy drainage to cover an operation for hypospadias may require loose wrist bands to the bedside to restrain his hands from being able to reach the perineum and pull out the tube, though these need not be so tight as to prevent all movement. However well-behaved the child is during the day he is likely to pull at any such annoyance either in his sleep or when half awake. If these kind of restraints are applied sympathetically by the nursing staff who take the time to talk and play with the child frequently, and avoid having him lying for long periods with nothing better to do than brood on the annoyance, they are surprisingly well tolerated. This kind of activity on the part of a children's nurse is not to be looked on as a luxury but as an essential part of her care of the child.

Early ambulation is now considered of great value in a wide variety of adult surgical procedures because of the avoidance of postoperative prolonged weakness and convalescence, and because of its reduction in the risk of venous thrombosis from stasis. Fortunately, children are not at all prone to venous thromboses. Whilst early ambulation is encouraged as much as the child wants it there is usually no need to force the child against his will into early ambulation, as there may be in adult cases. The exhausted and weak child, recovering from peritonitis following appendicitis, can be relied upon in the majority of cases to make it clear when he is fit to get up by asking to do so, and there is no need to force him out of bed earlier than this. Even in children, however, the pain of an abdominal or thoracic incision is likely to discourage deep breathing, and the use of physiotherapy to encourage this in the early postoperative days is of great value. In elective surgery where this kind of treatment is likely to be required it is of great value for the child to be taught breathing exercises before his operation, so that he knows the physiotherapist and knows what she expects of him beforehand. Prompt co-operation will then be more easily obtained.

TRANSPORT OF THE NEWBORN

It should rarely be necessary to attempt surgery with inadequate facilities for these babies travel very well with correct precautions carried out by the accompanying nurse:—

1. Portable incubator to maintain body temperature. (These can be hired.)

2. Intestinal obstruction carries the risk of inhalation of vomitus. The baby is nursed head low on one side. A nasogastric tube is passed and the stomach is emptied. The tube is retained and aspirations are repeated during the journey.

3. Œsophageal atresia carries the risk of inhalation of saliva and of reflux of gastric contents through the fistula. The pharynx and pouch are aspirated repeatedly during the journey with a mucus catheter and the baby is nursed head high to reduce the tendency to gastric juice reflux.

4. Diaphragmatic hernia is the most difficult transport problem but also a condition in particular need of management in practised hands. An

endotracheal tube should be passed so that positive pressure insufflation can be performed throughout the journey. A nasogastric tube should also be passed to empty the stomach of swallowed air and prevent distension of the misplaced intestine.

5. Severe Pierre Robin syndrome carries a high risk of tongue swallowing and asphyxiation. The baby should be nursed prone with an oropharyngeal airway, and if necessary a temporary tongue stitch.

REFERENCE

Wilkinson, A. (1960) *Body Fluids in Surgery*, 2nd Editn. E. & S. Livingstone, Edinburgh and London.

INDEX